Integrating Religion and Spirituality into Clinical Practice

Conference Proceedings

European Conference on Religion, Spirituality and Health
2014/2016

Special Issue Editors

René Hefti
Arndt Büssing

MDPI • Basel • Beijing • Wuhan • Barcelona • Belgrade

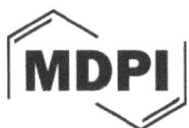

Special Issue Editors
René Hefti
University of Berne
Switzerland

Arndt Büssing
University Witten/Herdecke
Germany

Editorial Office
MDPI
St. Alban-Anlage 66
Basel, Switzerland

This edition is a reprint of the Special Issue published online in the open access journal *Religions* (ISSN 2077-1444) from 2014–2017 (available at: http://www.mdpi.com/journal/religions/special_issues/religions-health-care).

For citation purposes, cite each article independently as indicated on the article page online and as indicated below:

Lastname, F.M.; Lastname, F.M. Article title. *Journal Name* **Year**, *Article number*, page range.

First Edition 2018

ISBN 978-3-03842-930-2 (Pbk)
ISBN 978-3-03842-929-6 (PDF)

Cover photo courtesy of René Hefti

Table of Contents

Chapter 1: Religion and Spirituality in Patient Care

Chapter 2: Spirituality in Physical and Mental Disease

Chapter 3: Health Care Professionals and Spirituality

Chapter 4: Faith-Based Services and Programs in Health Care

About the Special Issue Editors

René Hefti, M.D., graduated from the Medical School of Zurich University in 1987; completed residencies in internal medicine and cardiology in Switzerland, Austria and Jemen from 1988–1998; did an additional training in psychosomatic medicine and existential psychotherapy from 1994–2002; and was the Head of the Psychosomatic Department of the Clinic SGM Langenthal, Switzerland, from 2006–2016. In 2005, Dr. Hefti founded the Research Institute for Spirituality and Health (www.rish.ch) and initiated the European Conferences on Religion, Spirituality and Health (www.ecrsh.eu). His research interests include religion as a stress buffering "agent", the integration of spirituality into an extended bio–psycho–social model and the impact of physician's beliefs on medical practice. Since 2006, Dr. Hefti has been a lecturer for psychosocial medicine at the University of Bern, Switzerland, also teaching clinical skills and the integration of spirituality into clinical practice (e.g., keeping a spiritual history).

Arndt Büssing (*1962) qualified as a medical doctor in 2010 and is now a full professor at the Witten/Herdecke University (Germany) for "Quality of Life, Spirituality and Coping". He was an Associated Cooperator and Relator of the Pontifical Council of Health Care Workers from 2012 to 2014. Further he was a senior research fellow of the "Freiburg Institute for Advanced Studies" (FRIAS) from 2012–2014, and has been an associated researcher at "IUNCTUS—Competence Center for Christian Spirituality", PTH/School of Theology Münster since 2016. He is on the board of directors of the International Society of Health and Spirituality (IGGS), an editorial board member of the German Journal of Oncology, of the journal Spiritual Care, and of the open access journal *Religions*.

European Conferences on Religion, Spirituality and Health: An Academic Initiative

The European Conferences on Religion, Spirituality and Health (ECRSH) are an academic and interdisciplinary initiative to establish a European Network of researchers, scholars and health care professionals investigating, discussing and implementing initiatives in the emerging field of Religion, Spirituality and Health in Europe (www.ecrsh.eu).

The primary initiative was taken by a cooperation of the Research Institute for Spirituality and Health (www.rish.ch) and the Institute of Complementary Medicine KIKOM, University of Bern, Switzerland, in 2007. The first Conference on Religion, Spirituality and Health (ECRSH) was held from May 1–3, 2008, at the University of Bern, Switzerland. As this conference proved to be very successful with excellent international participation and high quality of presentations and discussions, the founding institutions decided to establish ECRSH as a regular conference to be held every two years. The following conferences took place in 2010 and 2012 in the same university; in 2014, the conference was held at the University in Valletta, Malta; in 2016, at the University in Gdansk, Poland; and in 2018 at the University in Coventry, Great Britain (see also www.ecrsh.eu).

The overall aims of the European Conferences (ECRSH) and the European Network on Religions, Spirituality and Health (ENRSH) are:

1. To promote general awareness among researchers, scholars and professionals of the importance of religious and spiritual issues for the human being in all aspects of health, disease and suffering, and to work towards inclusion and application of this awareness in theory, research, education and practice in all health professions.

2. To provide an interdisciplinary forum within academic medicine and related academic health care disciplines for scientific exchange over questions of religion and spirituality in relation to matters of health and disease, and to foster high quality research.

3. To provide and secure an atmosphere of free intellectual exchange, true tolerance and mutual respect over questions of spirituality and religion in these areas, irrespective of personal faith, religious or spiritual affiliation and philosophical standpoint.

4. To promote a genuine European perspective on these issues, taking into account the varied religious, spiritual, cultural, philosophical and scientific European traditions and achievements, thus contributing to a re-humanization of modern medicine by integrating religious, spiritual and existential issues into health care.

To support these aims, ECSRH publishes conference proceedings and special issues such as this special issue book. We are grateful for the good collaboration with MDPI (open access journal *Religions*). Please note, there was also an earlier publication "*Spirituality and Health—Selected Contributions on Conflicting Priorities in Research and Practice*" (René Hefti und Jacqueline Bee, Peter Lang Verlag 2012), which is a collection of scientific articles from ECRSH 2008 and 2010.

Preface to "Integrating Religion and Spirituality into Clinical Practice"

This present collection of scientific articles is a fruitful collaboration of the European Network of Religion, Spirituality and Health (ENRSH), the Online Journal *Religions* and the academic authors. Therefore, we would like to sincerely thank the editorial office of *Religions* and all the authors for their contributions. It is a rich collection of articles representing the European Conferences of Religion, Spirituality and Health 2014 and 2016 (in part).

The first chapter of the book on "Religion and Spirituality in Patient Care" emphasizes the importance of addressing religious and spiritual needs and suffering in disease management. Specific tools such as the FICA Spiritual History Tool (Puchalski et al.) have been developed to support healthcare professionals (HCPs) in doing this. A survey from Poland (Pawlikoswski et al.) indicates that 88% of respondents (predominantly Catholic) share a belief in miraculous healing which supports pilgrimage to sanctuaries. A qualitative study by Esperandio and Ladd examined the health–prayer experience of Christian believers in the United States showing that prayer is used as a "spiritual tool" for dealing with physical suffering (spiritual-religious coping). The experience of prayer sustains hope, enables self-transcendence and provides personal empowerment. The last contribution in this first chapter links spirituality and creativity in the context of transformative coping (Corry et al.).

The second chapter on "Spirituality in Physical and Mental Disease" starts with a cross-sectional study from Austria (Gäbler et al.) showing a positive association between religious affiliation and health behavior in adolescents. The next two contributions originate from Thailand and explore spiritual well-being (Cheawchanwattana et al.) and quality of life (Saisunantararom et al.) in patients with chronic kidney disease. The fourth contribution is a cross-sectional study carried out in Poland which found that spirituality was associated with both a positive and negative interpretation of illness (Büssing et al.) The last contribution in this second chapter (Zagozdzon et al.) reviewed literature on the relevance of religious beliefs for treatment adherence in mental illness, an important topic in clinical practice.

The third chapter focuses on the training and practice of health care professionals ("Health Care Professionals and Spirituality"). In the first contribution provided by Baldacchino et al., creative and innovative ways of spiritual care education for nursing students are outlined. Spiritual care is defined as recognizing, respecting and meeting patients' spiritual needs. Role-modeling is used as an important tool in supporting nursing student's integration of spirituality into clinical practice. In the second paper, Koenig presents a project aiming to form spiritual care teams for in- and out-patient settings. The training provides health professionals with resources necessary to practice whole person healthcare, including spiritual care. The training has the potential to increase the quality of patient care and health professional's satisfaction with their work. In the last contribution of this chapter, Lee and co-workers present a survey comparing psychiatric staff's perception regarding their approach towards religious/spiritual issues, under the observation of clinical chaplains', revealing significant differences between the two perspectives.

The fourth and final chapter outlines the integration of religion and spirituality into the clinical context through the use of faith-based services and programs. In the first study, Sørensen et al. evaluated value-based addiction treatments in Norwegian rehabilitation clinics. Sermons and rituals helped patients to change their attitudes and find confidence, meaning and peace. For several patients, private confession was a turning point in their recovery from addiction. The second contribution is a qualitative study of participants' experience of a UK Christian-based intuitive eating program for obesity (Patel et al.). Participants found the program took them on a journey where they began to use faith as a resource, addressing 'more than just a weight problem' and found freedom in their relationship with food. The last paper of this chapter reports on a descriptive qualitative study that explored the value of a program of Serenity Spirituality Sessions for older nursing home residents in Ireland, which were tailored to a predominantly Christian population. The program had a calming influence on the clients and helped create a sense of belonging (Timmins et al.).

René Hefti and Arndt Büssing

Special Issue Editors

Chapter 1
Religion and Spirituality in Patient Care

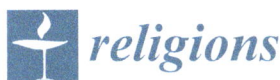

Article

Integrating Spirituality as a Key Component of Patient Care

Suzette Brémault-Phillips [1,*], Joanne Olson [2], Pamela Brett-MacLean [3,4], Doreen Oneschuk [5], Shane Sinclair [6], Ralph Magnus [7], Jeanne Weis [8], Marjan Abbasi [9], Jasneet Parmar [9] and Christina M. Puchalski [10,11]

[1] Department of Occupational Therapy, Faculty of Rehabilitation Medicine, 2-64 Corbett Hall, University of Alberta, Edmonton AB T6G 2G4, Canada
[2] Faculty of Nursing, 4-299 Edmonton Clinic Health Academy (ECHA), University of Alberta, Edmonton AB T6G 1C9, Canada; joanne.olson@ualberta.ca
[3] Arts & Humanities in Health & Medicine (Undergraduate Medical Education Program), Faculty of Medicine & Dentistry, 1-001 Katz Group Centre, University of Alberta, Edmonton AB T6G 2E1, Canada; pbrett@ualberta.ca
[4] Department of Psychiatry, Faculty of Medicine & Dentistry, 1E1 Walter Mackenzie Health Sciences Centre, University of Alberta, Edmonton AB T6G 2B7, Canada
[5] Division of Palliative Medicine, Department of Oncology, Faculty of Medicine & Dentistry, University of Alberta, Edmonton AB T6L 5X8, Canada; doreen.oneschuk@albertahealthservices.ca
[6] Faculty of Nursing, University of Calgary, Calgary AB T2N 1N4, Canada; sinclair@ucalgary.ca
[7] Spiritual Care, Covenant Health, Edmonton AB T6L 5X8, Canada; ralph.magnus@covenenthealth.ca
[8] Faculty of Health and Community Studies, NorQuest College, Edmonton AB T5J 1L6, Canada; weis@ualberta.ca
[9] Department of Family Medicine, Faculty of Medicine & Dentistry, University of Alberta, Edmonton AB T6G 2C8, Canada; mabbasi@ualberta.ca (M.A.); jasneet.parmar@albertahealthservices.ca (J.P.)
[10] The George Washington Institute for Spirituality and Health, School of Medicine and Health Sciences, The George Washington University, Washington, DC 20036, USA; cpuchals@gwu.edu
[11] Division of Geriatrics and Palliative Medicine, School of Medicine and Health Sciences, The George Washington University, Washington, DC 20037, USA
* Author to whom correspondence should be addressed; suzette.bremault-phillips@ualberta.ca; Tel.: +1-780-492-9503.

Academic Editor: Arndt Büssing
Received: 30 January 2015; Accepted: 2 April 2015; Published: 17 April 2015

Abstract: Patient care frequently focuses on physical aspects of disease management, with variable attention given to spiritual needs. And yet, patients indicate that spiritual suffering adds to distress associated with illness. Spirituality, broadly defined as that which gives meaning and purpose to a person's life and connectedness to the significant or sacred, often becomes a central issue for patients. Growing evidence demonstrates that spirituality is important in patient care. Yet healthcare professionals (HCPs) do not always feel prepared to engage with patients about spiritual issues. In this project, HCPs attended an educational session focused on using the FICA Spiritual History Tool to integrate spirituality into patient care. Later, they incorporated the tool when caring for patients participating in the study. This research (1) explored the value of including spiritual history taking in clinical practice; (2) identified facilitators and barriers to incorporating spirituality into person-centred care; and (3) determined ways in which HCPs can effectively utilize spiritual history taking. Data were collected using focus groups and chart reviews. Findings indicate positive impacts at organizational, clinical/unit, professional/personal and patient levels when HCPs include spirituality in patient care. Recommendations are offered.

Keywords: spirituality; spiritual care; healthcare professionals; spiritual history; patient care; interprofessional

1. Introduction

Spirituality, broadly defined as that which gives meaning and purpose to one's life and connectedness to the significant or sacred [1], is often an imminent and central issue for patients experiencing a serious or chronic medical condition, advancing in the aging process, or at the end of life. Puchalski [2] describes spiritual care as attending to the whole person, including physical, emotional, social, and spiritual dimensions of their experience. Broadly conceived, spiritual care is understood as "the foundation of whole person, patient-centred care" [3]. This component of quality care is heightened during illness, throwing into sharp relief compassionate clinical care as an inherently spiritual intervention. When conceptualized as a distinct domain of care, patients have consistently identified addressing spiritual issues as being among the most important and under-addressed end of life need [4–6]. Just as patient-centred care has been linked to healthcare outcomes [7,8], literature has begun to demonstrate the importance of spirituality to patients when making healthcare decisions [9] and coping with end of life distress [10].

Despite being recognized as a vital component of palliative care by patients and policy makers [11], care providers struggle to find ways to address spirituality in patient care [5,12]. Caring for patients with life limiting conditions has primarily taken a biomedical approach focused on cure orientated outcomes and/or physical symptom management [13]. Numerous studies have reported that the majority of patients facing the end of life, whether their spirituality is expressed through religious or secular means, desire to have their spiritual issues addressed by their healthcare providers [4,14,15]. Seriously ill patients have also identified spiritual suffering as contributing to patient distress [16], and likewise desire that this be attended to. Addressing spirituality at such significant times in life has been noted to buffer against spiritual pain and distress, which was reported at 44% of patients in one study [17] and 61% of patients in a separate study [18].

Evidence demonstrates that attending to this important component of patient care can help HCPs more fully understand their patients. Yet, a variety of organizational and structural, as well as professional and personal factors, have been identified that interfere with the provision of spiritual care. At a professional and personal level, some HCPs do not feel competent to engage patients around spiritual issues. Discussion of religious and spiritual issues is often described as a highly advanced communication skills area. Tools to help facilitate such discussion may be helpful. A recent survey of research priorities in spiritual care identified the evaluation of screening tools to address patient spiritual needs as the number one priority amongst an interprofessional (IP) sample ($n = 807$) of European palliative care providers [19]. HCPs have also noted that knowledge gaps can exist, making it difficult for them to meet patients' spiritual needs [20]. Initiating a conversation regarding emotional and spiritual care can be challenging for some HCPs [21], and concerns that engaging in such conversations will require a substantial time commitment [22] are at times a deterrent. When such conversations occur, however, they are often profoundly meaningful to patients, and informative and rewarding for HCPs [14,23]. Given the increasing awareness of the responsibility of all team members to address spirituality [1], professional programs are increasingly offering courses or integrating spirituality within curricula to support the development of HCPs' competencies in this area.

An Inpatient Spiritual Care Implementation Model [ISCIM] was developed to integrate spiritual history and ongoing spirituality-related discussions, as well as assessment of spiritual distress into routine care and treatment planning by IP team members [1]. One of the spiritual history tools suggested is the FICA Spiritual History Tool (FICA) [24–26], developed by Puchalski and Romer [25] as a practical, simple approach for taking a spiritual history within the context of clinical practice (See Box 1 for the FICA Spiritual History Tool).

The FICA (Faith, Importance, Community, Address) includes questions that help to identify the presence of Faith, belief, or meaning; the Importance of spirituality in relation to a patient's life and healthcare decision-making, their spiritual Community; and explore interventions that may be helpful in Addressing the patient's spiritual needs. It also offers a flexible interview guide to help HCPs engage in conversations and invite patients to share their spiritual beliefs and concerns in relation to their illness experience. Borneman *et al.* [27] conducted an early assessment of the FICA with cancer patients and found the tool to be helpful in identifying the depth and breadth of spirituality-related issues of patients, as well as opportunities for addressing these concerns. The FICA was helpful in ensuring respectful, patient-centred care, supporting the importance of determining spiritual needs in relation to treatment planning, and enhancing quality of life of patients in clinical settings. Borneman *et al.* recommended further use of the FICA in other practice settings.

Spiritual history taking and assessment are increasingly important activities in contemporary healthcare practice. The goal of the current project was to improve person-centred care by integrating spirituality as a key component of care in the context of IP healthcare teams. The following assumptions guided the current study: (1) education about use of the FICA by members of IP teams within palliative and geriatric care would increase the willingness of HCPs to engage in discussions about spiritual issues with patients; (2) taking a spiritual history would improve communication between patients and HCPs (as indicated by chart documentation and integration of spiritual issues in treatment planning and care, including increased referrals to spiritual care professionals (SCPs)), and enhance quality of care and outcomes for patients.

Box 1. FICA spiritual history tool [24–26].

FICA©—A Spiritual History

An acronym which can be used to remember what to ask in a spiritual history is:

F: Faith /Beliefs or Values/Meaning
I: Importance and Influence
C: Community
A: Address

Some specific questions you can use to discuss these issues are:

F: Do you consider yourself spiritual or religious?

Do you have spiritual beliefs or values that help you cope with stress (or what you are going through)?

What gives your life meaning?
I: What importance does your faith or belief have in your life?

Have your beliefs influenced how you handle stress or difficult times?

Do you have specific beliefs that might influence your healthcare decisions?
C: Are you part of a spiritual or religious community (Communities include church, temple, mosque, likeminded friends, family or other groups)?

Is this of support to you and how?

Is there a group of people you love or who are important to you?
A: How would you like me, your healthcare provider, to address these issues in your healthcare?

Notes: © C. Puchalski, 1996. Please contact Dr. C. Puchalski for permission to use the FICA tool; the "A" can also indicate "Assessment"—spiritual diagnosis, issue or resource of strength and then plan in a treatment/care plan.

---

2. Methods

This descriptive, qualitative exploratory project aimed to examine how use of a spiritual history tool affected provision of patient care. Study objectives were to (1) explore the value of including spirituality in clinical practice; (2) identify facilitators and barriers to incorporating spirituality into person-centred care; and (3) determine ways HCPs can utilize a spiritual history when giving person-centred care. The University of Alberta Health Research Ethics Board approved the study protocol. This pilot intervention generated data, which will inform further proposals for collaborative multisite intervention studies.

2.1. Setting and Participants

Three inpatient hospital units in Alberta, Canada operated by Covenant Health (a faith-based health care organization), served as the setting for this research: a hospice unit, a tertiary palliative care unit, and a geriatric assessment unit. The hospice unit is a 24-bed unit serving both advanced cancer patients and patients with life limiting illnesses, who have an estimated prognosis of less than four months. The tertiary palliative care unit is a dedicated 20-bed inpatient unit serving advanced cancer patients and those with life limiting illnesses. A 15-bed inpatient unit, the geriatric assessment unit provides an IP approach to assessment and rehabilitation of frail elderly with complex needs. Patients generally have multiple co-morbidities, some of which would be considered life limiting. Patients receive team-based care from a complement of HCPs working on the units.

2.2. Project Phases

The project unfolded in three phases over a six-month period. First, we recruited HCP participants and engaged them in a half-day workshop. The importance of spirituality in person-centred care was discussion and use of the FICA introduced. In the second phase, we conducted an intervention to assess the impact of introducing the FICA as part of patient care on three IP hospital-based units. The third phase focused on data analysis and knowledge translation.

Phase 1: Recruitment and education of HCPs. Recruitment occurred through poster solicitation and invitation by an individual at arms-length from the research team. Three clinical unit managers (one from each site) agreed to facilitate the study. They each designated a member of the IP team to screen clients for inclusion/exclusion criteria, liaise with the Research Assistant (RA) regarding potential study participants, and facilitate access to patient charts. Following recruitment, HCP participants attended a half-day education session during which both the ISCIM and the FICA were introduced. The HCPs had an opportunity to practice taking a spiritual history using the FICA. Written consent to participate in the study was obtained at the beginning of the education session and a pre-education survey was administered to participants. As a follow up to the education, research team members met face to face with HCPs on each of the three units for two focus groups (each 90 min in length) during which HCPs offered preliminary findings related to inclusion of spirituality in patient care and recommendations pertaining to the research protocol.

Phase 2: Data Collection. Patients were screened for eligibility for the study during routine intake, following which the study was described and consent was obtained from those interested. HCP participants conducted a spiritual history during routine patient intake by integrating the FICA into their patient interactions. Findings were documented in patient charts and shared with the IP team. A spiritual care plan was formulated and appropriate referrals were made. Spiritual Care Professionals (SCPs) were available to HCPs for support and guidance. At the end of data collection, HCPs participated in two focus groups: a site-specific focus group and a focus group with all HCPs participants, unit managers and SCPs from the three sites. (See Box 2 for End of Project Focus Group Guiding Questions). Focus groups were audio-recorded and professionally transcribed. Additionally, retrospective chart reviews of study patients were conducted to retrieve all notes regarding HCP inclusion of spirituality in patient care.

Phase 3: Data Analysis. Qualitative data analysis was completed for the focus group transcripts, survey questions, and chart review data. Thematic coding was conducted by three members of the research team (SBP, JW, and RB) using inductive content analysis and NVivo 10 software. To ensure the integrity of the research process, the four criteria of *trustworthiness*, detailed in Lincoln and Guba's [28] model were addressed throughout the analysis processes. Promoting *credibility* involved ensuring the study's conceptual description represented the participants' preferences. This study included focus groups in which the HCPs discussed key ideas and reactions to inclusion of spirituality in patient care. Also, research team members cumulatively bring many years of qualitative research, as well as clinical experience and expertise. Maintaining *transferability* involved using a purposeful and theoretical sampling strategy to identify key informants and satisfy the theoretical needs and comprehensiveness of the conceptual description. Ensuring *dependability* required examining whether the study process was consistent over time. Over a series of meetings, themes were checked and re-checked, using auditing notes as a source of clarification and to trail decisions made in collapsing themes together. Finally, *confirmability* was ensured through prolonged engagement, including during data collection and analysis, and the extensive use of memos and consultation with co-authors. Techniques of reflexivity and bracketing (researchers' reflection on and articulation of experiences and perceptions related to the research topic) were used to render explicit any idiosyncratic perspectives and potential biases of the researchers. This approach assisted in identifying, hence mitigating bias, to help ensure heightened sensitivity to viewpoints and experiences shared with the researchers.

Box 2. End of project focus group guiding questions.

End of Project Focus Group Guiding Questions

What was your experience using a spiritual history tool?

- What was the process?
- How receptive were the patients? Families?
- How comfortable were you?
- How much time did it take?
- Did you modify it—in what way(s) and why?

Did the use of a spiritual history tool:

- Facilitate conversation about spiritual issues with:

  - Patients or families?
  - Colleagues?

- Inform your caregiving? If so, in what ways?
- Did the IP team use the information from the spiritual history tool? How?

Do you think that use of a spiritual history tool would be helpful in assisting other clinicians to integrate spirituality into their clinical practice? Why or why not?
What do you see as potential strengths/barriers of integrating a spiritual history tool:

- Into routine patient care at a clinical/unit level?
- At an organizational level?

What impact, if any, did using a spiritual history tool have on:

- Patient impact and satisfaction?
- You personally and professionally?
- Your clinical practice?
- Your perception of the importance of attending to the spiritual domain?
- Your perception of the role of SCPs?

---

3. Results

3.1. HCP Participant Characteristics

Participants recruited for the study across the three units included nine HCPs working on the units (a nurse practitioner, an occupational therapist, a physical therapist, a physician, four registered nurses, and a social worker). HCPs participating in the half-day education session ranged in age from 30 to 59 years and all but one was female. Prior to the session, 11 HCPs (nine of whom actively participated in the project) completed a survey regarding their perspectives on, and comfort with, spirituality in patient care. Survey responses are displayed in Tables 1 and 2. Following the education, HCPs completed a second survey regarding their readiness to administer the FICA and address patient spiritual issues (See responses in Table 3).

Table 1. Healthcare professional preparation, perspectives, and comfort regarding spirituality in patient care.

Question	Strongly Agree	Agree	Neutral	Disagree	Strongly Disagree	Total Responses
My professional education provided me with an appropriate level of training in the area of spiritual assessment	1	3	2	5	0	11
I have had many post-professional opportunities for training in the area of spiritual assessment	0	1	3	7	0	11
I am comfortable asking patients questions of a spiritual nature	3	4	1	2	1	11
I think that it is important to integrate patient spirituality into care planning	8	3	0	0	0	11
I am comfortable integrating patient spirituality into care planning	3	4	4	0	0	11
I frequently ask patients questions of a spiritual nature	2	5	2	2	0	11
I consider inclusion of spirituality in overall care of patients to be very important	8	3	0	0	0	11
I believe a chaplain is an essential component of the healthcare delivery team	9	2	0	0	0	11
I believe asking a patient about his/her spirituality or religious beliefs in unethical when practicing in a clinical setting	0	0	1	4	6	11
My spiritual beliefs and practices strongly influence my role as a healthcare practitioner	4	3	2	2	0	11
Throughout the course of my day, I feel a sense of thankfulness for what others bring to my life	9	1	1	0	0	11
Addressing a patient's spiritual beliefs can benefit his/her health	7	3	1	0	0	11
It is important for at least some healthcare professionals to talk to patients about his/her spiritual concerns in healthcare	8	2	1	0	0	11

Table 2. Perspectives regarding IP roles & responsibilities regarding spirituality.

I Believe that the Following HCPs are to Discuss a Patients' Spiritual/Religious Concerns	Strongly Agree	Agree	Neutral	Disagree	Strongly Disagree	Total Responses
Physicians	3	7	1	0	0	11
Nurses	2	9	0	0	0	11
Physical Therapists	1	8	2	0	0	11
Occupational Therapists	1	8	2	0	0	11
Social Workers	2	9	0	0	0	11
Psychologists	2	8	0	0	1	11
Recreational Therapists	1	8	2	0	0	11
Music Therapists	1	9	1	0	0	11
Pharmacists	1	5	3	2	0	11

Table 3. Healthcare professionals preparedness to include spirituality in patient care (post-education).

Question	Strongly Agree	Agree	Neutral	Disagree	Strongly Disagree	Total Responses
The training prepared me to ask questions of a spiritual nature	1	10	0	0	0	11
Having had the training, I am more comfortable asking patients questions of a spiritual nature	0	9	2	0	0	11
Having had the training, I am more comfortable identifying spiritual distress	0	8	3	0	0	11
I feel prepared to use the FICA with patients	1	9	0	0	0	10
Having had the training, I feel more adequately prepared to engage with patients regarding spirituality	0	8	3	0	0	11
Having had the training, I feel better prepared to include spirituality in the overall care planning of patients	0	9	2	0	0	11
Having had the training, I feel better prepared to identify spiritual issues in patients	0	10	1	0	0	11

3.2. Patient Characteristics

Twenty-four patients were recruited for the study: 10 patients (three male and seven female) ranging in age from 71 to 92 years on the geriatric assessment unit; one 53 year old male on the tertiary palliative care unit; and 13 patients (seven male and six female) ranging in age from 54 to 84 years on the hospice unit. Patients had various diagnoses and symptoms: metastatic cancer ($n = 12$), pain and/or weakness ($n = 3$), dementia ($n = 1$), falls or injury ($n = 2$), gastrointestinal bleed ($n = 2$), COPD ($n = 2$), rehabilitation needs ($n = 1$), and flu-like illness ($n = 1$). Length of hospital stay ranged from 11 to 219 days, while the length of enrolment in the research study was 6–119 days. See Table 4 for a list of patient spiritual issues identified by HCPs and patients, and Table 5 for spiritual interventions offered by the HCPs, and reasons for referral to SCPs.

Table 4. Spiritual issues and interventions.

Spiritual Issues of Patients Identified by Patients and HCPs
Need for empowerment, courage, hope, meaning in suffering
Grieving, anxiety, lament or protest over loss
Sense of being overwhelmed by suffering and uncertain about their ability to endure
Difficulty expressing feelings about the situation
Expressing guilt, concerns, grief and/or difficulty reflecting on joys, hopes and values
Concerns regarding how significant others are coping with illness, loss/changes
Coming to acceptance of illness and mortality
Fear of dying
Abandonment by God and others
Religious/spiritual struggles

Spiritual Interventions Identified by HCPs to Address Patient Spiritual Issues
Referrals to Spiritual Care Professionals
Explore issues related to bereavement and loss
Active listening, emotional support and emotional expression
Allowing sharing of self in discussion, art, music and/or prayer
Acknowledgement of the family and its importance in the patient's life
Activity and exercise
Humour
Examination and encouragement of spiritual practices
Exploring what is sacred and Divine
Spiritual rituals and practices such as prayer, communion, Church attendance
Guided visualization, relaxing, breathing

Table 5. Interventions offered by IP team members and reasons for referral to SCPs.

Interventions Provided by HCPs	Reasons for Referral to SCPs
Supportive listening	Explore issues related to:
Provision of emotional support	Bereavement and loss
Being a compassionate presence	Hope/forgiveness and reconciliation
Prayer	Meaning of what is sacred and Divine
Inclusion of and engagement with family	Examine and encourage religious practice
Facilitation of patient:	Affirm strengths
Self-expression through conversation, art, music	Facilitate reception of blessings, rituals and
Participation in practices and rituals	sacraments specific to particular faith expressions
(e.g., meaningful activities, exercise, Church	
attendance, communion, or hymn sing)	

3.3. Key Findings

The overall purpose of this project was to explore what transpired when HCPs were introduced to a spiritual history tool and given the opportunity to incorporate spiritual history taking into routine patient care. The analysis: (1) explored the value of including spiritual history taking in clinical practice; (2) identified facilitators and barriers to incorporating spirituality into person-centred care; and (3) determined ways in which HCPs can effectively utilize spiritual history taking. The emergent findings include strengths, challenges, and opportunities regarding the inclusion of spirituality in patient care at the organizational, clinical/unit, HCP professional/personal, and patient levels.

3.3.1. Strengths of HCP Inclusion of Spirituality in Patient Care

Many strengths related to HCP inclusion of spirituality in patient care were identified. The main strength at the organizational level was the mission, vision, and values of the faith-based institution that served as the study setting. Its guiding documents state that the organization is "committed to serving people of all faiths, beliefs, cultures and circumstances", and caring for the "whole person—body, mind and soul". Another strength was that organizational and clinical leaders, as well as staff, felt aligned with these organizational commitments.

The organization's employment of Spiritual Care Professionals (SCPs) to offer support to patients and staff was identified as a strength at a clinical/unit level. One research participant shared "...our unit actually has spirituality and spiritual assessment very much integrated . . . so chaplains would be the ones who are doing the spiritual assessment more in-depth and they would get a referral" [29]. SCPs also provide coaching and support to HCPs, thereby cultivating a person-centred culture of care and fostering a "healthy spirituality" on some units.

On a clinical/unit level, staff in some cases were supported by clinical leaders who attended to and role modelled ways of providing care in the spiritual domain. Further, the HCPs functioning on the units were personally and professionally committed to a person-centred approach to care that inherently viewed spirituality as an essential component. Taking a spiritual history supported this approach to care:

> It validated why we're here...It makes you more joyous about being able to do your work in this way". [30]

> "It's just on my radar even more. So that's really wonderful just to tap into those needs of people". [31]

> "I think of it as having a conversation, getting to know the patient. If there are any issues, they will get uncovered". [32]

> "When we started to incorporate it into our assessment, it just flowed...people talk about community and their family. It was much easier for them to share. [29]

HCPs recognized the importance of getting to know, and establishing and maintaining trust with patients and families. One stated, "That person was actually quite happy that we had asked because there were a number of things going on in her life that she really had no one to talk to about. It enabled her to actually ask for help about things that were impeding upon her spiritual state" [33]. Another commented, "It's amazing what people will share with you, their vulnerabilities and everything" [30]. While HCPs were aware of their professional competencies around spirituality, use of a spiritual history tool allowed them to continue to develop, gain confidence with and incorporate it into care. "I see huge value in using a tool and I think this is the core of what we do" [34]. "Just an incredible experience. I'm hoping that this will stay with me. I think it will because I've already had encounters with patients who weren't part of the study with whom I discussed spirituality" [32].

Strengths also emerged at the patient level. Patients and families recognized that spirituality is an essential component of care and they were desirous of having their spiritual issues addressed and integrated into treatment. Inviting patients to share their spiritual perspectives and concerns enhanced their comfort level in the established relationship with the HCP. Patients appreciated that HCPs acknowledged what was meaningful to them and the ways in which this was integrated into their care (e.g., spiritual rituals, liturgy, prayer, art, reflection). Examples included: "A tile named 'A Road Less Travelled' has themes of perseverance, acceptance, not giving up and gratitude." "Intent on completing the tile today, in case something happens to him, at least there will still be the tile" [35]. These spiritual discussions also provided an opportunity for the patient to reflect upon feelings related to their illness and personal experiences. It is also an opportunity for the clinician to diagnose spiritual distress or patient inner resources of strength. Documentation in patient charts indicated, "He struggles with his wish to live and get better and the knowledge that he will not get better", and "It is hard to think of his mortality, finds it scary—is afraid to die" [35]. HCPs were able to find meaning in patient experiences: "Rain drops falling on his face as he smiled stating, 'It is a blessing from God. Ahhhhh, this is so good.' As we talked about his faith, the patient thanked the writer for taking him outside" [35]. Discussing what was meaningful to patients also changed how the HCPs interacted with them, enhancing the provision of both spiritual and emotional support. One HCP stated, "I've only done five of them [spiritual screens], but it's amazing how many deep, hurtful things people have to share, because you're listening" [29]. Patients would actively participate in spiritual interventions even at times when they were physically weak and compromised: "Joined in singing hymns and communicating when previously was considered unresponsive" [35].

3.3.2. Challenges of HCP Inclusion of Spirituality in Patient Care

HCPs identified a number of challenges at the organizational, clinical/unit, professional/personal, and patient levels when incorporating spirituality into patient care. While using a spiritual history tool was an effective means for eliciting the spiritual issues of patients, participants noted the need to develop follow up interventions. Identification of spiritual issues required that time, preparation, and resources were in place to subsequently address them.

A recurrent theme throughout the majority of the interviews was a strong emphasis on patient's physical needs and care. Because patients are often acutely ill, delirious, or cognitively or perceptually compromised, it was difficult to attend to spiritual care needs during hospitalization. Furthermore, there was pressure to discharge or transfer patients prior to spiritual concerns being addressed. Little consideration was given to consistency and continuity of care in this area post-discharge, "...consistency of care ... if one unit retains the spiritual information and a patient is transferred, the receiving facility has to start again. In the same way that we work to be consistent with medications during transfers, information about spirituality needs to be shared" [36]. Participants felt that discharge planning was mainly focused on physical issues such as whether the patient was mobile, physically stable, and asymptomatic, "She can walk. She can talk. She can eat. She can drink. Why can't she go home?" [37]. While the mission of the organization clearly supports a whole person focus, the provision of support for spiritual needs seemed to be viewed as extending beyond both essential health care needs and priorities, and the resource capacity of the organization. Overall, fiscal constraints and competing priorities seemed to impede the incorporation of spirituality into patient care. These findings provide rationale for a shift toward the use of the ISCIM [1] in inpatient care environments so as to ensure that spiritual needs are not overlooked.

Recognition of the importance of integrating spirituality into person-centred care requires leadership at the clinical/unit level. Such support makes it more likely that IP team members will address this aspect of care, and that adequate staffing will be in place to meet patient needs. Competing clinical demands—with physical care needs most often taking precedence over spiritual care needs—can result in spiritual needs not being addressed, particularly when time is at a premium,

> "It's not that we're trying to deny that patient or their family support in that area, it's just that there's a wealth of pressure on each of us to deliver on what we're being asked to do. So we really do need more spiritual care team members in our settings because I don't know that we can all individually take that on". [38]

"We may not have the time or ability to go into the depth of all the religious issues that a patient wants to bring up". [39]

"The barriers were purely logistical and were completely independent of the tool itself which was easy to use". [32]

Even if HCPs were able to find time within their schedules, there was an underlying feeling that using their time to address spiritual needs was not viewed by other IP team members as efficient and productive, "And I just felt like I couldn't justify the time even though I felt it was very important. I felt privileged to be able to be sitting and spending this time with the patient. But I just couldn't relax because I kept thinking I've got to be doing this, this, and this" [40]. At the same time, HCPs noted that taking time to address patients' spiritual needs often facilitated person-centred care.

Communicating patients' spiritual needs to other members of the IP team both verbally and through documentation was noted to be a challenge, "I struggle with the communication of my own plan of care. This is a conversation I've had and how does that then filter through so that the next nurse following me or the next team member doesn't have to repeat that whole conversation?" [34]. Without appropriate charting mechanisms or time allocated at a clinical/unit level to communicate findings, issues of inconsistency of approach can arise, "All these sacred moments that I have with patients and with families ... how do I capture their essence in the chart? Is that even the place for them? I don't want the moment to be dulled, tarnished, not capturing its beauty in this legal document called a chart" [32].

While addressing spirituality is a core competency, some HCPs felt that they required more knowledge and skills to confidently address spiritual issues, "A lot of information comes out that I'm not trained to deal with and I don't know how to respond to it" [41]. "There's other skills that need to be taught in terms of how to maintain professional boundaries" [39]. HCPs noted a difference between their professional training and that of the SCPs: "She [the SCP] seems to be able to just pile it all on and just keep going about life. And she seems like she's trained and skilled in separating it. These are your issues, this is your path and I'll walk with you down it. But I don't go there" [42]. In the absence of such formation, HCPs may experience more stress/distress, or intentionally or unintentionally cross professional boundaries. Engagement in conversations rather than in a formal process, while potentially indicative of comfort addressing spirituality, also risks diversion away from a patient-centred perspective or imposition of one's personal spiritual views on patients.

The possibility of HCPs experiencing moral/spiritual distress or vicarious suffering was also identified. Moral distress was experienced by HCPs at points when they perceived discord between their morals and values, and the demands placed on them by work, colleagues, families and patients. It also arose when discussing with a patient or family a prognosis, news of impending death, the dying process, or the impact that their illness would have on their quality of life,

"I think I had increased discomfort with this patient's death because of feeling guilt. Did not we, the professionals, hasten her death? By telling her she would move to LTC (long term care)...certainly it appears that the decision made a huge difference. The patient's condition changed drastically. After that she essentially gave up". [32]

Patient understandings of spirituality and their ability to speak about it impacted both their level of engagement in this area and the degree to which spirituality was integrated into their care. Patients who did not consider themselves to be "spiritual" refrained both from engaging in this area and involvement in the study, "(Patient) did not want to be part of 'anything big', and requested to be left alone" [43]. "I mentioned the research project and asked if I could talk with him. I got the same response again: 'Oh, I am not very spiritual, I do not know why I signed up for this'" [35]. Other patients were very private regarding their spirituality, "(She) said her spirituality was only her business and didn't wish to share" [43]. Some patients also became defensive when spirituality was raised, "I started to explain that spirituality is whatever is important to him. He looked at me and said, 'To hell with it, I'm out'" [32]. Language barriers further limited engagement with some patients, "I did find a challenge with one woman who didn't speak very much English. I couldn't get words out of her at all" [31]. Patient engagement around spiritual issues at times resulted in patients having a false perception of connectedness with and attachment to an HCP, "I had one negative experience where I didn't spend enough time with an individual after conducting the spiritual history. They felt I didn't love them anymore and that's what they told me, and so it actually turned kind of negative, which was unfortunate" [29]. The discussions brought a sense of closeness. When the HCP did not continue to engage in the same manner, the patient experienced distress.

A final challenge of note related to continuity of spiritual care upon transition to another clinical unit or discharge into the community. Spiritual resources were not consistently available at the time of transition and HCPs did not know how to access them, "I don't know what a treatment plan is for referring on for community follow up regarding spirituality" [39]. Further, the relationship with the HCP(s) who had engaged a patient on a spiritual level ended, leaving some patients feeling devastated, ambiguous and unsure of the future,

> "They gain a trust with the team, they feel comfortable, they gain that sense that I'm going to be alright, this is going to be OK, I am at the end of my journey, I'm safe. And then when we throw in that mix 'no, you've stabilized and you no longer need us', their world is turned upside down. Patients feel rejected. Often we see patients will just give up". [44]

HCP engagement in the spiritual domain is not without its challenges.

3.3.3. Opportunities for HCP Inclusion of Spirituality in Patient Care

There were many opportunities related to inclusion of spirituality in patient care at the organizational, clinical/unit, professional/personal, and patient levels. The funding of this research study—provided by an organization to explore ways to more explicitly include spirituality in patient care—is one example of an opportunity seized upon by an organization. Research days supported by this organization that are specifically focused on themes such as spirituality in healthcare, provide vehicles for dissemination of research findings and examination of clinical best practices. Further, the organization's openness to ongoing work with researchers on this topic, as well as financial and professional support to staff who decide to further their learning in this area, are additional examples of an approach that can be used to align an organizational mission with practice.

At the clinical/unit level, a more systematic and integrated approach to inclusion of spirituality in patient care may enhance patient and family satisfaction. Patients and families may perceive that the IP team is more attentive to and respectful of the patient as a person rather than as a constellation of physical symptoms. As well, satisfaction among HCPs could increase as their awareness of the central role of spirituality in the provision of healthcare increases, "It's a positive component. Being able to be part of the project and using this tool is just great. There's a framework which helps my confidence with patients, and gives me greater awareness again" [45]. Some HCPs were of the opinion that spirituality at the clinical/unit level would be more likely and consistently addressed if a specific tool were incorporated on an ongoing basis. HCPs felt that this would facilitate patient engagement around spiritual matters within the context of routine care, such as while walking with a patient, or during a therapy sessions. Some HCPs also questioned whether patients, on return admissions, would continue to want to address their spiritual concerns, "I think what's piqued my curiosity is when these patients that took part in the study come back (because they always do), will they be more willing to talk about their spiritual needs?" [46].

At the professional/personal level, HCPs have many opportunities to more intentionally include spirituality in patient care and become comfortable addressing this area,

> "I found that at first administering the tool was very awkward. It was just very rehearsed—bringing the tool in with me, going over it with the patient. But then you develop a game plan and you learn what to listen for". [36]

"As time progresses, you hear those keywords that the patients are saying and you can pick up on that because you're more familiar with the tool". [36]

"I think this allowed other components to be looked at. I think it really brought some enlightenment to some of the team, it opened up questions, and dialogue". [29]

An opportunity for increased job satisfaction was identified, with HCPs being better able to meet patient needs, "So it always is helpful to go deep because then you find out more and you get to know the person. You could work with them that way" [47]. As well, attending to the spiritual component of patient care validated the HCPs' professional role/vocation, "I think I boiled it down to this connection with people. So even if I couldn't have a conversation with someone because they were too ill, just the spark in their eyes, there's a connection. I'm connecting with this person and this person is connecting with me and we both know it, we can just feel it in the air. And I think I've had that before, but going through, doing the whole spiritual history, it just became so very present in my mind again. It wasn't at the back in my mind, it was at the forefront again" [48]. "I think it gives us an identity too. Because traditionally this institution is faith-based. But what do people see when they walk through the door that distinguishes us? So I think asking these questions kind of tells patients that we are different. We're actually interested in your spiritual needs at this time . . . during your moment of crisis when being admitted to hospital" [46].

Addressing spiritual issues also affords HCPs opportunities for professional growth. Some HCPs were better able to establish therapeutic relationships,

"I think my interactions with patients and families has just been so enriched . . . just getting to that connection, that core . . . I see the patient as a human being, not just as a frail, ill cancer patient. I see a person and a soul, the essence of them shining through, connecting on that level". [48]

Other HCPs were able to improve their communication and empathic capacity,

"I think we're here to try to provide care and comfort and quality to the remaining days that an individual has. So, it adds that ability because we're looking at that individual person and asking what matters to them . . . it could be as simple as taking that individual up to the roof top for fresh air". [45]

Finally, there is an opportunity for greater IP collaboration. Inclusion of spirituality provides common ground upon which all members of the IP team can collaborate. Some HCPs seemed surprised to learn that other disciplines have the ability to address the spiritual dimension,

"As the nurses were reading the charts, especially the spiritual histories that got put into the charts, a lot of them commented to me, 'Oh, I never really thought of an occupational therapist addressing spirituality, or a physiotherapist addressing spirituality as part of their role. So I think that was kind of an eye opener'". [49]

This finding presents a rich opportunity for IP learning and collaboration.

Attending to patient needs inclusive of spirituality presents opportunities to enhance the patient experience of care. Patients, families and HCPs recognized an overall increase in satisfaction when spiritual concerns were integrated as part of patient care planning. When patients were invited to share what they consider to be personally meaningful to them, HCP's were able to incorporate these components into their care plan,

"He was young. He just said 'I just want to feel the sunshine on my face one more time'. So somebody listened. It was five minutes. But what a beautiful bag to open instead of 'It's not medical so it doesn't fit within my framework or my context or my priorities'". [50]

HCP's also indicated that there have been fewer call bells heard on the unit since use of the FICA was introduced, and believed that the quality of care offered to patients was enhanced,

"In my mind, there is improved quality, care and comfort for our patients". [29]

"Spirituality should be practical and visible. He sees staff caring for him as representation of this". [35]

Participants felt that an opportunity existed for inviting family members to share their perspectives, and believed that there could be additional value in having both the patient and their family involved in completing a spiritual history. HCPs noted that families have good insight into a patient's spiritual values and concerns, and felt that they could assist in facilitating better spiritual care for the patient,

"I find I spend more time with the family than with the patient because it's the families that seem to have more of the questions. The patients seem to be, well, some of them, are not able to speak. So it's the families that I feel I'm more valuable to regarding the whole connection thing". [40]

The discussions provided an opportunity for patients to find meaning, grow, express themselves, and be empowered. As an example,

"Had image on a tile: a rock with a flower growing out of it. Patient found it awkward to share what symbol/image means to him. More comfortable in speaking of what it means to people. Words used were renewal and beginning of a cycle. Resonated with the idea that people have unique perspectives on the world and there is value in sharing it". [35]

Engaging in spiritual discussions can enhance the patient's experience, foster connectedness, and promote opportunities for further spiritual growth.

Patients reportedly appreciated being treated with dignity and respect, and connecting with what is most meaningful to them,

"I have worked on quite a lot of the units in the hospital and so I really do see a value, especially with patients that are facing end of life issues, who are dealing with significant health issues that are changing their abilities to manage. It is a valuable way to look at coping skills, your support systems, and how you draw on your faith to strengthen you to get through some of these moments". [51]

Having an awareness of what is meaningful to a patient enables HCPs to better help patients cope with their current and future circumstance,

"It was stormy out so the patient suggested that writer take him to another area of interest, looking at art. He was interested in color and texture. He spoke of his image of the flower in the rock on the tile. Meaning to him was a hopeful image of strength, surprise and gratitude". [35]

Discussions such as this can help a patient draw on spiritual resources in a time of crisis.

The inclusion of spirituality in care allowed for both the identification and reduction of existential suffering, and an opportunity to support patients in addressing unresolved spiritual issues, "The patient is so willing to share his feelings, his vulnerabilities. What a gift!" [32]. With each subsequent meeting, the HCP/patient relationship developed further and spiritual sharing continued, "Told HCP she wanted to die and that she has had enough. Things are changing and she is at peace. She spoke of her feelings about dying" [35]. Often referrals to SCP's were made as concerns were identified by the HCP's, which provided patients with additional spiritual and emotional support as they journeyed through their illness. Patients shared feeling at peace as they faced their illness and future passing, "Patient's reflections on death are very cathartic and thoughtful" [35].

The opportunity to explore additional spiritual resources, especially those that are community-based, arises when patients transition to another clinical unit or are discharged from hospital-based care. So as to ensure continuity of care, spiritual information gathered in one setting needs to be integrated into the next, "I think it helps as people near the end of life that they can actually have all those little pieces put together. It helps with advanced planning and future directions" [52].

4. Discussion

This study examined the effect of integrating spirituality into patient care within in-patient care settings by IP teams. Specifically, this project was undertaken to: (1) explore the value of including spiritual history taking in clinical practice; (2) identify facilitators and barriers to incorporating spirituality into person-centred care; and (3) determine ways in which HCPs can effectively utilize spiritual history taking. It yielded initial findings to support proposals for future collaborative multisite intervention studies. Overall, findings from this study contribute to a growing body of knowledge and evidence supporting the inclusion of spirituality in person-centred care by IP team members. HCPs indicated that the study facilitated a greater awareness of the need for all HCPs to possess the ability to recognize and respond to spiritual needs whenever and wherever they might arise. They also acknowledged ways in which attention to spirituality facilitated connection with patients, improved person-centred care, and enhanced their sense of job satisfaction when meeting patient needs. These findings suggest that, in addition to positive outcomes associated with improved patient care, attending to spiritual concerns may potentially also help to reduce rates of burnout among IP team members. Further, the study offered new insights into requirements that would support more intentional inclusion of the spiritual component in patient care at a variety of levels, including organizational, clinical/unit, professional/personal, and patient levels.

4.1. Incorporation of Spirituality

Incorporation of spirituality at a unit level was accomplished by integrating the tool into routine professional practice. This was found to be helpful in initiating and guiding spiritual conversations. More education and greater support for HCPs is required so that they can more competently, confidently and intentionally attend to the spiritual dimension of patient care. This education might include opportunities to (1) enhance self-awareness; (2) improve the ability to differentiate patient distress from one's own spiritual discomfort; (3) develop competencies and skills in spiritual history taking, interviewing and interventions; (4) explore ways to adhere to professional boundaries; and (5) practice responding to and reflecting on spiritual issues using a team-based, collaborative approach consistent with the ISCIM. Such education would be beneficial in undergraduate and graduate level curricula, and continuing education course offerings.

Facilitators (strengths) and challenges related to the incorporation of spirituality in person-centred care were explored. Findings suggest that, while inclusion of spirituality can be inherent in an organization's mission and vision, competing priorities, increasing fiscal constraints, urgency to discharge patients, and limited resources can compromise attention given to this area of patient care. There is potential for greater impact if the organization's mission, vision and values are followed up by explicit initiatives to help to advance the mission. These could include pilot studies, ongoing professional education offerings, supportive communication including introduction of change, as well as change management. HCPs identified a challenge regarding documentation following inclusion of spiritual history taking and intervention. Such an issue would best be addressed at the organizational and clinical/unit levels, as well as in education around spiritual history taking and intervention.

4.2. Study Limitations and Lessons

Limitations of the study include (1) gaps in HCP knowledge regarding inclusion of spirituality in patient care; (2) the small number of HCP and patient study participants; (3) participants being drawn exclusively from a single faith based healthcare organization; (4) brevity of the training sessions for HCPs; (5) limited follow-up with HCP participants regarding integrity of use of the FICA tool (e.g., which questions were asked and how the tool was used); and (6) challenges with the consenting process when working with vulnerable patients. Barriers to recruitment of HCPs were related to competing priorities and self-perceived inappropriateness for this type of study due to their limited understanding of, and confidence in, the area of spirituality. Some patients were reluctant to participate due to their perceptions of spirituality, while others did not consider themselves as "spiritual", and therefore did not see themselves as appropriate for the study. Declining health further precluded patient involvement in the study, as did unfortunate timing of engagement with patients around spiritual issues. Clients also often required immediate engagement in the area of spirituality once the conversation was initiated. Delays in provision of spiritual history taking and support at times resulted in patients not being open to engage further in this area. While the faith-based setting was considered to be a strength in that it facilitated and provided spiritual support from certified SCPs and other HCPs, results may vary in other institutions, including secular healthcare organizations that have differing missions, visions, and values.

Based on the experience of the research team and the findings of this study, we have learned that careful planning, collaborative consultations, and responsive adjustments are required when conducting research with HCPs caring for vulnerable populations. Further research in this area would require: (1) more extensive education for HCPs around use of the spiritual history tool; (2) evaluation of HCP fidelity to assessment protocol when using the spiritual history tool with various vulnerable populations; (3) larger numbers of participants; and (4) a longer trial period for HCP engagement and follow up with patients; Furthermore, we recommend (5) engagement with diverse IP teams working with various patient populations; and (6) inclusion of settings that are guided by both faith- and non-faith-based missions. Additional contributions to the growing body of knowledge in this area could be made through such research, thereby providing further evidence to support inclusion of spirituality in the provision of patient care.

5. Conclusions

This paper has highlighted research study findings related to the integration of spirituality in patient care within in-patient care settings by interprofessional teams. Such integration was found to enhance person-centred care, foster connection with patients, improve HCP job satisfaction and reduce burnout among IP team members. It also facilitated awareness of the need for recognition of and a response to patient spiritual needs in a timely manner. More intentional inclusion of the spiritual component in patient care at organizational, clinical/unit, professional/personal, and patient levels might be better supported through the mission and vision of an organization, support from leadership, provision of education and support for HCPs in the development of competencies and confidence addressing the spiritual domain, and consistent use of spiritual history tools in routine practice.

While inclusion of spirituality in patient care was found to have a significant impact on both patients and HCPs alike, competing priorities, fiscal constraints, urgency to discharge, documentation-related challenges and limited resources risk compromising attention given to this important area of patient care. Such a reduction has the potential to negatively effect patient care offered by IP teams, and the ability of HCPs to both relate to patients as people, and effectively help those reliant on them for care. Addressing the spiritual domain of individuals in care clearly has a positive influence on patient care, IP team members, and overall organizational culture. Its inclusion is therefore important when considering ways to effectively deliver high quality healthcare services.

Acknowledgments: The authors thank Roopa Belur (Research Assistant) and Brent Watts (Chaplain Specialist in Spiritual Care with Alberta Health Services/University of Alberta Hospital) for their contributions to the data analysis and formulations of recommendations for this project. We thank Covenant Health for funding this project, and the HCPs and patients who made this study possible through their participation. Covenant Health is committed to its faith-based vision and mission, a person-centred care approach, interprofessional teamwork, and research, all of which were critical to this project. Their willingness and desire to open their doors to researchers provides an opportunity to examine effective ways in which spirituality can be included in patient care.

Author Contributions: All authors substantively contributed to the research project that informed the findings reported in the article. Suzette Brémault-Phillips was the P.I. of the study. She along with Joanne Olson, Pamela

Brett-MacLean, Doreen Oneschuk, Shane Sinclair, Ralph Magnus, Marjan Abbasi, Jasneet Parmar, and Christina M. Puchalski developed the proposal for funding. Christina M. Puchalski developed the spiritual history tool utilized in this project, and provided permission for its use. Suzette Brémault-Phillips, Joanne Olson and Shane Sinclair wrote the application for ethical approval of the study. Suzette Brémault-Phillips, Joanne Olson, Shane Sinclair, Ralph Magnus and Christina M. Puchalski participated in the education day. Suzette Brémault-Phillips, Joanne Olson, Pamela Brett-MacLean, Doreen Oneschuk, Shane Sinclair, Ralph Magnus, Jasneet Parmar, and Christina M. Puchalski participated in the research project meeting that followed. Mid-project follow-up focus groups with HCP participants were conducted by Suzette Brémault-Phillips, Ralph Magnus, and Jeanne Weis. Marjan Abbasi attended one follow-up focus group. Final focus groups were conducted by Suzette Brémault-Phillips, Pamela Brett-MacLean, Doreen Oneschuk, Ralph Magnus, and Jeanne Weis. Jasneet Parmar attended a team meeting that followed. Patient consenting was done by Jeanne Weis and Suzette Brémault-Phillips, and chart reviews were done by Jeanne Weis. Suzette Brémault-Phillips, Jeanne Weis, and Joanne Olson were involved in data analysis. The manuscript was drafted by Suzette Brémault-Phillips, Joanne Olson, Pamela Brett-MacLean, Shane Sinclair, Doreen Oneschuk, and Jeanne Weis. All team members contributed to revising the final manuscript and provided their approval for authorship.

Abbreviations

HCP	Healthcare Professional
IP	Interprofessional
FICA	FICA Spiritual History Tool©
RA	Research Assistant
RN	Registered Nurse
SCP	Spiritual Care Professional

Conflicts of Interest: Ralph Magnus is an employee of the funding organization, while Doreen Oneschuk, Marjan Abbasi, and Jasneet Parmar conduct clinical practice within the funding organization. Christina M. Puchalski developed the spiritual history tool utilized in this project.

References

1. Christina M. Puchalski, Betty Ferrell, Rose Virani, Shirley Otis-Green, Pamela Baird, Janet Bull, Harvey Chochinov, George Handzo, Holly Nelson-Becker, Maryjo Prince-Paul, and *et al.* "Improving the quality of spiritual care as a dimension of palliative care: The report of the consensus conference." *Journal of Palliative Medicine* 12 (2009): 885–904.
2. Christina M. Puchalski. "Spirituality and health: The art of compassionate medicine." *Hospital Physician* 37 (2001): 30–36.
3. Mark Cobb, Christopher Dowrick, and Mari Lloyd-Williams. "What can we learn about the spiritual needs of palliative care patients from the research literature? " *Journal of Pain and Symptom Management* 43 (2012): 1105–19.
4. Karen E. Steinhauser, Nicholas A. Christakis, Elizabeth C. Lipp, Maya McNeilly, Lauren McIntyre, and James A. Tulsky. "Factors considered important at the end of life by patients, family, physicians, and other care providers." *The Journals of American Medical Association* 284 (2000): 2476–82.
5. Daren Heyland, Peter Dodek, Graeme Rocker, Dianne Groll, Amiram Gafni, Deb Pichora, Sam Shortt, Joan Tranmer, Neil Lazar, Jim Kutsogiannis, and Miu Lam. "What matters most to patients." *Canadian Medical Association Journal* 174 (2006): 627–33.
6. Shane Sinclair, Jose Pereira, and Shelley Raffin. "A thematic review of the spirituality literature in palliative care." *Journals Palliative Medicine* 9 (2006): 464–79.
7. Moira Stewart, Judith Belle Brown, Allan Donner, Ian R. McWhinney, Julian Oates, Wayne W. Weston, and John Jordan. "The impact of patient-centred care on outcomes." *Family Practice* 49 (2000): 796–804.
8. Moira Stewart, Bridget L. Ryan, and Christina Bodea. "Is patient-centred care associated with lower diagnostic costs? " *Healthcare Policy* 6 (2011): 27–31.
9. Tracy A. Balboni, Lauren C. Vanderwerker, Susan D. Block, M. Elizabeth Paulk, Christopher S. Lathan, John R. Peteet, and Holly G. Prigerson. "Religiousness and spiritual support among advanced cancer patients and associations with end-of-life treatment preferences and quality of life." *Journal of Clinical Oncology* 25 (2007): 555–60.

10. Harvey Max Chochinov, Thomas Hassard, Susan McClement, Thomas Hack, Linda J. Kristjanson, Mike Harlos, Shane Sinclair, and Alison Murray. "The landscape of distress in the terminally ill." *Journal of Pain and Symptom Management* 38 (2009): 641–49.

11. Christina M. Puchalski, Robert Vitillo, Sharon K. Hull, and Nancy Reller. "Improving the spiritual dimension of whole person care: Reaching national and international consensus." *Journal of Palliative Medicine* 17 (2014): 642–56.

12. Shane Sinclair, and Harvey Max Chochinov. "Communicating with patients about existential and spiritual issues: SACR-D work." *Progress in Palliative Care* 20 (2012): 72–78.

13. Christina M. Puchalski. "The role of spirituality in health care." *Proceedings (Baylor University Medical Center)* 14 (2001): 352–57.

14. John W. Ehman, Barbara B. Ott, Thomas H. Short, Ralph C. Ciampa, and John Hansen-Flaschen. "Do patients want physicians to inquire about their spiritual or religious beliefs if they become gravely ill? " *JAMA Internal Medicine* 159 (1999): 1803–06.

15. Shane Sinclair, Shelley Raffin Bouchal, Harvey Chochinov, Neil Hagen, and Susan McClement. "Spiritual care: How to do it." *BMJ Supportive and Palliative Care* 2 (2012): 319–27.

16. Gallup International Institute. *Spiritual Beliefs and the Dying Process: A Report on a National Survey*. Princeton: Gallup International Institute, 1997.

17. David Hui, Maxine de la Cruz, Steve Thorney, Henrique A. Parsons, Marvin Delgado-Guay, and Eduardo Bruera. "The frequency and correlates of spiritual distress among patients with advanced cancer admitted to an acute palliative care unit." *American Journal of Hospice & Palliative Medicine* 28 (2011): 264–70.

18. Caterina Mako, Kathleen Galek, and Shannon Poppito. "Spiritual pain among patients with advanced cancer in palliative care." *Journal of Palliative Medicine* 9 (2006): 1106–13.

19. Lucy Selman, Teresa Young, Mieke Vermandere, Ian Stirling, and Carlo Leget. "Research priorities in spiritual care: An international survey of palliative care researchers and clinicians." *Journal of Pain and Symptom Management* 48 (2014): 518–31.

20. Mark Ellis, James D. Campbell, Ann Detwiler-Breindenbach, and Dena K. Hubbard. "What do family physicians think about spirituality in clinical practice? " *Journal of Family Practice* 51 (2002): 249–54.

21. Anita Molzahn, and Laurene Shields. "Why is it so hard to talk about spirituality? " *Canadian Nurse* 104 (2008): 25–29.

22. Christina M. Puchalski, Beverly Lunsford, Mary H. Harris, and Rabbi Tamara Miller. "Interdisciplinary spiritual care for seriously ill and dying patients: A collaborative model." *The Cancer Journal* 12 (2006): 398–416.

23. Shane Sinclair. "Impact of Death and Dying on the Personal and Professional Lives of Palliative Care Professionals." *Canadian Medical Association Journal* 183 (2011): 180–87.

24. FICA Spiritual History Tool, © C. Puchalski, 1996. Please contact Dr. Puchalski for permission to use the FICA tool at cpuchals@gwu.edu

25. Christina M. Puchalski, and Anna L. Romer. "Taking a spiritual history allows clinicians to understand patients more fully." *Journal of Palliative Medicine* 3 (2000): 129–37.

26. Christina M. Puchalski. "The FICA Spiritual History Tool #274." *Journal of Palliative Medicine* 17 (2014): 105–06.

27. Tami Borneman, Betty Ferrell, and Christina M. Puchalski. "Evaluation of the FICA Tool for Spiritual Assessment." *Journal of Pain and Symptom Management* 40 (2010): 163–73.

28. Yvonna S. Lincoln, and Egon G. Guba. *Naturalistic Inquiry*. Beverly Hills: Sage, 1985.

29. Interviewee S-FG-b (Covenant Health, Edmonton, Alberta). Interview, 2014

30. Interviewee S-FG-A-4 (Covenant Health, Edmonton, Alberta). Interview, 2014

31. Interviewee JN-FG-A-2 (Covenant Health, Edmonton, Alberta). Interview, 2014

32. Interviewee S-FG-E (Covenant Health, Edmonton, Alberta). Interview, 2014

33. Interviewee S-FG-B-2 (Covenant Health, Edmonton, Alberta). Interview, 2014

34. Interviewee JN-FG-A-3 (Covenant Health, Edmonton, Alberta). Interview, 2014

35. Interviewee (Covenant Health, Edmonton, Alberta). Chart Documentation, 2014

36. Interviewee S-FG-A-3 (Covenant Health, Edmonton, Alberta). Interview, 2014

37. Interviewee J-FG-b-2 (Covenant Health, Edmonton, Alberta). Interview, 2014

38. Interviewee S-FG-B-3 (Covenant Health, Edmonton, Alberta). Interview, 2014

39. Interviewee JL-FG-B-2 (Covenant Health, Edmonton, Alberta). Interview, 2014
40. Interviewee JN-FG-A-5 (Covenant Health, Edmonton, Alberta). Interview, 2014
41. Interviewee S-FG-B-1 (Covenant Health, Edmonton, Alberta). Interview, 2014
42. Interviewee JL-FG-b-2 (Covenant Health, Edmonton, Alberta). Interview, 2014
43. Interviewee (Covenant Health, Edmonton, Alberta). Patient Declines Note, 2014
44. Interviewee S-FG-B (Covenant Health, Edmonton, Alberta). Interview, 2014
45. Interviewee JL-FG-A-3 (Covenant Health, Edmonton, Alberta). Interview, 2014
46. Interviewee JL-FG-B-1 (Covenant Health, Edmonton, Alberta). Interview, 2014
47. Interviewee JL-FG-B-3 (Covenant Health, Edmonton, Alberta). Interview, 2014
48. Interviewee S-FG-b-3 (Covenant Health, Edmonton, Alberta). Interview, 2014
49. Interviewee S-FG-B-4 (Covenant Health, Edmonton, Alberta). Interview, 2014
50. Interviewee JL-FG-A-1 (Covenant Health, Edmonton, Alberta). Interview, 2014
51. Interviewee S-FG-b-2 (Covenant Health, Edmonton, Alberta). Interview, 2014
52. Interviewee (Covenant Health, Edmonton, Alberta). Reflection 7, 2014

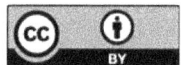

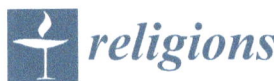

Article

Beliefs in Miraculous Healings, Religiosity and Meaning in Life

Jakub Pawlikowski [1,*], Michał Wiechetek [2], Jarosław Sak [1] and Marek Jarosz [2]

[1] Department of Ethics and Human Philosophy, Medical University of Lublin, Aleje Racławickie 1,
20-950 Lublin, Poland; jaroslaw.sak@umlub.pl

[2] Institute of Psychology, John Paul II Catholic University of Lublin, Aleje Racławickie 14,
20-950 Lublin, Poland; wiechetek@kul.pl (M.W.); mjarosz@kul.pl (M.J.)

* Author to whom correspondence should be addressed; jpawlikowski@wp.pl; Tel.: +48-81-4486-850.

Academic Editors: Arndt Büssing and René Hefti
Received: 1 June 2015; Accepted: 9 September 2015; Published: 17 September 2015

Abstract: Throughout centuries, many interpretations of miraculous healings have been offered by philosophers, theologians, physicians and psychologists. Different approaches to miracles originate from the differences in understanding of causative factors, concepts of nature and the relationship between God and nature. Despite many skeptical arguments, a vast majority of people (approximately 70%) in modern Western societies share a belief in miracles and millions of sick people pilgrimage to sanctuaries seeking their occurrence. The aim of the research was to describe the social perception of miraculous healings, and the relationship between beliefs in miraculous healings, religiosity and meaning in life. A survey was conducted on a group of 178 respondents aged 18 to 30 (M = 21.5; SD = 2.31), 90% Catholics. The obtained results show that it is possible to describe the perception of miraculous healings in category of the essence of the causative factors (natural/supranatural) and definiteness (defined/undefined). The majority (88%) of the respondents believed in miracles and most frequently associated them with God's action/intervention, less often with the still undiscovered possibilities of the human organism or the nature, and the least with medical biases. Respondents with stronger religiosity more often understood miraculous healings as an act of God than the activity of unspecified supernatural powers. Moreover, higher religiosity and understanding of miraculous healings as an effect of the supernatural specified determinant was connected with higher meaning in life.

Keywords: miraculous healings; religiosity; meaning in life

1. Introduction

Beliefs in miracles, among them in miraculous healings, have been present in human culture since its origins. They have attracted the attention of ordinary people, artists and thinkers. For centuries, many philosophers, theologians and scientists offered their interpretations of miraculous healings. In contemporary times we can also observe the debate about miraculous healings in the medical society [1–8]. The last official confirmation of an inexplicable healing in Lourdes occurred in 2005 [9]. The Vatican Congregation for the Causes of Saints proclaimed 347 decrees about miracles between 1983 and 2004 [10,11]. The majority of Polish physicians and medical students (approximately 70%) believe in miracles defined as supernatural phenomena caused by God [12]. A great majority of people in modern Western societies (including physicians) share a belief in miracles. According to Mansfield it may be as much as 80% of the Western population. The faith in miraculous healing is stronger among women, African-Americans, Evangelical Protestants, the poorer, sicker, and less educated and majority of respondents understand that God acts through the hands of the physicians [13]. Beliefs in miraculous healings are the part of beliefs in miracles, and miraculous healings are the most popular examples of miracles. However, in many studies it is difficult to determine how respondents perceive or define miracles.

There have been numerous definitions of miracles, and it is difficult to present a detailed and commonly accepted one. The word "miracle" comes from the Latin *miraculum*, which is derived from *mirari* (to wonder). Thus, the most general epistemological characterization of a miracle is an event that causes wonder and is in some way unusual or contrary to our expectations [14–16]. Ontological aspects of miracles to which many definitions point to treat miracles as extraordinary and in some sense beyond (above, contrary to) nature. A subjective conviction of a divine intervention also seems to be very common for the miracle (miraculous phenomena).

A detailed history of philosophical thinking about miracles was described by J. Pawlikowski [8]. Different approaches to miracles originated from the differences in understanding the notion of God (personal or impersonal, transcendent or immanent), nature (deterministic or indeterministic) and the relationship between God and nature. If one perceive laws of nature as relative and God as personal and transcendent but acting, usually one believes in miracles. It is also possible to be open to the transcendent interpretation of the miraculous phenomena but has not the personal concept of God and understand miracles as the effect of supernatural powers. If one perceives nature as a deterministic system and denies the existence of God or His ability to act in nature, usually there is no space for theistic interpretation of miracles, thus miracles are understood as the effects of unknown supernatural factors, still undiscovered possibilities of the nature, the effect of a medically ambiguous diagnosis, medical error or bias. It is possible to determine the typology of understanding of miraculous healings based on the essence of the causative factors (natural or supernatural) and their definiteness (defined/undefined). Referring to the philosophical concepts presented above it can be assumed that belief in miraculous healings can be described in two categories: the essence (nature) of the causative factor as natural *vs.* supernatural and its definiteness as undefined *vs.* defined-miraculous healings can be explained as a result of supernatural defined (SD, in other words transcendent specified cause, e.g., God) or undefined factors (SU, transcendent unspecified, e.g., unknown supernatural powers). They can also be understood as an effect of natural defined (ND, in other words immanent specified cause, e.g., the effect of medical biases) or natural undefined factors (NU, immanent unspecified, e.g., still undiscovered possibilities of the human organism, unknown natural energies and laws). Some examples are listed below. This theoretical concept is present in the model TMMHB in later part of the manuscript ().

We can provide many examples of supernatural interpretations of miracles. According to the Bible, God created the world, and thus all the phenomena are directly related to Him. Consequently, miracles could be treated as a special sign (Hebr. *Oth*, Gr. *semeion*, Eng. *sign*) given by God to Man (SD) [17]. According to St. Thomas Aquinas (1225–1274) "Those events then are properly to be styled miracles, which happen by divine power beyond the order commonly observed in nature" (*Summa Contra Gentiles*, 3.101). In his concept, the cause of the miracle is external to the world, it surpasses nature, and therefore that could be only God (SD). Some modern and contemporary thinkers also defended the understanding of miracle as the act of God (SD), e.g., Blaise Pascal ([18], lines 803–55) or C. S. Lewis [19]. The belief in mysterious powers that could influence nature and human life is also present in New Age literature, but is understood as the effect of cosmic energy or spiritual powers (SU), or as unknown laws of nature or mysterious human mind powers (NU) [8].

It is also possible to enumerate many examples of natural interpretations of miracles. Ancient philosophers such as Pythagoras or Empedocles were believed to be thaumaturges, although they themselves denied performing miracles and said that they simply knew nature (ND). Celsus (2nd c.) claimed that the gods were not interested in human affairs and miracles could only be the effect of an error in diagnosis (ND) [20,21]. In the Middle Ages thinkers distinguished between the *miraculum*, understood as God's work (SD), and the *mirabile* perceived as an exceptional, curious event, that could not be the work of God but that of a magician or trickster (ND or NU). In modern times there were many ideas concerning miracles as natural phenomena. Baruch Spinoza, Immanuel Kant, representatives of deism (e.g., John Toland) stated that the immutability of laws of nature excludes the possibility of God's intervention in the natural world, however they did not define the causative factor—for them a "miracle" was an incomprehensible natural fact (NU) [22,23]; ([24], chapter 6, lines 1–134). David Hume (1711–1776) believed that the invariability of laws of nature and weak human evidence spoke against miracles and only the faith gave people power to believe in things that are against experience (NU) (*Enquiries*, p. 114)[1] [25]. In the 19th century J.M. Charcot, believed that healings in Lourdes had a natural explanation—hysteria and hypnosis (ND) [26], but A. Carrel (1873–1944), Nobel Prize laureate (1912), acknowledge the mysterious character of the place and understood miracles as an effect of unknown powers of nature (NU)[2] [28]. From the perspective of the process philosophy (A.N. Whitehead) miracles are a very rare phenomena and can neither be confirmed nor excluded using modern scientific methods (NU) [29–31]. Most theoretical disputes on the possibility of miracles concentrate on the concept of a miracle perceived as contrary to laws of nature (an event that is *contra naturam*); comprehending miracles as signs, manifestations of nature's powers at God's command or subjective experience is not so controversial.

Referring to the philosophical concepts presented above and in Pawlikowski's work [8], it can be assumed that beliefs on miraculous healings can be described on two categories: the essence (nature) of the causative factor as natural *vs.* supranatural and its definiteness as undefined *vs.* defined (Theoretical model of miraculous healings beliefs, TMMHB; see). Vertical axis describes the belief that miraculous healings are caused by factors associated with natural *vs.* supranatural (transcendental) elements. In turn, the horizontal axis refers to understanding miraculous healings using defined (specified) and undefined elements (difficult to define, specify or identify). On the quadrants of the scheme the authors propose hypothetical names relating to the perception of miraculous healings.

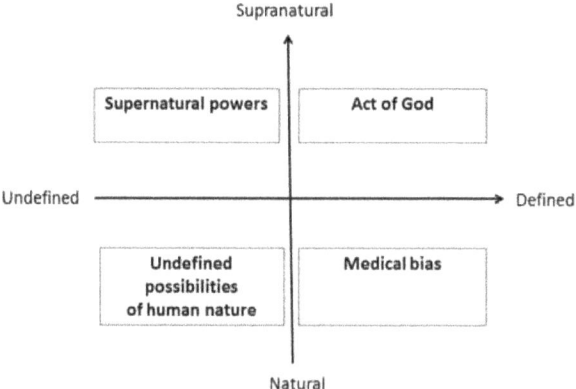

Scheme 1. Theoretical model of miraculous healings beliefs (TMMHB).

Analyses conducted by contemporary philosophers (e.g., Ch. Hartshorne, R. Swinburne) underlines that the perception of miracles is an outcome of metaphysical presuppositions and not scientific data [32,33]. It is interesting to know how people understand miraculous healings and how this belief interacts with other personal, sociological and psychological factors, such as: age, gender, ethnicity, household incomes, level of experienced stress, life satisfaction, religiosity and beliefs [34].

---

[1] C. S. Lewis arguing for theistic interpretation of miracles and analyzing the Humean critique of miracles wrote: "we know the experience against them [miracles] to be uniform only if we know that all the reports of them are false. And we can know all the reports to be false only if we know already that miracles have never occurred. In fact, we are arguing in a circle." [19].

[2] A. Carrel as a young physician traveled to Lourdes with a group of sick people, saw the inexplicable recovery of one of his patients [27].

It seems that religiosity may be of particular importance as to a large extent it shapes ideas about the relationship between the material and spiritual world and is connected with life's meaning [35].

The premise for interconnections between the belief in miraculous healings, religion and the meaning of life can be the Concept of Personal Meaning. According to it, the meaning of life is defined as "the awareness of an order, coherence, purpose in life of an individual and the accompanying sense of accomplishment" [36]. This multidimensional reality is created by structural components of sense, which include the source, scope and depth of meaning. Within the framework of this concept, four main levels of meaning's development and discovering its depth are distinguished. They are divided in accordance with the degree of transcendence of the "I". The first level is characterized by the focus of the individual on him/herself, his preoccupation with hedonistic pleasures and caring only for his/her needs. The second level is reflected by devoting time and energy for implementing one's own potentiality, using one's own skill and self-improving. On the other two levels, individuals in their actions, decisions and activities go beyond his/her own "I", transcendence occurs and the individual begins to be opened and sensitized to other people and the supernatural. Level three is thus associated with serving others and belonging to a larger community, becoming engaged in political affairs and pro-social activities. The last level (4) is connected with receiving values, which go beyond the individual and the recognition of the ultimate goal—the highest level of transcendence of the "I". Current studies indicate that people experiencing meaning from the last two levels have a greater sense of accomplishment and feel higher life satisfaction compared with those experiencing meaning from the Reker's lower levels [37].

The above theoretical arguments and studies indicate that transgression, being open for eternal values and towards the supernatural reality helps to increase a sense of purpose and satisfaction with life [38]. It has also been indicated that the sole acceptance of God's existence and religious involvement (one of the aspects of religiosity) help to find the meaning of life. It seems that the meaning will be greater, if the greater the openness to the Absolute is, especially in terms of the belief in the possibility of "His" intervention in the world. Thus, the level of the acceptance of the transcendent reality depends not only on the belief in God but also in the conviction of his intervention in the real world e.g., by miraculous healings.

The aim of the research was to describe the perception of miraculous healings, verify the TMMH, and analyze the relationship between beliefs in miraculous healings, religiosity and meaning in life. It was hypothesized that perception of miraculous healings is heterogeneous (we propose four dimensions) and that the different perceptions of miraculous healings are associated with religiosity and the meaning in life in different way (positive or negative).

2. Materials and Methods

The study was conducted using an online questionnaire distributed voluntarily via e-mail to students of psychology. During the research, data from 200 participants had been collected, but only 178 (89%) questionnaires were accepted. The respondents' ages were: 18 to 30 (M = 21.5; SD = 2.31). The majority of the respondents were women (69.7%) and people of Roman Catholic religion (90%). Respondents completed three research tools and short demographics. In order to determine the perception of miraculous healings an experimental version of the Beliefs about Miraculous Healings Scale (BMHS) was applied. It allows for subjective assess of miraculous healings as: Act of God (1 item), Undefined possibilities of human nature (3 items), Supernatural powers (1 item) and Medical bias (2 items). This method consists of 7 claims (e.g., a miraculous healing is a result of supernatural forces") rated on a scale from 1 to 4 where 1 strongly disagree and 4 strongly agree [39]. The results in multi-items dimensions are computed as mean scores. Religiosity was measured using the Duke University Religion Index (DUREL) [40]. It is a self-administered five-items measure allows us to assess three aspects of religiosity: Organizational Religious Activity (one item, ORA), Non-organizational Religious Activity (two items, NORA), Intrinsic Religiosity (three items, IR). The results of the method are sum of points obtained from questions assessed on six-point (ORA, NORA) and five-point (IR) scales. The level of life's meaning was analyzed using the Meaning in Life Questionnaire (MLQ) [41]. MLQ is a 10-items tool that investigates two dimensions of meaning in life: the presence of meaning (five items) and the search for meaning (five items). Each statement was assessed on five-point Likert's scale.

3. Results

The collected data were statistically analyzed using the SPSS v.22. A vast majority (89%) of the respondents declared the belief in miracles, as a phenomenon or event that for various reasons does not have scientific explanation. The starting point of the basic analyses was to determine in what dimensions the statements included in the methods capturing the perception of miraculous healings were located. In accordance with the literature mentioned in the introduction part, the existence of categories which will arrange themselves on the axis of Natural *vs.* Supernatural and Undefined *vs.* Defined was assumed. The results of the factor analysis (Varimax method) revealed the existence of four dimensions describing the belief in miraculous healings (Table 1). These dimensions include unknown possibilities of the human nature, supernatural powers, medical bias and act of God. The solution explains 88.6% of variance. The obtained results are coherent with the above-mentioned theoretical considerations and may point to the diversity in understanding and the interpretation of miraculous healings.

Table 1. Results of the factor analysis for the Beliefs about Miraculous Healings Scale (BMHS) *.

	Dimension			
	Undefined possibilities of human nature	Supernatural powers	Medical bias	Act of God
Consequence of still undiscovered human organism potentials	0.876			
Effect of unknown natural laws	0.778			
Effect of human psychic action	0.754			
Effect of supernatural powers		0.994		
Effect of medical data manipulation			0.885	
Result of medical biased diagnosis			0.822	
Act of God				−0.860

* Only factor loadings > 0.5 are displayed.

Respondents obtained the highest indicators in the dimension that describes miracles as an act of God (Figure 1), the lowest, in the dimension which treats miracles as the manipulation of medical data and medical bias.

The majority of the distinguished dimensions of BMHS is associated with the variables taken into consideration during the research (Table 2). Explaining miracles through natural factors negatively correlates with all the categories of religiosity. Those more religiously involved to a lesser extend treat miracles as a result of undiscovered possibilities of the organism, unknown laws of nature, the effects of the human psyche, medical data manipulation and diagnostic errors. These dimensions are also associated with the level of satisfying the sense of life. In case of treating miracles in terms of a supernatural defined factor (God) the correlation is positive. A miracle as the result of God's activity coexists with both the religious commitment as well as with the sense of meaning in life. Interestingly, none of the religious variables included in the study and describing the aspects of meaning in life correlates with the belief that miracles are an effect of undefined supernatural forces. Additionally, no statistically significant relations were found between the interpretation of miraculous healings and the search for meaning in life.

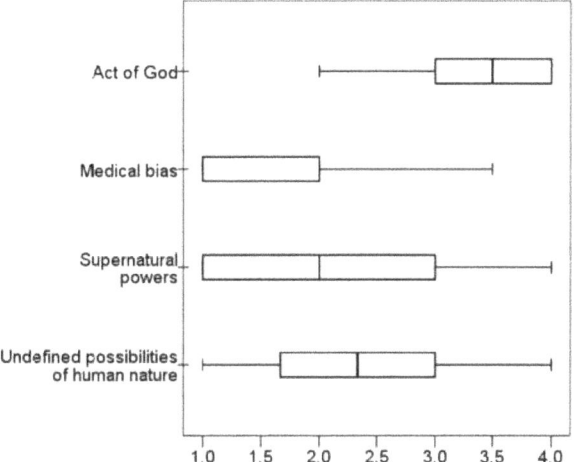

Figure 1. The distribution of results for various beliefs on miraculous healings (On the figure are presented minimum, maximum, median and interquartile range in each dimension).

Table 2. The relationship between perception of miraculous healings, religiosity and aspects of the meaning of life (Spearman's rank correlation coefficient).

	(1)	(2)	(3)	(4)	(5)	(6)	(7)	(8)	(9)
Act of God (1)	-								
Medical bias (2)	−0.600 **	(α = 0.87)							
Supernatural powers (3)	−0.007	0.144	-						
Undefined possibilities of human nature (4)	−0.630 **	0.667 **	0.122	(α = 0.87)					
Organizational religious activity (5)	0.655 **	−0.478 **	−0.025	−0.526 **	-				
Non-organizational religious activity (6)	0.469 **	−0.378 **	−0.024	−0.415 **	0.676 **	-			
Intrinsic religiosity (7)	0.680 **	−0.472 **	−0.037	−0.574 **	0.793 **	0.707 **	(α = 0.86)		
Presence of meaning (8)	0.171 *	−0.248 **	−0.057	−0.168 *	0.145	0.326 **	0.281 **	(α = 0.84)	
Search of meaning (9)	0.024	0.093	0.089	0.038	0.059	−0.081	0.000	−0.391 **	(α = 0.85)

* $p < 0.05$; ** $p < 0.01$; On the diagonal are presented Cronbach's alpha reliability coefficients for multi item dimensions.

4. Discussion

Results indicate the existence of a relationship between the perception and understanding of the miraculous healings, religiosity and the respondents' meaning of life. Such a relationship is confirmed by few previous reports, which not always specify the definition of events reported as miraculous [42,43] or place general description [7,13,44]. In the interpretation of the relationship between the acceptance of miracles and the religiosity and the meaning in life it seems essential to establish the respondent's beliefs on the cause of miraculous phenomenon. Such assertion is possible through the application of a BMHS (Beliefs about Miraculous Healings Scale) based on Theoretical Model of Miraculous Healings Beliefs (TMMHB). This research tool shows correlations between the understanding of a miracle as a phenomenon of a supernatural origin (SD, e.g., God), religiosity and the sense of meaning in life occur. The credibility of this observation is confirmed by the existence of a negative correlation between understanding miraculous healings as natural phenomenon (ND, NU) and religiosity and the sense of meaning in life. The lack of a relationship between understanding miracles as phenomenon resulting from the activity of undefined supernatural causes (SU) is interesting.

Perhaps this is due to the double ambiguity of the described category connected to transcendence and indeterminacy. Because of a metaphysical distance (transcendence) and epistemological indeterminacy, this category cannot create religious behaviors nor influence the meaning in life. This observation requires further in-depth research.

Obtained results seem to confirm the validity of the Theoretical Model of Miraculous Healings Beliefs (TMMHB) proposed in the introduction. Different perceptions of the essence of causative factor of miraculous healings (natural/supernatural) and his definiteness (defined/undefined) relevantly differentiate the attitudes and correlate with religiosity and meaning in life in different way. A negative correlation has been observed between the understanding of miracles as phenomenon belonging to the sphere of nature, religious activity and the sense of meaning in life, and at the same time a positive correlation was visible within the supernatural sphere. It is coherent with other researches which show that religiosity and believing in miracles have protective effect in terms of being exposed to stress and trauma, e.g., Manglos [34], in his study conducted on a group of American teenagers (aged 13–17) identified the protective effect of believing in miracles understood as a God's intervention in relation to various types of traumatic experience. On the other hand, the influence of traumatic experience on the level of acceptance of the relationship between supernatural events and the intervention of the divine factor should also be analyzed.

The Beliefs about Miraculous Healings Scale may be useful tool in the research focused on perception of miraculous healings. Despite certain limitations it may contribute to conducting further research on the correlations between understanding of the miraculous healings and variables characterizing the existential situation of a person in various life periods. It may be also useful for comparative studies in communities shaped by different religious traditions concerning the understanding of transcendence, e.g., comparing various groups of followers of monotheistic religions, Buddhism and animistic beliefs. An interesting perspective is the compilation of perceptions of miracles with religious thought styles. Analysis of the content of the dimensions found in the Beliefs about Miraculous Healings Scale indicates that such a way of perceiving miracles is close to the perspective of religious cognitive styles proposed by D. Wulff [45]. According to him it is possible to enumerate four styles of thinking about religion (Orthodoxy, External Critique, Relativism, Second Naiveté) located on two axes; Exclusion *vs.* Inclusion of Transcendence and the Literal *vs.* Symbolic way of interpreting the content of religious beliefs [46–48]. From this perspective it seems reasonable to conduct research not only within the Polish culture but also in other European countries, experiencing secularization processes.

The task that should be undertaken in further evaluation of the hermeneutical possibilities of the theoretical model of beliefs in miraculous healings (TMMHB) is the broadening of the scope of age groups, and their diversity in terms of existential experience and religious traditions. The research presented in this article was conducted in a religiously homogenous group of Polish students, who were shaped by the Catholic tradition. A certain limitation of the used research tool is determining its psychometric properties given a limited group (young people) and a small number of items in each of the dimensions. The short form is the advantage of this research tool and it can be used among advanced age groups of respondents. In subsequent studies it would also be beneficial to take into consideration the sense of control localization and superstition as two aspects, which indicate the existence of an external reality, which could affect the actions of an individual.

5. Conclusions

Vast majority of respondents understand miraculous healings as a result of God's action and not the effect of natural unknown factors. Respondents with lower religiosity more often believe that miraculous healings are the activity of unspecified supernatural powers or results of medical biases than an act of God. Higher religiosity and understanding of miraculous healings as an effect of the supernatural specified determinant was connected with higher meaning in life.

Religions **2015**, *6*, 1113–1124

Conflicts of Interest: The authors declare no conflict of interest.

Author Contributions: Jakub Pawlikowski: designing research, analyzing data, writing paper; Michal Wiechetek: designing research, performing research, analyzing data, writing paper; Jaroslaw Sak: analyzing data, writing paper; Marek Jarosz: analyzing data. All authors read and approved the final manuscript.

References

1. Virginia Morell. "No Miracles." *Science* 19 (2014): 1443–45. [CrossRef] [PubMed]
2. Andrus Viidik. "Medical miracles in fact and fiction." *Lakartidningen* 111 (2014): 1194–95. [PubMed]
3. Dan P. Sulmasy. "What is a miracle? " *Southern Medical Journal* 100 (2007): 1223–28. [CrossRef] [PubMed]
4. Richard Lakeman. "Talking science and wishing for miracles: Understanding cultures of mental health practice." *International Journal of Mental Health Nursing* 22 (2013): 106–15. [CrossRef] [PubMed]
5. Julian Savulescu, and Steve Clarke. "Waiting for a miracle. miracles, miraclism, and discrimination." *Southern Medical Journal* 100 (2007): 1259–62. [CrossRef] [PubMed]
6. Horace M. DeLisser. "A practical approach to the family that expects a miracle." *Chest* 35 (2009): 1643–47. [CrossRef] [PubMed]
7. Eric W. Widera, Kenneth E. Rosenfeld, Erik K. Fromme, Daniel P. Sulmasy, and Robert M. Arnold. "Approaching Patients and Family Members Who Hope for a Miracle." *Journal of Pain and Symptom Management* 42 (2011): 119–25. [CrossRef] [PubMed]
8. Jakub Pawlikowski. "The history of thinking about miracles in the West." *Southern Medical Journal* 100 (2007): 1229–35. [CrossRef] [PubMed]
9. Anonymous. "The cures at Lourdes recognised as miraculous by the Church." Available online: http://www.lourdes-france.org/upload/pdf/gb_guerisons.pdf (accessed on 20 April 2015).
10. Wiesław Bar, and Dariusz Blicharz. "Charakterystyka cudów do beatyfikacji i kanonizacji uznanych po reformie prawa kanonizacyjnego w 1983 roku (The Characterization of Miracles Confirmed in Beatifications and Canonizations Processes after the reform of the Canonization Law in 1983 year)." In *Cuda w Sprawach Kanonizacyjnych (Miracles in Canonizations Processes)*. Edited by Wiesław Bar. Lublin: WDS, 2006, pp. 153–206.
11. Kenneth Woodward. *Making Saints: How the Catholic Church Determines Who Becomes a Saint, Who Doesn't, and Why*. New York: Touchstone, 1996, pp. 191–220.
12. Jakub Pawlikowski, Jarosław Sak, and Krzysztof Marczewski. "The belief in miracles among students of medicine." *Annal UMCS Section D Medcine* 61 (2006): 373–379.
13. Christopher J. Mansfield, Jim Mitchell, and Dana E. King. "The doctor as God's mechanic? Beliefs in the Southeastern United States." *Social Science and Medicine* 54 (2002): 399–409. [CrossRef]
14. Edward Craig. *A Routledge Encyclopedia of Philosophy*. London and New York: Taylor & Francis, 1998.
15. Simon Blackburn. *The Oxford Dictionary of Philosophy*. Oxford and New York: Oxford University Press, 1996.
16. Michael Levine. "Miracles." In *Stanford Encyclopedia of Philosophy*. Edited by Edward N. Zalta. Stanford: Stanford Online Media, 2002, Available online: http://plato.stanford.edu/entries/miracles/ (accessed on 20 April 2015).
17. Charles Francis D. Moule. "The vocabulary of miracle." In *Miracles. Cambridge Studies in Their Philosophy and History*. Edited by Charles Francis D. Moule. London: A. R. Mowbray & Co Ltd., 1965, pp. 235–38.
18. Blaise Pascal. *Thoughts*. Garden City: Doubleday, 1961.
19. Clive S. Lewis. *Miracles. A Preliminary Study*. New York: The MacMillan Company, 1947, pp. 121–30.
20. Wendy Cotter. *Miracles in Greco-Roman Antiquity. A Sourcebook*. London: Routledge Taylor & Francis Group, 1999.
21. Howard C. Kee. *Miracle in the Early Christian World: A Study in Socio-Historical Method*. New Haven and London: Yale University Press, 1983, p. 89.
22. John Toland. *Christianity Not Mysterious*. New York: Garland Pub, 1978.
23. Immanuel Kant. *Religion within the Limits of Reason alone*. Translated by Theodore M. Greene, and Hoyt Hudson. New York: Harper, 1960, pp. 80–85.
24. Baruch Spinoza. "Tractatus Theologico-Politicus." In *The Chief Works of Benedict de Spinoza*. Translated by Robert Harvey M. Elwes. New York: Dover Publications, 1955.
25. David Hume. *Enquiries Concerning Human Understanding*. Oxford: Oxford University Press, 1975, pp. 109–31.

26. Robert B. Mullin. *Miracles and Modern Religious Imagination*. New Haven and London: Yale University Press, 1996, pp. 119–37.

27. Alexis Carrell. *Voyage to Lourdes*. New York: Harper, 1950.

28. Alexis Carrel. *Man, The Unknown*. McPherson: ADP Gauntlet, 2014.

29. William Lane Craig. "The Problem of Miracles: A Historical and Philosophical Perspective." In *Gospel Perspectives*. Edited by D. Wenham and C. Blomberg. Sheffield: JSOT Press, 1986, pp. 9–40.

30. Colin Brown. *Miracles and the Critical Mind*. Grand Rapids: William B. Eerdmans Publishing Company, 1984.

31. William E. Stempsey. "Miracles and the limits of medical knowledge." *Medical Health Care Philosophy* 5 (2002): 1–9. [CrossRef]

32. Charles Hartshorne. "A Reply to My Critics." In *The Philosophy of Charles Hartshorne*. Edited by Lewis E. Hahn. La Salle: Open Court, 1991, pp. 569–731.

33. Richard Swinburne. *The Concept of Miracle*. New York: St. Martin's Press, 1970.

34. Nicolette D. Manglos. "Faith Pinnacle Moments: Stress, Miraculous Experiences, and Life Satisfaction in Young Adulthood." *Sociology of Religion* 74 (2013): 176–98. [CrossRef] [PubMed]

35. Crystal L. Park, and Donald Edmondson. "Religion as a source of meaning." In *Meaning, Mortality, and Choice: The Social Psychology of Existential Concerns*. Edited by Phillip R. Shaver and Mario Mikulincer. Washington: American Psychological Association, 2012, pp. 145–62.

36. Gary T. Reker, and Paul T. Wong. "Aging as an individual proces: Toward a theory of personal meaning." In *Emergent Theories of Aging*. Edited by James E. Birren and Vern L. Bengtson. New York: Springer, 1988, pp. 214–46.

37. Gary T. Reker. "Theoretical perspective, dimensions, and measurement of existential meaning." In *Exploring Existential Meaning: Optimizing Human Development across the Life Span*. Thousand Oaks: Sage Publications, 2000, pp. 39–55.

38. Yung-Jong Shiah, Frances Chang, Shih-Kuang Chiang, I-Mei Lin, and Wai-Cheong Carl Tam. "Religion and Health: Anxiety, religiosity, meaning of life and mental health." *Journal of Religion and Health* 54 (2015): 35–45. [CrossRef] [PubMed]

39. Michał Wiechetek, and Jakub Pawlikowski. *Beliefs about Miraculous Healings Scale*. Lublin: The John Paul II Catholic University of Lublin, 2012, Unpublished manuscript.

40. Harold Koenig, and Arndt Büssing. "The Duke University Religion Index (DUREL): A Five-Item Measure for Use in Epidemiological Studies." *Religions* 1 (2010): 78–85. [CrossRef]

41. Michael F. Steger, Patricia Frazier, and Shigehiro Oishi. "The Meaning in Life Questionnaire: Assessing the Presence of and Search for Meaning in Life." *Journal of Counseling Psychology* 53 (2006): 80–93. [CrossRef]

42. Michele A. Schottenbauer, Benjamin F. Rodriguez, Carol R. Glass, and Diane B. Arnkoff. "Religious coping research and contemporary personality theory: An exploration of Endler's (1997) integrative personality theory." *British Journal of Psychology* 97 (2006): 499–519. [CrossRef] [PubMed]

43. Shayesteh Salehi, Arash Ghodousi, and Khadijeh Ojaghloo. "The spiritual experiences of patients with diabetes-related limb amputation." *Iranian Journal of Nursing and Midwifery Research* 17 (2012): 225–28. [PubMed]

44. Rodney Stark, and Jared Maier. "Faith and Happiness." *Review of Religious Research* 50 (2008): 120–25.

45. David M. Wulff. *Psychology of Religion: Classic and Contemporary Views*. New York: Wiley, 1991.

46. Rafał Bartczuk, Beata Zarzycka, and Michał Wiechetek. "The Internal Structure of the Polish Adaptation of the Post-Critical Belief Scale." *Annals of Psychology* 16 (2013): 539–61.

47. Bart Duriez, Johnny R. J. Fontaine, and Dirk Hutsebaut. "A further elaboration of the Post-Critical Belief Scale: Evidence for the existence of four different approaches to religion in Flanders Belgium." *Psychologica Belgica* 40 (2000): 153–81.

48. Dirk Hutsebaut. "Post-critical belief. A new approach to the religious attitude problem." *Journal of Empirical Theology* 9 (1996): 48–66. [CrossRef]

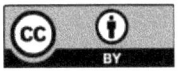

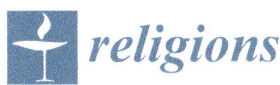

Article

"I Heard the Voice. I Felt the Presence": Prayer, Health and Implications for Clinical Practice

Mary Rute Gomes Esperandio [1,†,*] and Kevin L. Ladd [2,†]

[1]   Postgraduate Program in Theology/Postgraduate Program in Bioethics, Pontifícia Universidade Católica do Paraná, Rua Imaculada Conceição, 1155, Prado Velho, CEP 80215-901 Curitiba, Paraná, Brazil

[2]   Department of Psychology, Indiana University South Bend, 1700 Mishawaka Ave, South Bend, IN 46601, USA; kladd@iusb.edu

*   Author to whom correspondence should be addressed; mary.esperandio@pucpr.br; Tel.: +55-41-3039-5779.

†   These authors contributed equally to this work.

Academic Editors: René Hefti and Arndt Büssing

Received: 7 April 2015; Accepted: 3 June 2015; Published: 11 June 2015

Abstract: Research concerning the relation between physical health and prayer typically employs an outcome oriented paradigm and results are inconsistent. This is not surprising since prayer *per se* is not governed by physiological principles. More revealing and logically compelling, but more rare, is literature examining health and prayer from the perspective of the participants. The present study examines the health–prayer experience of 104 Christians in the United States. Data were collected through recorded video interviews and analyzed by means of content analysis. Results show that prayer is used as a context nuanced spiritual tool for: dealing with physical suffering (spiritual-religious coping); sustaining hope and spirituality via a sacred dimension; personal empowerment; self-transcendence. These findings demonstrate that practitioners primarily engage prayer at a spiritual rather than a physical level, underscoring the limitations of a biomedical or "Complementary and Alternative Medicine" perspective that conceptualizes prayer as a mechanism for intentionally improving physical health. In clinical practice, regarding the medical, psychotherapeutic, or pastoral, the challenge is to understand prayer through the framework of the practitioner, in order to affirm its potential in healthcare processes.

Keywords: prayer; spirituality; religion; health; clinical practice

---

1. Introduction

Studies have demonstrated that in the Western world, many people turn to religion in difficult times, especially when facing illness [1,2]. According to an American survey on use of prayer ($N = 2055$), 35% of respondents used prayer for health concerns; 75% of these prayed for wellness, and 22% prayed for specific medical conditions; of those praying for specific medical conditions, 69% found prayer very helpful [3]. What is not at all clear from this or similar work, is the extent of the respondents' histories of prayer practice. If, for instance, this 35% represents a group of people trying prayer for the first time as a "last resort" the interpretation of the findings would be radically different that if the group had a lifetime discipline of fervent prayer.

In other words, understanding the relation between prayer and health appears deceptively simple if one has in mind solely that prayer has been shown in research to be one of the main religious coping strategies within the health-illness context. However, prayer is much more than merely a tool for promoting "positive religious coping". According to Ladd and Spilka, prayer is a way of connecting with the self, others, and the sacred [4]. These connections can occur in a variety of ways. For instance, they concluded that in relation to the self, prayers may evoke deeply troubling concerns (tears) or they be more linked to broad evaluations (examination). Some people pray for others to receive support (intercession), or for themselves to actively *become* the support for others even though it will be a great challenge to endure (suffering). On occasion, prayers can be very forceful, stating one's personal position (radical), or requesting tangible forms of assistance (petition), while at other times, the prayers are seeking peace and stillness (rest). Still other prayers are often linked to traditional texts (sacrament) ([5], p. 59).

In sum, prayer is multi-faceted and therefore will be useful to people in a wide variety of ways when it comes to dealing with difficulties, whether chronic or acute. In addition, the quality and conditions of the context matter because prayer can have both negative and positive effects; however, the multi-faceted negative aspects of prayer have been minimally explored with regard to coping [6].

To discuss more comprehensively the relation between prayer, health, and clinical practice, it is necessary to shed light on the varied roles of prayer in one's life and the quality of the relationships it allows one to establish. Thus, the discussion of this topic will be based on a study of the prayer experiences reported by 104 participants and will present several considerations regarding the relation between prayer, health, and clinical practice. The purpose of this discussion is not to delineate all the possibilities and/or risks of integrating prayer into the clinical context, or even to address the effects of prayer on specific health outcomes. Rather, the aim is to contribute to the theoretical studies on the psychology of prayer, taking into consideration what the participants themselves state about their prayer experiences, beyond the utilitarian question effects of prayer.

Initially, some aspects of the relation between prayer and health revealed by major studies on this topic will be discussed. Then, the results of the above research will be presented and, finally, some implications of the relation between prayer and health for clinical and pastoral practice will be indicated. In the concluding paragraphs, suggestions for further studies will be provided.

2. Prayer and Health: A Tenuous Relation

In a recent review of the literature about prayer and health, Ladd and Spilka [6] raised the question of why one should assume there is any relation between these two topics. The authors argue that the expected relation between prayer and health is ambiguous and certainly cannot be taken for granted based on any theological presumptions. From both a theological and a clinical perspective, there is not necessarily a consistently predictable relation between prayer and its results. Most religious traditions state only that the deities will hear the prayers, and no specific consequences, whether positive or negative, are absolutely guaranteed from the practice of prayer. Ladd and Spilka [6] caution that studies drawing the conclusion that there are positive relations between faith and health can have the unintended consequence of implying that those who do not experience positive benefits from prayer are somehow personally at fault; likewise it is imperative to avoid framing of the potential effects of prayer on health in terms of divine response, as this goes beyond the scientific nature of studies on prayer. These authors [6] also observe that studies correlating prayer and cardiovascular diseases, cancer, spirituality and health outcomes studies often failed to consider other variables that may have affected health outcomes not directly related to prayer, but relate to a broader context, such as lifestyle, work, *etc.* With regard to intercessory-type prayer and health in particular, the authors are adamant about the disappointing state of the literature.

The observations of Ladd and Spilka [6] and other authors [7,8] who have criticized the relation between spirituality and health are relevant. It is also apparent that the basic theoretical foundation of many studies is unclear (or not presented in any substantive fashion), just as the notions of health and prayer used in such studies often are unclear.

Given the above caveats, we believe that exploring the perceptions of practitioners on their own personal prayer experiences may represent a useful subject matter for further research. It may also support reflections concerning the possible implications of prayer in clinical practice. By delving into practitioner's stories, we may extract clues concerning how and why prayer is employed in dire circumstances. This approach will help us at least partially determine the extent to which the ideas of researchers and participants align.

3. The Practice of Prayer from the Perspective of Practitioners

The data presented here were collected between 2009 and 2011. A set of 104 participants, 73 women and 31 men, with an average age of 51 years (ranging from 17 to 79 years), mostly Americans, but also Latinos and Africans, residing in various regions of the United States were interviewed on video. As part of a larger study about prayer practices, participants answered the following request: "If you feel comfortable doing so, please describe in as much detail as you can do, one of the most powerful experiences you have had with prayer."

The participants interviewed represented ten faith communities distributed as follows: three Roman Catholic churches (44 participants representing 42.31% of the sample), five mainline Protestant churches (43 participants: one Anglican church, one Presbyterian church, two United Methodist denomination churches, and a Seventh-Day Adventist church, totaling 41.35% of the sample), and two Pentecostal churches (17 participants from the Assembly of God, representing 16.34% of the sample). With regard to economic class, 9.5% participants belonged to the lower class, 24.2% to the lower middle class, 17.9% to the middle class, 21.1% to the upper middle class, and 27.3% to the upper class[1]. As for the level of education of the study group, only 1% reported having dropped out of high school; 10.2% completed high school; 25.5% attended but did not complete higher education; 6.1% completed technical school (two-year technical degree); 22.4% completed higher education; and 34.7% completed graduate school.

Based on the Content Analysis[2] [9,10], the material was organized into four categories to describe the use of prayer by these practitioners. For the participants of this sample, prayer was used as a spiritual tool to deal with suffering (religious/spiritual coping strategy; 64.5%); as an access channel to the sacred (discipline which keeps the spirituality alive; 15.3%); as a way of strengthening relationships (technique to promote mutual empowerment; 8.6%); and as a means of self-transcendence ("turning point" in the existential process; 13.4%). We next employed the Ladd and Spilka [6] framework to identify different ways of praying that were prevalent in each of these four categories.

Although the data presented here have been used in a previous study published in Portuguese by the authors [11], the current analysis focuses a different and not yet explored angle: the relation between prayer, health and its clinical implications.

3.1. A Spiritual Tool to Deal with Suffering—Prayer as A Religious/Spiritual Coping Strategy

Of all participants, 62.5% reported prayer experiences that characterize its use as a religious-spiritual coping method. Coping here refers to the behavioral and cognitive efforts to dominate, reduce, or tolerate internal and/or external demands originating from stressful operations [12,13]. For example, Lazarus and Folkman [13] note that after a cognitive appraisal of a stressful event, people often have two major types of coping responses: emotion focused coping strategies or problem oriented coping strategies.

Pargament [14] applied the coping theory of Lazarus and Folkman to the sphere of religion, thereby creating the notion of religious coping. For this author, religious/spiritual coping refers to the introduction of sacred elements in responding to stressor events, in which religious coping methods can be "positive" or "negative". Positive coping encompasses a secure relationship with God, the belief that there is meaning in life, and the sense of connection with others. It consists of a pattern of the following positive coping methods: benevolent religious appraisal; collaborative religious coping; and

---

[1] The American reference for the classification of economic class is as follows: lower class: annual income of less than $32,000; middle class: annual income between $32,700 and $45,000; and upper class: annual income of more than $45,000.
[2] The Content Analysis aims to critically understand both the sense of communications as well as its explicit and implicit content [9]. Bardin [10] suggests three phases in the process of content analysis: 1. pre-analysis: where the material is organized in order to make it operational by systematizing the initial ideas; 2. material exploration: defining categories (coding system), identifying recording units (content), and identifying the context units; and 3. processing of results, inference and interpretation (moment of intuition, of reflective and critical analysis).

a search for spiritual support, life transformation, *etc.* In contrast, negative coping is characterized by a less secure relationship with God, a fragile and threatening worldview, and spiritual conflicts in the search for meaning [15].

In situations when the practice of problem-focused coping is not feasible, (mourning, for instance), religious-spiritual coping assumes significant importance.

The current participants described experiences of profound stress and suffering and how prayer helped them face the following situations: divorce; the mourning process for the death of friends and family; various physical illnesses; family relationship problems; problems at work or unemployment; difficulty in forgiving; anxiety of various origins (situational or as an individual disorder); abuse; spontaneous abortion; and material needs. In this category, the types of prayer employed were those of Petition and Tears. The connectivity modalities that are benefited by this type of prayer are inward and upward.

Ladd and Spilka [16] identified the following content in Tears prayer: bereavement, loss, and agony, which are typical in situations of personal turbulence, characterizing a form of inward prayer to alleviate personal feelings of unrest and agony. In several interviews, participants reported that prayer was used as a successful coping method to deal with this sort of personal, intense suffering. Approaching God via prayer enables the transformation of emotion, especially in uncontrolled or irreversible situation, such as the death of a significant person and other similar situations. Through Petitionary or even Tears prayer, the participants describe their experience as the care and comfort received from God.

> I have come to pray when a horrible, horrible, horrible thing happened to my family and it was going to get worse, as a result. And I went to the chapel at my church (…) where we have Blessed Sacrament exposed. (…) And normally you would spend an hour there. But it was my lunch hour and I couldn't work...and I went in there because I was just...it was such a horrible thing that happened...and it was so fresh that I couldn't sort through it yet (it had to do with my brother and different things that happened) and I went in there and-and knelt in front of the Blessed Sacrament, cause I knew there was nowhere else I could go … and just said "Lord, I don't have an hour. I have five minutes. That's all I have that you've got to take this terror away from my stomach, cause I can't function. I have a family and I have to work. I need help right now and I could just immediately feel it all just drain away. All of it drained away, and the situation did not change...which it wasn't going to, I just needed to be able to be present...so that I could function whatever way I was supposed to in this situation. And I'll never forget that, cause it was an immediate response. And I'm sure I've had immediate responses before. But I remember that one very, very, very, very well. The power of prayer (...) it's just the strongest there is.
>
> (Female Participant 710123)

Several studies have demonstrated that in situations of poor health, one of the main religious coping strategies is prayer. In such contexts, prayer is not restricted to requests for restoring physical health. It is also used as a source of strength to deal with the suffering, as a coping strategy focused on emotion, as exemplified by one of the current participants:

> Almost ten years ago, I was diagnosed with breast cancer … and sitting in the surgeon's off-office, and- and he said to me: "Mrs. [X] your left breast is fine, but we found cancer in your right breast."...and I said to him: "don't say anything else to me, talk to him." My husband was with me, and I didn't say a word … from then, we got in the car, we drove home, he turned to me, and said: "are you alright?" and I flung open the door and I said, "hell no: I'm not alright! I have breast cancer!" and I went just tearing down our driveway (we live in the woods, thank goodness), I went out into the woods, and screaming and running around. I was an absolute crazy woman and at some point, I was: "you're alright.

It will be alright." and you know, it wasn't a Pollyanna, kind of thing. There was...*I heard the words, I felt the presence* (. . .) that was, for me pretty powerful.

(Female Participant 07086133)

The respondents reported using prayer not only when their physical health was impaired, but also as a way to maintain physical and mental health, as stated by this person:

I believe my day-to-day life is guided by God. And if I miss a day or I don't talk to God, I feel like I'm lost. And most of the times, even when I'm going through problems, or frustrations, just like the experience of my father—it was more frustrating distress. You're angry, everything every emotion runs through you, you're not happy but uh, the minute I pray, it enables me to lift off and take the load off my shoulders and I feel relieved so I believe that every day, if I don't talk to God, even through (my experience) whether I'm happy or not, whether I'm sad or not, I'll be the most depressed person on Earth because I would not have anybody to help me carry through the whole thing or walk with me.

(Female Participant 07091636)

Such reports exemplify the use of positive religious coping. The participants have no doubts about the benefits of prayer in their emotions in daily life, and its use as a coping tool. Despite the fact that such situations are not modified by the practice of the petitionary-type prayer, or even when the person reports a lack of an immediate response from God, the benefit is perceived to be manifested as a change in the emotion as a result of the consolation.

However, prayer does not only favor positive coping. The interpretation of an answer to prayer may lead to a negative coping outcome, manifesting as the presence of some type of *spiritual conflict*:

Well recently I asked God for something for some help, and well a year ago probably for some help and the direction I was going, and then I had a major life change and I think I've been upset ever since . . . so I'm trying to, to figure it all out, but I think it's connected and I'm trying to seek what it is. It was just the beginning I think, the changes that occurred, I think it's all related to my request. So. . . . .

(Female Participant 0710125)

Empirical studies show there is a strong relation between spiritual conflict and distress, including poorer psychological functioning and more debilitated physical health [17]. The interview above indicates a *spiritual conflict* involving beliefs and feelings about God, such as anxiety and fear. Pargament [18] notes there are three types of *spiritual conflicts: interpersonal, intrapersonal,* and *divine*: "(a) interpersonal struggles involving conflicts and tensions with family, friends, clergy, or church around spiritual issues; (b) intrapersonal struggles that focus on internal questions and doubts about matters of faith, as well as intrapsychic conflicts between higher and lower aspects of oneself; and (c) divine struggles that involve negative emotions toward God, such as anger, anxiety, fear, and feelings of abandonment" ([17], p. 265).

Although the example above indicates the presence of *spiritual conflict* as resulting from the use of prayer as a negative coping method, most practitioners reported decreased anxiety and improved overall functioning capacity. They also reported a search for more assertive behavior and the realization of a more meaningful life.

3.2. An Access Channel to the Sacred—Prayer as a Discipline to Sustain Spirituality

Rest- and Sacramental-type prayers (Sacred Traditions) are predominantly upward, directed toward a divine listener. Thus, in addition to a coping mechanism, prayer is a channel for connection with the sacred, a form of spiritual discipline with a view to spiritual maturity:

When I pray I relax. It's important for me to relax my body so I can be more attentive...and so *I can hear better*...I do body relaxation meditation. I walk into complete darkness...and the

> darkness is the presence of God that surrounds me. So God surrounds me in the darkness (...) a powerful experience for lack of a better word...I'm enveloped by that mystery...and so darkness for me is not is a negative thing.
>
> (Male Participant 0710167)

Ladd and Spilka [16] characterize the prayer of Rest as stillness, tranquility, serenity, and silence in search for connecting with the sacred. A total of 15.3% of the participants interviewed conveyed experiences that can be interpreted as having a purpose of spiritual connection:

> It's more like a daily thing for me though sometimes I forget ... so it's like if I forget like something goes wrong ... and I need to pray or something so, it is like I'm attached basically. That's like my way of more like comfort after....
>
> (Female Participant 07091631)

The German theologian, Heiler [19] states that the effort to strengthen, enhance, and improve one's own life is the reason that leads people to pray. For him, this is the reason behind all prayer, "but the discovery of the deepest root of prayer does not disclose its peculiar essence. In order to get to the bottom of this, we should not ask for the psychological motive of prayer; we must rather make clear the religious ideas of him who prays in simplicity, we must grasp his inner attitude and spiritual aim, the intellectual presuppositions which underlie prayer as a psychical experience" ([19], p. 355). The theologian argues that the person who prays makes a vital spiritual exchange with the divine and that there are three elements that form the internal structure of the prayer experience: faith in a personal God, faith in his real immediate presence, and a real communion in which the person enters into relationship with God—conceived as a presence ([19], p. 356).

> For me prayer is communicating with God. So and- and after you connected with God spiritually,...has to have communication. In every relationship where there's no communication that relationship dies. Even a husband and wife, if the husband is not communicating with the wife, that relationship cannot hold. So it's the same with me and God, so if- if I stop praying, I feel that I have broken a relationship with my creator...and if I'm not connected with him through communication, I won't understand what he want to tell me to do on a daily basis ... because I believe he made me and he has purpose certain thing for me (in my life), so I have to keep connection with God. So, prayer to me is being in connection with God, being communication with God...so I anytime I'm not praying, I feel that I'm not in communication with God, and that my life is on my own, and I don't want to be on my own.
>
> (Male Participant 07091637)

While the prayer of Rest is more personal, held in a private context, and allows for a direct connection between the individual and the sacred, Sacramental-type prayer generally, though not exclusively, occurs in the collective space of worship, and employs religious traditions to establish this form of connectivity. Some people seem to identify more with the structure, the teachings, and the environment the institution provides. As argued by Heiler, the prayer rituals, liturgical hymns, and the liturgical prayers that are commonly used by worship institutions are the crystallization of phenomena that formerly occurred in personal life, but may subsequently morph into an objective, impersonal, and routine form ([19], p. 354). However, even in the most institutionalized form of prayer, as is characteristic of sacramental prayer, the individual frequently performs it with the clear intention to keep the spiritual dimension alive:

> I should say that some of the best-loved hymns of the church have had fragments that have had an impact on my own prayer life, in regard to confession and affirmation, and commitment, fellowship.
>
> (Male Participant 9091004)

> It's hard to say just one experience [*Editor:* constitutes prayer]. Every Sunday I go to church and I receive communion. That's really powerful.
>
> (Female Participant 0710168)

As an access channel to the sacred, prayer is also commonly practiced as a discipline to maintain personal spiritual health, with potentially visible downstream effects on general health as a whole. In addition to the absence of disease, health concerns the creative process of a meaningful existence and a life worth living. From this perspective, prayer is perceived by its practitioners as vital to maintaining healthy spirituality and in a continuous process of maturation.

3.3. A Way to Strengthen Relationships—Prayer as A Technique of Mutual Empowerment

For 8.6% of the sample, Intercessory-type prayer was the most significant prayer experience. Predominantly outward and upward, intercessory prayer is one of the most studied prayer types in the United States of America. Ladd and Spilka [4] cite four reviews about the link between intercessory prayer and health, concluding that " . . . the empirical evidence that intercessory prayer has an effect on the health of those for whom the intercessory prayer was held is minimal" ([4], p. 299). Masters and Spielmans ([7], p. 332), advise researchers interested in studies on the effects of prayer on health to avoid this type of study and it likely that a substantial number of "file drawers" are filled with similar projects that failed to show significance and hence did not go forward to publication or presentation [20].

Moreover, from a theological point of view, intercessory prayer is inherently confusing. The theologian Vincent Brümmer [21] points out the dilemma brought forth by this type of prayer: a God who is perfectly good could not depend on the intercession of human as a necessity to exercise his benevolence. However, if one denies that the benevolence of God toward some person or situation depends on the intercession of others, what would be the point of intercessory prayer anyway? Even to argue that intercession somehow influences the otherwise independent action of God presents significant theological challenges: Why would one prayer influence God but another prayer not? A full discussion of this theological conundrum is beyond the scope of this paper, and we have noted in another study [11], "from the standpoint of physical health, this type of investigation could lead the researcher into a difficult situation. If we consider the self-reported appraisal on the benefits of intercessory prayer they point out the mutual care and empowerment as the greatest benefit they have from this intercessory prayer" ([11], p. 647).

From the perspective of the participants who pray, intercessory prayer both enables the practice of mutual care and has an empowering effect on the parties involved, with a significant impact on the spiritual dimension.

> Recently having a prayer time with one of my members of my church, and they were struggling with their uh terminal illness, struggling with their sense of prayer, and their relationship with God, and I remember having a moment where we were praying that if their condition could be reversed that would be what we'd pray for, that's what we would desire. But if that physical condition could not be changed, then their need FOR that healing to be changed, so that what we were really praying for is that if healing could happen, that's what we pray for, and if healing was not physical healing was not to come, then to be healed of the need to be healed. And I found both of us found that to be, powerful moment.
>
> (Male Participant 09091010)

As noted by Brümmer [21], intercessory prayer activates the role of cooperation of the believer seeking God's benevolence. "God acts through the actions performed by us", states the theologian ([21], p. 65). For this author, the person who intercedes on behalf of a person or cause stands available as a "secondary cause" through which God could act in answer to the prayer. In other words, "'intercession is a cooperation with that transcendent will of God which is none the less immanently at work in and through man's relationships with one another', and therefore involves both God and the petitioner as partners in realizing what is being asked." ([21], pp. 65–66). Thus, for the believer, petitionary-prayer on behalf of others seems to be understood as a way to enter into God's purposeful activity [21].

Beyond just an individual context, " . . . corporate prayer is more effective than individual prayer, not because it brings more pressure to bear on God but because it enlists more people in the realization of God's will" ([21], p. 66). One of the interviewees expresses himself in terms that are aligned with this type of understanding:

> I believe that prayer does work and it works much more in groups, sometimes, than it does individually, but it-prayer does definitely work.

> (Male Participant 09091003)

Another aspect expressed by intercessory prayer is empathy for the suffering of another. Consequently, prayer in favor of another does not only create bonds of fellowship among those who pray. It is, for its practitioners, a community access channel to the sacred:

> Just standing there with the family or without the family and praying for that person, I just feel like that it is bringing God closer to me, and closer to them even though God knows that they're there.

> (Female Participant 0710174)

3.4. A Self-Transcendence Route—Prayer as Turning Point in the Existential Process

This category consisted of 13.4% of the sample. The participants reported the following outcomes of prayer: Conversion, Calling, and Movement of the Spirit. The set of these three types of prayer characterize a phenomenon in the subjective process we can name as *epiphany*. From the Greek, the word *epiphaneia* means an appearing, a remarkable manifestation. The term has its origin in religion and refers to revelation—for example, the revelation to the wise men about the incarnation of Christ as son of God; the revelation of the Holy Spirit who descends upon Jesus during his baptism by John; the Pentecost (descent of the Holy Spirit reported in the biblical book of Acts); the work of the spirit in the process of awareness and recognition of the human being on its state of alienation from God.

The sense of epiphany is not restricted to the boundaries of the religious sphere and can be also found in secular contexts such as Brazilian literature. The term indicates a sudden moment of enlightenment, a new understanding, a new perception of a state of affairs, and a profound change in the subjectivity of those who experience it. Sometimes, such experience may be marked by a great spiritual distress.

The description of this experience by the participants in this study suggests the character of "occurrence" at the time of prayer. Unable to explain "how" or "why" this occurred, the participants realized such experiences as extraordinary or unusual. Referred to as "conversion", "calling", "glossolalia" (speaking in tongues) or as a "movement of the Spirit", these experiences have in common a sense of revelation, enlightenment, joy, hope, trust in God, or excitement. Above all, the individuals reflect on this experience as something that has no obvious initiative in their inner selves, or in their minds, but as something that comes from outside, from a more distant dimension and fulfill them, gives them direction and insight, gives them a new meaning and purpose in life. This experience is, therefore, understood as originating in the sacred dimension, as a divine initiative ([11], p. 650).

Thus, the types of prayer described above feature a connection experience that is distinct from the previous (inward, outward, upward), as such initiative originates from an exogenous dimension towards the person who prays. For one who believes, *Conversion* prayer represents a return to God. It is the acceptance of salvation offered by God

> [It] is when I felt a need to pray to God for myself to forgive me for my sins and how that burden was totally lifted, so it's called conversion . . . Which you may be aware of, so to me that's the most powerful experience I've had when I knew that my life had been

totally changed in a moment when God did what He promised to do...when I confessed my sins, when He forgave me for them and when they were thrown into the depths of the sea and when I didn't have that burden to carry around anymore and that truly gave me the lightheartedness, a pep in my step when I knew that nobody could ever down with anything from my past.

(Female Participant 07091243)

Prayer as a *Calling* is characterized by a belief in a divine calling to engage, and to devote oneself to religious work.

My daughter was six to nine months old. I was got into the habit of praying for her each evening...I always prayed for (...) God watch over her: help her to grow happy, healthy, and strong. One evening while praying that *I heard the voice* (...) "I have her, but I wanted you." And, that like, really scared me, but it was a very powerful experience, and, it was something that'll, stay with me for the rest of my days.

(Male Participant 09091008)

The *"Movement of the Spirit"* type prayer refers to the strong experience that is revealing in character, whether or not accompanied the phenomenon of glossolalia (the Angel's language or speaking in tongues):

(. . .)When I was praying, the Lord dropped me to my knees, the Lord dropped me to my knees. I wasn't gonna, I—I forgot all about that, um the Lord dropped me to my knees twice in that week, I didn't get on my knees just like that, the Lord dropped me to me knees and I mean, felt like an earthquake when He dropped me to my knees, I mean it was forced, I mean then I started crying out to God and I won't say what I said, I don't remember at all what I said, but just the Lord dropped me to my knees.

(Male Participant 07091628)

It seems that the *epiphanic experience* of connectivity (described above) activates a sort of "mystical psychological function", in order to promote a sense of human unity with what one considers sacred. It triggers a subjective transformation process where participants report positive effects on spiritual and mental health. It marks a turning point loaded with deep meaning and purpose in life, joy, and subjective wellbeing—a discovery. The practitioners understand such experience as being part of a *theophany* (manifestation of God) in their existential process, and it becomes clear that the existential reorganization from such experience has effects on mental health and spiritual dimensions, especially when one considers the theological notion of health as advocated by Tillich [22]. For this theologian, health has to do with healing and salvation. In this sense, health is a state of self-integration of the being with the ultimate foundation of existence ([22], pp. 408–23).

4. Prayer and Health—Implications for Clinical Care Practice

The analysis of the prayer experience from the point of view of practitioners leads one to reflect on several issues regarding the relation of prayer to health/illness, as well as its possible implications for clinical practice in its variety of contexts: medical, psychotherapeutic, or pastoral.

4.1. Need to Understand Health beyond a Biomedical Perspective

The main revisions in the literature about prayer and health [4,6–8] indicate a lack of a consistent theory to sustain the quantitative research studies on prayer and health. It is often assumed that everyone knows what is being discussed when one refers to health and prayer. One forgets that such notions are always related to the current mode of knowledge construction. Presently, with the predominance of the biomedical model, "health is understood as the absence of disease, and health care, therefore, it focuses on disease, diagnosis, drug therapy, with an emphasis on the biological aspect, and with health management that reaches the sphere of a political government of life itself" ([11], p. 634). An understanding of health that fails to take into account the environment, the family, social relationships, and the potential of the individual restricts the notion of health to the absence of symptoms and to the physical sphere. Winnicott [23], a highly influential British psychiatrist between the 1960s and the 1980s, assumes a notion of health as necessarily related to the maturational process and the ability of the person to create his/her own style. Tillich, an existential theologian who advocates a theology emanating from the process of existence, supports the idea of health as a process of self-integration of the being in all dimensions of existence (physical, chemical, biological, psychological, mental, spiritual, and historical). In addition, as it is socially produced, the notion of health is not static. Instead it varies according to the normative processes that define the normal and the pathological. In the biomedical model, one easily forgets that the dimensions of mental and spiritual health are as important as physical well-being and the absence of symptoms. In this sense, a clinical practice from a holistic perspective, as proposed Hefti [24,25], favors the approach of religious and spiritual matters in a more integrated manner.

Hefti [24] expands the three-dimensional clinical practice proposed by George Engels, the Biopsychosocial Model, suggesting the inclusion of a fourth dimension: that of religion and spirituality. Assuming that religion and spirituality influence both mental and physical health, Hefti argues that "the 'Expanded Biopsychosocial Model' explains that a holistic approach to mental health has to integrate pharmacotherapy, psychotherapy, sociotherapy and spiritual elements" ([24], p. 612). The clinical application of the Expanded Biopsychosocial Model takes into account the spiritual history, the support for religious beliefs, and the practice of the spiritual care model (interdisciplinary and subject-centered care—with needs/spiritual resources). Hefti argues that religion can be a causative, mediating, or moderating factor in any biological, psychological, or social outcome, as exemplified by the physiological reaction to psychological stress ([25], p. 121). In this sense, the author points out that one cannot overlook the potential influence of religion and spirituality on disease progression, the doctor-patient relationship, and the treatment process itself. Therefore, spiritual needs and conflicts, as well as the distress and resources of the patient, should be accessed by taking a spiritual history in order to integrate them into the treatment plan ([25], p. 121).

The emotional and spiritual well-being practitioners experience through prayer is evident in the overall perception of practitioners regarding their personal health and well-being. In other words, the effectiveness of prayer does not necessarily reside in the positive outcome of a petitionary (or intercessory) prayer for physical healing. Healthcare professionals could better assist their patients, beyond the biomedical model, by considering religious and spiritual matters during the process of diagnosis and treatment.

4.2. Prayer Cannot Be Seen Simply as Complementary and Alternative Medicine for Improving Physical Health

From the practitioner's point of view, prayer is a spiritual tool used for spiritual purposes. However, even though its practice promotes mental and spiritual well-being, understanding it as "complementary medicine" is at least a misconception. Even in situations when Petitionary-type prayer is used, what is most important for the practitioner is not the divine response to the request made, but what it enables as a connection with oneself, with others, and with what they consider sacred. In other words, prayer is a means of transcending the physical world, not necessarily "fixing" it. Indeed, participants claimed that "prayer always works!"

> I pray more for good health and understanding, you know, (. . .) some good friends of ours lost a son thirty years old, you know, to cancer and, you know, you pray about those things.

> I feel that prayer is a conversation with God, and he does respond to us not necessarily immediately, and so you know, that's—that's just my life experience is a continual thing

and again it seems to be tied into the health, it's how long are we here? You know, and prayer is sorta what keeps us—what keeps us going while we're here, you know so (....).

(Male Participant 0710102)

I was on massive drugs because of a back problem and could not get doctors to really address the issue, everybody seemed to think it was in my head until I finally found a sports-medicine doctor but that's way beside the point. When I was deeply involved in the drugs I felt unable to pray. Not because I didn't think God was there but just I couldn't-I couldn't get to that place inside of me where I had the assurance that God even heard me anymore...and I ask faith people around me to pray for me for that issue not for my health because that was even more important than my health to me.

(Female Participant 0710177)

Studies that examine the issue of whether prayer works—in a solely biomedical perspective of eradicating disease—suppose an understanding of prayer that does not match the use of those who practice it. This discrepant understanding of the role and meaning of prayer should give pause to scholars regarding such investigations. As mentioned above, the studies on the effectiveness of prayer (especially intercessory prayer) with regard to effecting physical healing are not supported in a consistent fashion. Although prayer is known to be an influential factor in the overall health of practitioners, as can be seen in this study, its role as an alternative physical medicine lacks firm empirical support. The integration of a spiritual dimension into clinical practice is intended to provide better care to patients. This goal can only be met by developing a thorough understanding of the patients' perspectives.

Beyond the biomedical context, understanding prayer as a spiritual tool with a spiritual purpose requires a psychotherapist to position him/herself regarding matters related to spirituality and clinical practice. If the psychotherapist assumes that spiritual issues not only constitute the subject's subjectivity, but also affect his/her emotional and mental health, the clinic may represent a privileged space to investigate and work with the patient on the positive and negative effects arising from his/her spiritual-religious understandings.

For the pastoral counselor, it is also important to understand the way in which the individual uses this prayer resource in order to ascertain religious beliefs that lead to potential emotional and spiritual struggles, such as: "God has forsaken me"; "This is punishment from God." Such interpretations are typical of a negative religious coping style, which is characterized by spiritual conflicts and predicts symptoms of depression and anxiety [17].

5. Conclusions

The reflection on the relation between prayer and health and the implications for clinical practice leads one to realize just how much advancement is still needed in the studies on the topic. The practice of prayer is a living and dynamic reality in the existential process of the person who believes in God or some form of a higher power. It offers several elements that express the subject's psychic and behavioral functioning. In this sense, a consistent analysis of the experience of prayer described by the individual may indicate not only the healthy or symptomatic functioning of the subject, but also offer clues for clinical intervention and point out aspects to be addressed in the practice of holistic health care.

The volume of research on religiosity/spirituality and prayer, and their use in clinical practice, is still small [26]. The present article only mentions various aspects, which deserve an in-depth investigation, with an aim to further our understanding of the religious experience of the contemporary subject, and to discuss the validity, necessity, and challenges involving the integration of religious/spiritual dimensions into health care and clinical practice. A key issue that warrants investigation is the development of theory-based intervention models beyond the biomedical model that consider the influence of *spiritual struggles*, *attachment behaviors*, and *religious-spiritual coping*, particularly in countries other than the United States and Europe.

Research on these topics, especially from an interdisciplinary perspective with the participation of experts in medicine, nursing, sociology, psychology, and theology, can contribute greatly to a more refined understanding of contemporary subjectivity and health care practices, as well as the way and degree to which the religious/spiritual dimension acts upon these processes.

Prayer can be a powerful spiritual resource available to health care professionals (psychologists, physicians, nurses) and pastoral counselors in the assisting of people who seek health care: "I'd be lost without prayer [...] peace and strength are two major things that I get from my life of prayer" (Female Participant 0710173). Listening attentively to the way a person who believes in a higher power experiences and recounts his/her practice of prayer is necessary for a holistic-care-based clinical practice. Prayer can be a means of expressing a person's psychological dynamics, as well as an ally in the process of clinical interventions that seek to use this important dimension of human life—spirituality—for the promotion of holistic health. *"Hearing the voice and feeling the presence"* does not have to be a statement that is exclusively spoken by believers regarding their prayer experience; it may also be an expression used by health professionals and pastoral counselors when describing how they listen to their patients and feel their presence as a whole (in all its dimensions) in the exercise of a clinical practice focused on the affirmation of life and health processes.

Acknowledgments: We are grateful to the anonymous participants of this study as well as to the student members of Kevin L. Ladd's Social Psychology of Religion Lab at Indiana University South Bend: Briana Becker, Wanakee L. Brown, Cara A. Cook, Kaitlyn M. Foreman, Melissa Lentine, Sarah C. Mertes, Kyle J. Messick, Alison Niemi, Brice Petgen, Erik A. Ritter, Amelia Sinnott, and Erin Tracey who collected and transcribed the data. The study was supported, in part, by a Post-Doctoral Fellowship from CAPES—Coordination for the Improvement of Higher Education, Proc. nr. 10484-12-4 to the first author and grants #12282 and #34837 from the John Templeton Foundation to the second author.

Author Contributions: Kevin L. Ladd designed the research and supervised the data collection. Mary R. G. Esperandio supervised the qualitative analyses and crafted the first draft of the paper. Both authors read, revised, and approved the final manuscript.

Conflicts of Interest: The authors declare no conflict of interest.

References

1. Harold G. Koenig, Michael E. McCullough, and David B. Larson. *Handbook of Religion and Health*. New York: Oxford University Press, 2001.
2. Jeremy P. Cummings, and Kenneth I. Pargament. "Medicine for the Spirit: Religious Coping in Individuals with Medical Conditions." *Religions* 1 (2010): 28–53. [CrossRef]
3. Anne M. McCaffrey, David M. Eisenberg, Anna T. Legedza, Roger B. Davis, and Russell S. Phillips. "Prayer for Health Concerns: Results of A National Survey on Prevalence And Patterns of Use." *Archives of Internal Medicine* 164 (2004): 858–62. [CrossRef] [PubMed]
4. Kevin L. Ladd, and Bernard Spilka. "Prayer: A Review of the empirical literature." In *APA Handbook of Psychology, Religion, and Spirituality*. Washington: American Psychological Association, 2013, vol. 1, pp. 293–307.
5. Bernard Spilka, and Kevin L. Ladd. *The Psychology of Prayer: A Scientific Approach*. New York: Guilford, 2013.
6. Kevin L. Ladd, and Bernard Spilka. "Prayer and Health Research: Proxies, Missed Targets, and Opportunities." *Revista Pistis Praxis* 6 (2014): 33–50. [CrossRef]
7. Kevin S. Master, and Glen I. Spielmans. "Prayer and Health. Review, Meta-Analysis, and Research Agenda." *Journal of Behavioral Medicine* 30 (2007): 329–38. [CrossRef] [PubMed]
8. David R. Hodge. "A systematic review of the empirical literature on intercessory prayer. Research on Social Work Practice." *Research on Social Work Practice* 17 (2007): 174–87. [CrossRef]
9. Antonio Chizzotti. *Pesquisa qualitativa em Ciências Humanas e Sociais*. São Paulo: Cortez, 2006.
10. Laurence Bardin. *Análise de conteúdo*. Lisboa: Edições 70, 2006.
11. Mary R. Esperandio, and Kevin L. Ladd. "Oração e Saúde. Questões para a Teologia e para a Psicologia da Religião." *Horizonte-Revista de Estudos de Teologia e Ciências da Religião* 11 (2013): 627–56.

12. Susan Folkman. "Personal Control and Stress and Coping Processes: A Theoretical Analysis." *Journal of Personality and Social Psychology* 46 (1984): 839–52. [CrossRef]

13. Richard S. Lazarus, and Susan Folkman. *Stress, Appraisal, and Coping.* New York: Springer, 1984.

14. Kenneth I. Pargament. *Psychology of Religion and Coping. Theory, Research, Practice.* New York: Guilford Press, 1997.

15. Kenneth Pargament, Bruce W. Smith, Harold G. Koenig, and Lisa Perez. "Patterns of Positive and Negative Religious Coping with Major Life Stressors." *Journal for the Scientific Study of Religion* 37 (1998): 710–24. [CrossRef]

16. Kevin L. Ladd, and Bernard Spilka. "Inward, Outward, Upward Prayer: Scale Reliability and Validation." *Journal for the Scientific Study of Religion* 45 (2006): 233–51. [CrossRef]

17. Julie J. Exline, and Eric D. Rose. "Religious and Spiritual Struggles." In *Handbook of the Psychology of Religion and Spirituality.* Edited by Raymond F. Paloutzian and Crystal L. Park. New York: Guilford Press, 2005, pp. 315–30.

18. Kenneth I. Pargament. "Searching for the Sacred: Toward a Nonreductionistic Theory of Spirituality." In *APA Handbook of Psychology, Religion, and Spirituality.* Edited by Kenneth I. Pargament. Washington: American Psychological Association, 2013, vol. 1, pp. 257–69.

19. Friedrich Heiler. *Prayer: A Study in the History and the Psychology of Religion.* Oxford: One World, 1932.

20. Jeffrey D. Scargle. "Publication Bias: The 'File-Drawer' Problem in Scientific Inference." *Journal of Scientific Exploration* 14 (2000): 91–106.

21. Vincent Brümmer. *What Are We Doing When We Pray? On Prayer and the Nature of Faith.* Farnham: Ashgate Publishing, 2008.

22. Paul Tillich. *Teologia Sistemática.* São Leopoldo: Sinodal, 2002, pp. 409–23.

23. Donald W. Winnicott. *Maturational Processes and the Facilitating Environment: Studies in the Theory of Emotional Development.* London: Hogarth Press, 1965.

24. René Hefti. "Integrating Religion and Spirituality into Mental Health Care, Psychiatry and Psychotherapy." *Religions* 2 (2011): 611–27.

25. René Hefti. "The Extended Biopsychosocial Model: A whole-person-approach to psychosomatic medicine and psychiatry." *Psyche & Geloof* 24 (2013): 119–29.

26. Karin Jors, Arndt Büssing, Niels C. Hvidt, and Klaus Baumann. "Personal Prayer in Patients Dealing with Chronic Illness: A Review of the Research Literature." *Evidence-Based Complementary and Alternative Medicine* 2015 article 927973. (2015). [CrossRef]

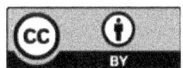

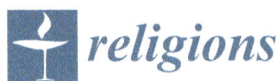

Article

Spirituality and Creativity in Coping, Their Association and Transformative Effect: A Qualitative Enquiry

Dagmar Anna S. Corry [1,*], Anne P. Tracey [2] and Christopher Alan Lewis [1]

[1] Department of Psychology, Glyndŵr University, Plas Coch Campus, Mold Road, Wrexham, LL11 2AW Wales, UK; ca.lewis@glyndwr.ac.uk

[2] School of Psychology, University of Ulster, Magee College, Northland Road, Londonderry BT48 7JL, UK; ap.tracey@ulster.ac.uk

* Author to whom correspondence should be addressed; d.corry@glyndwr.ac.uk; Tel.: +44-0-2881-658582.

Academic Editors: Arndt Büssing and René Hefti

Received: 27 January 2015; Accepted: 8 April 2015; Published: 17 April 2015

Abstract: While the beneficial effects on mental health of spirituality and creativity as separate entities have been well documented, little attention has been given to the interactive effect of the two constructs in coping. Recently, the *theory of transformative coping* and associated Transformative Coping Model have been developed and examined from both theoretical and quantitative perspectives. To extend this work, the present study critically examined the theory of transformative coping and associated Transformative Coping Model from a qualitative perspective. Ten interviews were conducted among Northern Irish and Irish artists, contemplative prayer group members, and mental health service users. Data were analysed using Interpretative Phenomenological Analysis. The results showed that the majority of participants had experienced stress and trauma, and have suffered mental ill-health as a consequence. Most defined themselves as both creative and spiritual, and resorted to a spiritual attitude along with creative expression in order to cope with traumatic events and ongoing stressful situations. Most participants believed that their creativity was rooted in their spirituality and that the application of both helped them to transform negative emotional states into positive ones. This, in turn, gave them increased resilience to and a different perspective of stressful events, which aided and improved their coping skills throughout the lifespan.

Keywords: creativity; spirituality; coping; transformative coping; stress; mental health; resilience; Interpretative Phenomenological Analysis (IPA)

1. Introduction

To facilitate the understanding and promotion of transformative coping, it is necessary that its components and their mutual association are explained. Eminent artists (e.g., [1,2]) and scientists (e.g., [3–5]) saw creativity and spirituality intrinsically linked in as much as creativity is understood as an aspect of spirituality. Tolstoy [2] and Kandinsky [1] believed that art was a means of emotional expression and communication, whereby the emotion is closely linked to the soul.

Recently, Corry, Lewis, and Mallett [6] presented a first introduction to the *theory of transformative coping* (TTC) which proposes the combined application of spirituality and creativity as a positive and pro-active coping strategy.

The TTC is based on the premise that both creativity and spirituality are aspects and expressions of the human spirit (e.g., [3,7]) and are thus connected (e.g., [1,2]). Coleman [3] and Jacobs [8] explained that creativity and spirituality mutually affect one another, and Bray [9] saw creative expression as an important step in the psycho-spiritual transformation of individuals.

Through the application of Interpretative Phenomenological Analysis ("IPA") [10] the present study was dedicated to qualitatively investigating how the phenomenon of transformative coping works for a sample of ten participants. The aim was to establish whether and to what extent individuals use their creativity as well as their spirituality in coping throughout their lifespan, how they are helped by resorting to them; and how important they are to them.

The research questions were:

(1)   Are creativity and spirituality used in coping and if so, how are people helped by resorting to them?

(2)   Are spiritual and creative coping used in conjunction? And, what is thus the lived experience of transformative coping?

(3)   What does it mean to the participants to apply creative and spiritual coping and how important is it to them?

Thus, in seeking to establish what it means to the participants to be able to resort to their combined inner resources of creativity and spirituality in an effort to cope with psychological stress, this study applied the *Transformative Coping Model* ("TCM-R"; for the original model, see [6]) as a conceptual framework for the TTC.

1.1. The Transformative Coping Model (TCM-R)

1.1.1. What is the TCM-R?

Figure 1 illustrates the TCM-R—the original model was introduced by Corry, Lewis, and Mallett [6]—which is based on the premise that creativity and spirituality are intrinsically connected and related [1,2] as they are both expressions of the human spirit [3,7]. At the interface of this connection lies the opportunity for positive transformation and personal growth [3,11]. Creativity [12] and spirituality [13] are both a search for the sacred, with creativity also being a search for the self [10]. Both creativity [11] and spirituality [14] have transformative power and are a quest for meaning and unity [3].

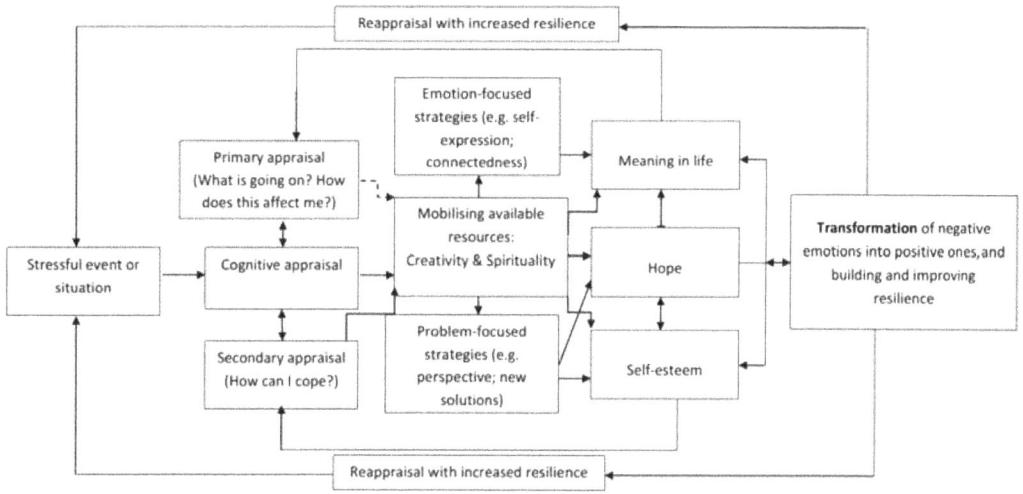

Figure 1. The revised transformative coping model ("TCM-R"; see [6] for the original model).

The TCM-R provides a new, efficient, accessible and universally applicable coping strategy. This model (see Figure 1) is rooted in Lazarus' [15] well-known *Stress and Coping Model* and links into

Fredrickson's [16] *broaden-and-build theory of positive emotions.* Lazarus and Folkman's [17] *Stress and Coping Model* includes problem-focused-, and emotion-focused strategies. When encountering a stressful event, an individual will appraise it cognitively. During the primary appraisal process the individual evaluates whether a situation is a threat to well-being. It is the subjective appraisal of an event which turns it into a stress-encounter rather than the event in itself. Individuals' responses to a specific occurrence can differ substantially depending on its inherent significance to them, irrespective of the extent of the loss, hurt or problem. Lazarus and Folkman [17] differentiate between harm/loss, (where the damage has already been sustained), threat, (harms or losses are anticipated, permits anticipatory coping, involves negative emotions like fear, anxiety, and anger), and challenge appraisal (also calls for mobilisation of coping efforts, but is growth-oriented and involves positive emotions, like excitement and exhilaration). During the secondary appraisal process individuals evaluate which of their own resources they could resort to in the coping process.

Fredrickson's [16] theory describes how through the repeated cultivated experiencing of positive emotions people transform themselves and become more creative, more resilient, increase their personal resources and become more socially integrated and healthy individuals. This enables them to cope with and counteract negative emotions.

Building on these models, the TCM-R describes how during cognitive appraisal problems are evaluated often leading to negative emotions (e.g., anxiety, fear, anger, guilt, despair, hopelessness, *etc.*) but that through combining creativity and spirituality as a positive and pro-active, life-long coping strategy these negative emotions are transformed into positive ones (e.g., joy, love, gratitude, inspiration, serenity, interest, *etc.*), bringing with it an increased sense of meaning in life, hope, and self-esteem. As a result, negative emotions are transformed into positive ones and resilience is improved, which leaves the individual in a position to more positively (re-)appraise stressful current and future events. So, on the one hand, the TCM-R works very much on the principle of emotion management because: "The bottom-line message is that people should cultivate positive emotions in themselves, but also as a means to achieving psychological growth and improved psychological and physical well-being over time." ([16], p. 1367). On the other hand, the TCM-R affords perspective and fosters innovative solutions to problems. Transformative coping can play a vital role in the promotion and maintenance of mental health, prevention of mental ill-health, and aiding of recovery.

Fredrickson's [16] theory was influential to, and fits neatly with the TCM-R as it suggests the broadening of the thought-action repertoire (the range of thoughts and actions that come to mind when faced with a problem) and the building of enduring personal resources. "Through experiences of positive emotions, then, people transform themselves, becoming more creative, knowledgeable, resilient, socially integrated and healthy individuals" ([16], p. 1369). As Fredrickson [16] points out, negative emotions, when they are either extreme, not appropriate, or enduring, produce severe problems for individuals and, consequently, society. These difficulties include mental problems like phobias, anxiety disorders, aggression and violence, eating disorders and sexual dysfunction, as well as depression and suicide. They also result in a multitude of stress-related physical illnesses.

In contrast, positive affect is related to flexible and creative thinking, increased attention, open-mindedness and efficiency; it broadens cognition and increases resilience. Fredrickson [16] suggests in her "undo" hypothesis that positive emotions can correct the effects of lingering negative emotions. This is where the TCM-R links in, proposing the transformation from negative emotional states into positive ones through the combined application of creativity and spirituality in coping.

1.1.2. How Does the TCM-R Work?

The TCM-R suggests that, to begin with, a traumatic event or ongoing stressful situation is cognitively appraised. This appraisal consists firstly of the primary appraisal [17], which serves primarily as an evaluation of the problem or situation. This evaluation is followed by the secondary appraisal process, during which individuals establish which resources they have available in order to first, cope with or manage the emotional effect the problem has on them and second, find an effective solution to the problem. As a result of the secondary appraisal process, individuals mobilise their creative and spiritual resources and put them into practice.

This takes the form of becoming spiritually aware by connecting with self, others and the world around them, and in many cases, with God or a higher power. They focus on positive human values, inner peace and finding meaning and purpose in life. They actively seek a new perspective by considering that life has meaning beyond their immediate problematic circumstances. They become aware of the metaphysical and transcendent dimension in the world and within their relationships.

Subsequently, individuals can mobilise their creative resources and express themselves—that is their spiritual meaning finding and meaning making—in whichever form and through whichever medium suits them best (cooking, drawing, gardening, music, painting, sewing, woodwork, *etc.*). They find relief in being able to express their thoughts and emotions through a creative medium; it affords them a new perspective, and through fostering their imagination, it enables them to find innovative solutions to problems.

This combined application of their spiritual and creative resources allows individuals to find and maintain a sense of meaning and purpose in their lives, it gives them hope and self-esteem, all of which have been shown to contribute to mental health. For instance, hope has been implicated as a source of resilience (e.g., [18]), positive affect [19], described as a vital coping resource (e.g., [20]), and a key psychological strength [21]. Self-esteem has been shown to be an effective buffer against stress (e.g., [10,22]), implicated in coping with chronic illness [23], and to support well-being [1], positive affect in chronic disease patients [22] and mental health [24]. Meaning in life, in particular, has been strongly associated with coping and mental health [12,13,25–32].

Hope, self-esteem, and meaning-in-life impact positively on the cognitive appraisal process and the individual is able to reappraise the situation or event from a new perspective which changes the perception of the stressful event. As a result, negative affect is diminished. For example, Juth, Smyth, and Santuzzi [22] showed that self-esteem influences secondary appraisal, and Snyder [19] demonstrated the association between hope, self-esteem and meaning in life. As Lazarus [15] points out, it is the meaning attached to an occurrence that shapes a person's emotional and behavioural response.

Lazarus and Folkman ([17], p. 375) emphasise "To be effective, any stress management program must stimulate the person to appraise situations and/or cope with their demands in new ways". The TCM-R represents a conceptual framework for positive, proactive and effective coping across the lifespan. By applying the tenets of the model individuals become aware of their inherent positive resources. They are thereby enabled to help themselves as and when they need to and in a manner that suits them personally.

2. Method

The methodology employed for this study was Interpretative Phenomenological Analysis ("IPA") [33–35], a qualitative research approach which is widely used in contemporary British psychology [32] and which aims to explore individuals' perceptions of the lived experience of particular phenomena and what personal meaning their experiences have for them. A core principle of IPA [32] is that all description constitutes a form of interpretation. It does not involve "bracketing" of presuppositions as they are necessary in the meaning-making process of understanding and interpreting of the phenomena under investigation. As such, analyses produced by the researcher are always an interpretation of the participant's experience. Using an idiographic approach IPA involves intensive and detailed engagement with individual cases, with insights integrated at later stages of the research.

2.1. Participants

Following ethical approval from the University Ethics Committee, a purposive (*i.e.*, criterion-based) sample of ten adult participants was recruited from three key groups in order to obtain a clear picture of the phenomenon of transformative coping, and to allow for greater transferability Three artists (in order to ensure inclusion of creative individuals) were recruited from Northern Ireland and the Republic of Ireland via the internet, along with three members of a contemplative prayer group (in an effort to ensure inclusion of spiritual individuals) in Northern Ireland via a priest as gatekeeper; and four members of a mental health support group (in order to ensure inclusion of individuals who have experienced mental health difficulties) in Northern Ireland via a member of staff as gatekeeper.

2.2. Procedure

Participants were contacted by the researcher and a suitable time and place for interview was agreed. No incentives were provided. All participants received a detailed participant brief and consent form prior to interview. They were informed that they may change their mind at any time and discontinue with the interview, and were supplied with a list of support organizations they could contact if they became distressed as a result of the interview. In order to ensure confidentiality and anonymity, no identifying information was made available. Identifiers assigned to participants in analysis and write-up consisted of random initials. The semi-structured interviews were recorded and transcribed verbatim. The transcripts were entered into NVivo-7 [36], a software package designed to afford analysis of qualitative data. The individual transcripts were analysed according to Smith, Jarman, and Osborn's [35] detailed method. The resulting theme structure is summarised in Figure 2.

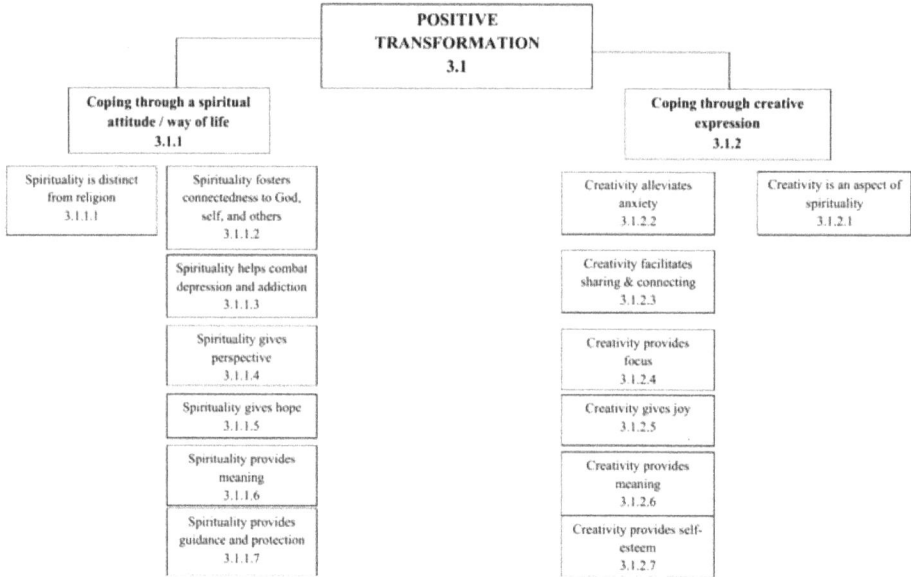

Figure 2. Theme structure for transformative coping.

Measures taken to ensure validity included participant triangulation, and the involvement of two further researchers to check the analysis and validate interpretations. To observe reflexivity the lead researcher (DASC) has examined the potential effects of her own beliefs, knowledge, and experiences of transformative coping on the current research. She acknowledged and retained an awareness of potential biases throughout the study, focusing on the participants' unique experience in a conscious effort to take an idiographic approach. Such biases include the researcher's knowledge of theoretical and empirical accounts of a positive association between creativity and spirituality, along with their salutogenic effect on wellbeing. The researcher also has personal experience of the beneficial effects of transformative coping.

2.3. Topic Guides

In order to ensure the richest data possible, semi-structured topic guides were used as a framework, which allowed the interviewees ample opportunity to elaborate as much or as little as they felt comfortable with and tell their story in their own words Typical questions, which were followed up with appropriate prompts, where applicable, were: "Do you resort to your spirituality in times of trouble?—Could you give me an example of this?", and: "Can you remember an instance where resorting to your craft has helped you overcome a problem?" The topic guides were constructed specifically with the view to ascertain whether the interviewees considered themselves spiritual and/or creative; whether they applied their creativity and spirituality in coping; what this meant to them, and how important it was to them. The interview guide can be requested from the corresponding author.

In line with recommendations by Smith and Osborn [34] a conscious effort was made to conduct every interview with the utmost respect for the participant and their unique story. This involved intense listening and observation, including "hearing" and noticing what was *not* said. Participants were not rushed through the questions but care was taken to allow them to take the lead within reasonable reach of the topic. Any information obtained was freely given by the participants rather than coerced from them.

3. Findings

This section presents and interprets interview excerpts illustrating the super-ordinate themes and their respective sub-themes as they emerged from IPA [35] and as summarised in the theme structure in Figure 2. Table 1 provides a brief summary of demographic details and findings. The gender distribution was even with five male and five female participants. Ages ranged from 29 to 70; six participants were single, three were married, and one was divorced.

Creativity (eight participants) and spirituality (seven participants) were used in coping, with six participants applying a combination of both capacities as a coping strategy. Two participants did not see themselves as creative, while three said they were not spiritual, with one of them being neither creative nor spiritual. The following quotes and interpretations illustrate the lived experience of transformative coping and demonstrate what it means to the participants to apply creative and spiritual coping. All initials used to denote particular participants are fictional.

Table 1. Participants' commonalities and differences.

	Artist	Artist	Artist	Mental Health Group Member	Mental Health Group Member	Mental Health Group Member	Mental Health Group Member	Prayer Group Member	Prayer Group Member	Prayer Group Member
ID	JB	LM	RN	HN	LO	SC	PT	KS	TC	MR
Gender	Male	Female	Female	Male	Male	Male	Female	Female	Male	Female
Nationality	Northern Ireland	Republic of Ireland	Republic of Ireland	Northern Ireland	Northern Ireland	Northern Ireland	Northern Ireland	Northern Ireland	Northern Ireland	Northern Ireland
Marital status	Single	Married	Divorced	Single	Single	Single	Single	Married	Married	Single
Age	29	54	57	37	52	41	44	55	70	48
Religion	Catholic	Catholic	Catholic	Catholic	Catholic	No denomination	Catholic	Catholic	Catholic	Catholic
Physical illness	None reported	None reported	None reported	None reported	Stomach problems	None reported	None reported	Obesity; Suspected heart attack	Hernia	none
Mental health problem	Anxiety	None reported but anxiety transpired	None reported but anxiety transpired	Depression and PTSD	Bipolar disorder; Suicidal ideation	Schizophrenia; Anxiety and fear are issues; Alcoholism	Paranoid schizophrenia; Anxiety is an issue	Depression, Addiction; Eating disorder; Suicidal ideation	None reported	Depression and anxiety
Trauma or stressful situation(s)	Adopted. Ran away from home at 16 (came back)	Alludes to difficult things having happened.	"Troubled childhood"; Divorce	Mother died aged 63 of motor-neuron disease	Not known.	Lost job	Not known.	Abuse; Death of a child	Allusions to marital strife	Death of nephew and sister
Creative	Sculpture	Painting	Singing; Creative writing	Not actively but appreciates creativity	Creative writing	Creative writing	Painting; Creative writing	Creative writing; Flower-arranging; singing/song-writing	Says no; yet proceeds to recite poetry	Flower-arranging; Interior decorating
Spiritual	Yes, but not religious. Eastern philosophy	Says no, yet demonstrates spiritual values	Silent prayer; Contemplative prayer	No: Paedophilia among clergy; Mother's death; Division in NI	Yes, but not religious. The "Troubles" in NI	Meditation	No	Contemplative prayer, reflection	Contemplative prayer, reflection	Contemplative prayer; Silent prayer

3.1. Positive Transformation

The superordinate theme established was that of positive transformation, with constituent themes being "Creative expression" and "Spiritual attitude/way of life", as well as the "Creativity is an aspect of spirituality". The theme of transformation was inherent in each main-, and subtheme. In other words, the application or attainment of the concepts which comprise the themes (*i.e.*, focus, connecting to God, self or others, perspective, *etc.*) each brought about a positive transformation within the interviewee and, consequently, transformed their lives, making them more resilient, and better able to cope.

JB's quote regarding the application of wool in his art refers to the comforting, soothing, and transformative effect this has on him. He talks about his environment of political and religious conflict and links this statement directly to the material he uses in his art. He feels that the negative emotions that were evoked in him as a result of the conflict surrounding him, are eradicated and transformed into positive ones.

> I'm from Northern Ireland and from the conflict that was here I would see that as a healing. In a way it's quite healing and therapeutic and very gentle. It has a transformative quality whenever you put it around hard, tough and rough surfaces so it has that transformative effect. (JB).

PT, who had lost a nephew in a tragic car accident, had to deal with her own grief while supporting her grieving sister, and mother of the young man. Together they resorted to refurbishing caravans as a way of coping with their sadness and despair. PT believes that this shared activity changed how they felt. It made them feel better: it transformed their outlook on the situation. "We done all that and it just changed things around and brought a bit of life and a bit of hope and maybe helped." (PT).

LM, who declared that her worst nightmare would be to have nothing to work with creatively, made a very profound statement when she said: "Life is change and an artist's work has to be about change. The nature of art is to push forward." (LM).

LM's quote captures the thinking behind, and the purpose of, transformative coping very well. Change, or transformation, is an intrinsic and fundamental part of life. Every change requires that we adapt to it. The more skillful people are in adapting, the better they cope. Tools that assist in this adaptive process are highly beneficial, and what LM is indicating here is that art is supremely suitable for supporting transformation.

3.1.1. Coping through a Spiritual "Attitude" or "Way of Life"

JB's quote captures the main theme of "spiritual attitude" very well. By taking a positive outlook on life in general, and towards oneself and other people in particular, a conscious choice can be made to view matters in a different light. Instead of focusing on negatives, a conscious and ongoing effort can be made to embrace any situation one finds oneself in and look for the good in it. Rather than perceiving oneself as terribly put upon, the same situation can be regarded as a challenge and thus take on different meaning.

> [It's about] increasing your base level of happiness and about dealing with issues, even the people that are difficult to get along with, because you get that in every situation. That they are actually a special gift that help you practice patience and tolerance. If you were always around people you got along with you would never actually be able to develop as a human being. So it teaches you a different perspective, to look at situations from a different point of view. People that represent challenges, you can see them as a gift. (JB).

Spirituality, as a subjective construct, means different things to different people. This view has found support in this study as will become evident throughout this section. For example, for JB, spirituality was about human connections. He shared this personal meaning mostly with participants HN and LO.

A further quote from JB demonstrates this very well, as he talks about the importance of making a positive contribution to peaceful relationships in one's immediate environment through practicing and applying desirable human qualities.

> I think it's in a very, very small part that you want to contribute to humanity , just in the little environment that you are in, that you are doing something positive towards compassion and kindness, and practice patience, tolerance and forgiveness, that would bring a sense of peace and harmony to whatever situation you are in. To try and bring that to dissolve where there are tensions and bring peace and when I say that I am not talking on about some huge global scale, I just mean the environment that you are in. (JB).

JB's sentiments are echoed in LO's quotation, where a spiritual person is also interpreted as someone who takes a benevolent attitude towards others. In addition, LO defines a spiritual person as someone who's meaning in life is not oriented towards the material.

> It's I think somebody that cares, cares about his fellow human beings, cares not to harm, particularly in terms of language and as well as physical, consideration and somebody who—it's very hard to do in this world—is not money-orientated. (LO).

3.1.1.1. Spirituality is Distinct from Religion

Despite the fact that there was no question on the interview guide with regard to religiosity, four participants made a distinction between religion and spirituality. One of them was MR, who was herself both spiritual and religious but was aware of a distinction between the two: "You know, there are people who could be spiritual but they might never go to mass or practice religion." (MR).

Three participants felt strongly about this distinction, declaring themselves to be spiritual only. LO implicated the religious conflict in Northern Ireland in his decision to abandon religion in favour of spirituality.

> The troubles had something to do with it as well, I would have rejected all types of organised religion and start thinking for myself but I would have still believed in God and that sort of thing. (LO).

LO, who had had a traditional Irish Catholic upbringing, probably wanted to distance himself from the religious element of the political conflict in Northern Ireland, when he moved to England in order to attend college in his twenties. He made it very clear where he stood: "I would never describe myself as religious, I prefer the word spiritual." (LO).

This theme is important because it highlights the importance of spirituality to the participants above and beyond organised religion. As such it once more underlines the intrinsic personal nature of spirituality. RN's quotation captures this aspect very well: "So that was the spiritual side, that was quite big and has accompanied my life rather than the religious, I had my own rules." (RN).

The associated excerpt illustrates perhaps why RN felt more drawn to spirituality than to religion. It seems an important aspect that could, again, be said to be related to meaning. Since RN felt excluded from her religion on the basis of her gender, this would have impacted profoundly on how significant religion was to her. As it was, it caused her to turn away from it and concentrate on her individual spirituality. "I was kind of rejecting the Romanised side of things and felt excluded really as a woman whereas in our own Celtic spirituality there are Goddesses, not Gods." (RN).

Lastly, JB's sense of spirituality appears to have jarred with his religious background:

> I have chosen my own path. My upbringing would have been from a Roman Catholic upbringing, but I felt that was, it just did not work for me. From what I consider spiritual, I didn't get a sense of the spiritual. (JB).

As a result, he distanced himself from religion and chose to live by his own definition of spirituality: "I mean I use the word spirituality here as opposed to religion because I am not religious." (JB).

3.1.1.2. Spirituality Fosters Connectedness to God, Self, and Others

Meditation and prayer were used by the interviewees as a means to connect with themselves or God. SC, for example, not only had made prayer a daily item on his agenda as part of his spiritual journey to improved mental health: "I would pray in the morning, I pray every morning", but also resorted to mediation when he felt particularly unwell: "Yeah. I meditate whenever I'm bad, I would meditate." (SC).

In difficult times, LO sought quiet time alone in order to reflect: "I would pray more. I would go into churches for some peace and quiet, to sort myself out and try to get a resolution to my troubles." (LO).

He shared this approach to dealing with difficulties with RN, who also resorted to quiet meditation in order to find answers: "If I am in a dilemma, then I would just go into that space, light a candle and just sit there, and, you know, listen." (RN).

The subtheme of "connecting through meditation and prayer" somewhat overlaps with that of "guidance" in that, in both themes, the interviewees looked for direction either from within themselves or from a higher power, and possibly both, as MR's quote shows:

> It would be in silent prayer...I wouldn't pray like Rosaries and stuff. I go to church and Holy Communion but my main thing would be to spend time alone with God. Just time alone basically, trying to cope with things. But I definitely would resort to it a lot. (MR).

MR recounted how, after her nephew's untimely death, she and her sister derived a deep sense of support from regular contemplative prayer meetings and so were able to maintain a reasonable level of good mental health during the grieving period that followed:

> But we had already been going to the meetings with Fr. B. for years. Only for that I think, otherwise I don't know how we would have survived it, both of us. Ehm [sic], that was the only thing that kept us going through that black time. (MR).

Like SC, KS's spiritual way of life was guided by daily prayer and a request for direction and guidance in her daily thoughts, words and actions concerning herself as well as others:

> I get on my knees every morning and I ask God or my higher power "Please God direct my day today, guide and protect me, help me with my abstinence around my food, guide my every thought, word and deed today, come into my very being and speak, use me as an instrument and speak your message to other people, your love to other people." (KS).

3.1.1.3. Connectedness to God: Positive God Image

It became evident during the interviews that those participants who considered themselves to be spiritual, had a positive image of God. SC, for example, saw God as a caring, understanding and forgiving power, who stood by him even during those times of his life which he was not proud of: "I mean I don't believe God ever really left me, even when I was a rogue, like." (SC).

RN developed a strong and very close relationship to God from very early on in her life. He is ever present in her life and she regularly connects with him through meditation. "Very early on I began to regard this transcendence or this God as my very best friend." (RN).

MR, who tragically lost two close family members within a short space of time, has found solace in contemplative prayer and believes that turning to God was her salvation: "I knew I couldn't survive without God. Without that help in me I couldn't have gone through it." (MR).

3.1.1.4. Connectedness to Self: Increased Self-Awareness

A spiritual way of life enabled the interviewees to become aware of their own weaknesses. As SC becomes more self-aware he learns to forgive himself which dispels his feelings of guilt and shame:

The best thing for me is that I can admit my faults, I can be honest and admit my faults and anything I done bad, I persevere and take it on the chin until its gone, until I'm more liberated all the bad things I done. (SC).

Having connected with herself at a deep level KS has learned to accept herself wholeheartedly, with all her strengths and weaknesses, and has achieved a high level of self-awareness.

I am still only a child, I make mistakes, I do know the difference. I have boundaries in my life today that I never had before, I have compassion and love and I do get angry. I am still a child, I get angry. I realise that sometimes other people's actions towards me actually stir up old behaviours but today I am aware of that. (KS).

On the other hand, HN did not seem to be in touch with himself and did not appear to know where he belonged. His own words were "I feel like I'm lost." He did not see himself as spiritual or religious and appeared to regard them as identical concepts. He had distanced himself from organised religion after the recent revelations of paedophilia within the Catholic Church, and after he lost his mother to motor-neuron disease at a relatively young age.

I couldn't tell, some people could say to you, well, I'm a Christian, or I'm a Humanist or I'm this or I'm that, but I don't feel as if I have a sort of clear focus where I wanna [sic] go or who I wanna [sic] be, you know. (HN).

3.1.1.5. Connectedness to Others: Positive Relations

HN's understanding of a spiritual way of life centred on respectful relationships with his fellow human beings. For him, spirituality meant mutual respect, which is of course, a tremendously important aspect of human relations and so a vital component of a spiritual outlook in life:

Ehm [sic], I think basically it's a sort of understanding towards people and if you listen to people and try to understand them and try and not belittle people and treat them as an equal ...Just treat people the way you want to be treated. Treat people with respect. (HN).

TC endeavoured to apply his spiritual values in daily life in his relationships with others. His quotation is an excellent example of applied spirituality, where transforming something potentially destructive into something constructive is key.

I'm thinking of this morning...with my wife and, frequently the conversations we have are difficult and I would go into just prayerful mode and that and just asking God to give me the wisdom and guidance to derive something constructive out of this. (TC).

Asked how his spirituality manifests itself, LO referred to his efforts of actively supporting others. "I would seek to help people, advising them or helping them, you know." (LO).

3.1.1.6. Spirituality Helps Combat Depression and Addiction

Spirituality was described by the interviewees as a crucial factor in combating addiction and depression. SC, for example, who suffered from severe alcoholism, gives witness to that when he recalls how joining the spiritual program of Alcoholics Anonymous helped him overcome his alcohol addiction:

It helped my drink problem. It helped my alcohol problems...I had to make a decision, because the drink would have killed me or something or I could have got locked up. I would have been in a rubber room, you know. (SC)

KS described how her spiritual beliefs helped her in finally beating her food addiction and losing half her body weight, thus overcoming obesity: "So that would be my, I have come from a person of 22 stone weight today to a person of 10 stone, 12 $\frac{1}{2}$ lb by the grace of God and a higher power. I am a miracle." (KS).

LO had suffered from suicidal ideation on a number of occasions throughout his life. In the following excerpt he makes reference to his belief that hope to carry on came from his own spiritual core:

> Well, yeah, like I've had my bad times, obviously with bipolar, I've had serious severe depression and a couple of times I've been suicidal...But there's always a spiritual core that sort of holds you back and if you hadn't that you would do it. (LO).

Lastly, here is another excerpt describing how KS's spirituality, which expressed itself in prayer, has prevented her from committing suicide which she describes as a miracle: "That was a miracle that I was brought away from the suicide that was an instant miracle." LO and KS were the two participants in the study who had contemplated suicide in the past and both of them reported that it was their spirituality which stopped them from carrying out their intentions.

> There was one stage where I was so, so distraught that I was on my knees, thinking about how I would commit suicide. I really didn't want to live and I had been conjuring up ways of how I commit suicide so that nobody would know. In the midst of all that I started to say the Hail Mary and just begged the mother of God, the mother of our Lord Jesus, to come and help me, ah, I went to my bed and I was in a really, really distraught, really distraught state and I went to sleep, I don't know how I done it, because normally I would have just been running tapes in my head and my tapes were very vivid films. And I went to sleep and I wakened in the morning with a calm that I hadn't known in a number of weeks, days, months. (KS).

3.1.1.7. Spirituality Gives Perspective

"Perspective" was one of the subthemes that the interviewees appeared to derive from both spiritual- as well as from creative coping, along with "connecting" and "increasing self-awareness": "It definitely helps you with the bigger picture, I think." (RM).

TC gave a splendid account of how he achieves perspective on things through consciously choosing to change his outlook on them and how he is thus able to transform his experiences of the daily grind from something stressful into something enjoyable and worthwhile:

> Reaching out and embracing these things as an essential part of your mission, your vocation, your story in life. The wee book of St Peter would have a few of those terms if not more. It would be down there as part and partial of life and when you embrace it in that way it actually, you know, threatens the concept of hassle and enables you to live in the present and to embrace these things and to elevate them onto a higher plain if you like and in that way would it help me to cope with some of the daily hassles. (TC).

TC considered spirituality to be "part of my negotiation, my truth" (TC). I believe that it was his intensely spiritual outlook on life combined with, possibly, the fact that he was the oldest interviewee, which accounted for him having achieved the highest level of acumen of them all. His next quote, again, demonstrated his efforts to arrive at a positive perspective on life and maintain it:

> Darkness isn't always maybe the enemy. It seems but an opportunity to push through to a new reality, to a new world or whatever, you know that type of possibility of coping with great, great difficulty. (TC).

Lastly, and importantly, TC emphasises the importance of the positive human virtue of gratitude. What he is saying is that rather than focusing on the negatives in life, by choosing to be grateful for the positives, the perspective changes, and life is transformed: "And then, to allow the attitude of gratitude ...and in that way negotiate the hassle and minimise the hassle and contextualise the hassle and making it a lot easier from that point." (TC).

LO's quote demonstrates the importance of perspective obtained through a spiritual outlook, as it has prevented him from committing suicide:

> There's always somebody worse in the world, African child, starving, so there's always something at the back of me. If you haven't got that spiritual conscience, you would take the easy option and take your own life, you know. (LO).

3.1.1.8. Spirituality Gives Hope

LO derived hope from his spirituality through his belief in a higher power and a higher purpose in life. In light of this he was able to change his perspective on his difficulties and contextualise them within a larger scheme of things, thereby making them seem less overpowering and more meaningful: "As I say, it gives you hope. To know that there's somebody up there looking after you. He's putting you through these challenges for a purpose." (LO).

LO's quote illustrates how his own spirituality prevented him from committing suicide. Importantly, he said that it was solely his spiritual core which stopped him from carrying out the act:

> Well, yeah, like I've had my bad times, obviously with bipolar, I've had serious severe depression and a couple of times I've been suicidal. But there's always been a sort of inner voice, a spiritual one, sort of saying, things will get better, this is only temporary, you know. (LO).

MR had made notes on her interview schedule, one of which, with regard to the question as to how spirituality helps her with life's difficulties, read: "Gives me hope to keep going". This theme of hope enabling her to keep going in dark and difficult times is revisited during the interview when she refers to the contemplative prayer meetings she and her sister regularly attended after her nephew's demise: "Ehm [sic], that was the only thing that kept us going through that black time." (MR).

3.1.1.9. Spirituality Provides Meaning

Spirituality held great significance for the participants. Some identified entirely with it as in RN's case: "It's my essence, I think." RN had a very spiritual outlook on life, a strong connection with a well-meaning and protective God, and resorted to meditation and reflection on a regular basis.

Others, too, made it very clear, how much spirituality meant to them. KS, for example, who made time for spiritual reflection every morning and whose personal development and self-awareness was greatly guided and advanced through her spiritual attitude, said: "So, I could not live my life today without a spiritual way of being." (KS).

Equally, MR, who attends regular contemplative prayer meetings and who has found great solace, comfort and hope in spirituality after the loss of her nephew and sister, sees spirituality as an intrinsic part of her life. As such, it is of great significance to her: "Well, it's part of my life now and I wouldn't want to do without it basically." (MR).

Her sentiments are shared by TC, who describes spirituality as part of "his truth", a phrase close in meaning to RN's "my essence". "No, no. It would be part of my negotiation, my truth." (TC)

JB, who declared that spirituality is more important to him than creativity and that spirituality flows through his art, expresses what spirituality means to him in the following quote. He is, in effect saying, that spirituality gives life warmth and colour and energy. In other words, it is, in itself, life-giving: "I think without being spiritual life would be very cold. I think it would be very black and white...I think it would take the sparkle out of life."

3.1.1.10. Spirituality Provides Guidance and Protection

The quotes illustrating the theme of guidance and protection are very powerful and really provide a snapshot into how their spiritual beliefs provide the participants with a strong feeling of being supported and protected, rather than feeling alone and helpless. RN's excerpt projects an image of spirituality as a shield in the strife: "Hm [sic], I suppose it surrounds you. Like a coat, like something for going out in the cold that gives you protection, that's around you, that you evoke." (RN).

KS's quote is quite striking: "It's just my total crutch, without God I am nothing, I can say that. That's just the bottom line." (KS).

KS' spirituality helped her in increasing her self-awareness and accepting the fact that humans do not have control over everything that happens in life. She had learned that trying to solve and fix everything and everybody in her life on her own all the time had often led to setting herself up for failure. This, in turn, led her into depression. She had also suffered from various addictions and contemplated suicide on one occasion. Through trusting in God she came to accept that not everything is her responsibility and she felt tremendous relief. She tellingly compared the time before she had this realisation ("When I ran on my own self-will") to the time when she learned to have faith, as: "Between insanity and sanity."

MR, who declared that spirituality is part of her life now and that she would not want to do without it, simply and powerfully put it like this: "It's a great source of help to me, I don't think I could survive without it." (MR).

3.1.2. Coping through Creative Expression

The multidimensional construct of creativity emerged as a mode of self-expression and was another constituent theme to the super-ordinate theme of "Transformation". As such, it contained the sub-themes of focus, perspective, sharing and connecting, purpose, self-esteem, joy, and self-awareness as well as that of alleviating anxiety. In addition, the participants perceived creativity to be an aspect of spirituality. Creativity, like spirituality, is a very subjective construct, meaning different things to different people.

RN captures the idea of creative potential in her quote and links it directly into the idea of opportunity. As a very creative person herself, she considers herself lucky to be able to use her creativity in her daily life: "I think we are all capable of so much creativity. It's just if you are lucky to find the expression." (RN).

TC, one of the two participants who was not actively creative, also made reference to the creative potential, as the following quote demonstrates. He demonstrated his interest in poetry with an ad-hoc recital of a poem. The impression during the interview was that TC had indeed the potential and interest to be creative but due to lack of nurture and opportunity had not found a way of expressing it: "I would acknowledge that yes, surely, there's a creative person in there, that just never took time or the energy or was too lazy to try the things."

Creative self-expression as an inner need is portrayed very well in PT's quote: "Someone who needs to express themselves through drawing or writing." (PT).

TC, who was not actively creative and was not given the opportunity for creativity in his earlier years, nevertheless displayed not only a propensity for creativity when he recited a poem ad hoc during the interview, but also a profound understanding of the concept of creativity which the following quotation demonstrates. He describes a creative person as someone who has a different perspective on life; a sense of awe and wonder; someone who not only sees things differently but is able to share what he perceives with others through creative expression.

> A person who is able to see all these aspects of beauty and truth and goes beyond that and is able to express them in a way that evokes a response from his public, his fellow man. (TC).

KS gives a good example of creative coping in action. When she feels unwell, she resorts to creative writing (poetry) in order to express her feelings. By writing about her feelings she is dealing with them and is able to manage them. This, in turn, helps her in her process of recovery from illness:

> Yes. In times of illness I would, I use my writing as well to just, to express my feelings today, to get my feelings...onto paper; to take my emotions and get them out of my system

and by removing the emotions from my being I am opening myself to new avenues of recovery. (KS).

3.1.2.1. Creativity is an Aspect of Spirituality

The participants who described themselves as both creative and spiritual, understood creativity as an aspect of spirituality. At the end of the interview, when asked whether she would like to add anything, MR said she felt that creativity and spirituality are mutually associated and that this combination provides a good coping strategy. "I feel both things kind of go hand in hand because one thing has come out of the other and they do, they link in. They link in in helping, both things help in different ways." (MR).

RN, when asked where she believes her creativity comes from, made a clear and direct link from spirituality to creativity, thereby supporting the idea of creativity being an aspect of spirituality:"[My creativity comes] From the ultimate spiritual, spirituality within me, the God within me. Or the spirit within me." (RN).

RN felt very strongly about this association and made repeated reference to it throughout the interview. In her view, both spirituality and creativity are rooted in the spirit. "So, I would believe that it's that elusive spirit that brings together the two, you know, and where the two can meet there and that they speak the same language." (RN).

JB, when asked whether he could imagine without creativity, said that whilst he would find it very hard not to be able to pursue ideas, he would find it harder still to live without spirituality. To him, spirituality was a higher order concept and expressed itself in his art. This, of course is a strong demonstration of the proposed association between creativity and spirituality, and more specifically, of the idea that creativity is, in fact, an aspect of spirituality.

I would still say that a spiritual outlook in life is still far more important than the creativity, as long as I still have the spiritual side, because it would be on the higher level, so I wouldn't put creativity on the top, I would still put it secondary to the spiritual things in the world, so I would say that in that sense my spirituality would actually flow through my art without a doubt. (JB).

KS said she could not imagine life without creativity, believing it to be a gift from God who was the central figure in her spirituality. She very clearly sees creativity as potential which serves the purpose of self-actualisation and personal growth and development. Again, the creativity—spirituality link is very powerfully expressed here. KS, like JB, also sees creativity as an aspect of spirituality:

I could not imagine life without being creative because to me creativity, in whatever form it comes, is a gift from God, and as a gift from God, it has been given to us to broaden our being, you know, to bring us out and help us to flower. You know, we are a seed and we are growing and our creativity has been given to us to enable us to blossom. (KS).

KS gave a very good description of transformative coping in action. She describes how she resorts to her creativity on a daily basis. In fact she says she *needs* to do that. She then explains how she combines her creative writing with mediation and how she puts the results of her reflections to use all day in order to deal with negative emotions or difficult situations.

I need to use my creativity every day of my life. I write in the morning, I pray, I meditate, I meditate on a word or a line or a maybe just a thought that I have. If the word's love, I write down you know, what love means to me. And then I just meditate for a period of time. I try to carry that word with me all through my day and I envisage whatever the line, whatever anger, it could be anger, and if the word's anger, then how I handle that through the day is that anger is not from the God of my understanding. (KS).

3.1.2.2. Creativity Alleviates Anxiety

A number of examples for creativity providing relief from anxiety were given by the participants, such as the following excerpt from PT's interview. It illustrates how she responds to tension and anxiety by resorting to her creativity, which makes her feel calmer.

> Yes, the more sort of nervy and edgy I would feel, the more creative I would be and the more I would sit down and do some writing, some painting...It sort of grounds me a bit. Being calmer. (PT).

SC who had suffered badly with fear earlier in his life, wrote poetry himself. He believed that reading others' poetry also helped to alleviate his anxiety: "Bit of poetry how you feel better, you know. I think that's mostly for beating fear." (SC).

JB, who had suffered severe anxiety in his younger years, describes his creative process as therapeutically beneficial to him. It provides him with a safe space he can withdraw to when faced with difficulty and where the repetitive nature of his creative work calms him and provides him with stability:

> You go into your own world whenever you are working on your art, but no matter what happens on the outside world, you'd still be contained in this cocoon, in your own little head space while you're making your art, whether its there's instability in your domestic life, you still go into this little place...It is a repetitive kind of process so in that sense it is quite therapeutic because it gives you a grounding and stability. (JB).

LM referred to anxiety and fear frequently during her interview and explained that the act of painting keeps her anxieties at bay. Her creativity is of such significance to her that she compares it to breathing. Even as she said this her voice and demeanour had a tormented quality.

> I am a painter. I paint every day. I work full time as a painter. When I stop I get absolutely full of anxiety. You've no idea. It's like breathing to me. (LM).

The phrase "when it's taken away from me" suggests a belief in external locus of control which would explain LM's intense and enduring feelings of anxiety. In the following quote LM also refers to difficult things having happened in her life. The interview did not shed any further light on this, however, as this remark was made alongside an implicit reference to external locus of control, and anxiety in the absence of creative expression, it stands to reason that the three things are somehow associated.

> Well, I know that when it's taken away from me I am full of anxieties, you know, so, it's the absence that creates a lot of anxieties. Obviously, there is other things in my life that have happened, that are...and part of that would be difficult. (LM).

The next quote is more explicit in as much as LM explains that her painting serves as a healing process. Her description is reminiscent of someone putting ointment onto a wound. Again, the mention of anxieties, fears and "things that happened":

> For instance the material I use, I tend to use layer upon layer so I think I probably cover up a lot. I cover up and cover up and cover up. In a sense there is this therapeutic healing and somehow covering up the hurt and dealing with anxieties, fears and things that happened, by the actual act of painting. (LM).

3.1.2.3. Creativity Facilitates Sharing and Connecting

Sharing with others and thus being able to connect with them was another sub-theme of creative expression. LM explains this in her quote; which illustrates that when it comes to the product of a creative expression; it is equally satisfactory for the spectator or reader; *etc.* to understand and connect with what the creator was trying to express; as the expression of it is for the creator.

> But you can share, I mean even being able to read a poem and get it. You know, when you get something, I mean that is being creative, because that's our combined...as human beings, this is what we share, this ability, this is what raises us above animals. (LM).

HN, who was himself not actively creative and did not appear to have been given the opportunity to get creative in his early days, was nevertheless very appreciative of creativity: "I admire people who are creative, you know." He also linked creativity with the sharing of emotions between the creator and the spectator:

> See human beings really have emotion, right, and like you could hear a piece of music that maybe is so beautiful that it makes you cry, you know. So, you need creativity; or people like to go and look at art and they can get lost in a piece of art and they can study it for ages and ages. (HN).

The quotations in this category have demonstrated that creativity fosters a positive connection between the creator and the spectator through the sharing of human emotions. KS gives another insight into the creator's perspective of this process. She describes how she derives satisfaction (self-esteem!) from the act of creating something, and joy about being able to share what she enjoys with other. "...and to feel good about the work you have done and then, in turn, be able to pass your experience of something very beautiful onto someone else." (KS).

3.1.2.4. Creativity Provides Focus

Coming back to the subjectivity of creative expression, the analysis has made it clear, that different interviewees derived different benefits from creative expression. Focus, for example is a benefit which was very important to MR. She and her sister started being creative in order to deal with their feelings of grief. They refurbished caravans as a way of coping with the difficult time after MR's nephew died. This activity allowed them to mentally focus on something productive which they perceived as enjoyable and rewarding: "I didn't realise it was creativity. Just thought it was something to focus on and something to put a different light on things." (MR).

In doing so, they were able to distance themselves from the negative emotions, so they did not become overwhelming but get a bit dispersed and could be managed a little easier: "It definitely was a different focus, to get away from the sadness." (MR).

In addition, MR and her sister took to flower arranging in response to their grief. Again, it is a powerful illustration of how creative expression can help to transform negative emotions into positive ones. The flower arranging provided them not only with focus but with a good deal of joy and satisfaction, thereby counteracting the intense feelings of sadness. "...the flower arranging started after Michael's death...me and my sister together and I think it helped us to focus on something else." (MR).

3.1.2.5. Creativity Gives Joy

The positive emotion of joy was another sub-theme of creative expression, which, in LM's case, she described as deriving from the excitement that her creativity provided and the opportunity of learning something new. "Yes, an excitement, an interest in discovery, in learning something." (LM).

LO described how he used to sit in a park, or on the underground in London and write poetry. He too, felt that writing poetry gave him joy as it made him feel better about himself and increased his self-esteem. This joyfulness was almost palpable in his voice and facial expression at this point in the interview. "Sitting there and writing a poem and coming away feeling happier. I mean it's an achievement." (LO).

MR described that sense of joy, too, which she felt she received as a result of her interior design and flower arranging which she started during her grieving process. "Well, I think it definitely puts the focus on something else, not even yourself and what you are going through and brings more joy into your life, definitely." (MR).

JB explained how his creative activity brings him joy. The excitement of a new idea forming in his mind and the anticipation of translating it into a finished product are themes in his quotation:

> But certainly, it releases endorphins, so I suppose in a sense there is something that happens creatively on an idea and you get that feel-good factor and you are making the idea sort of alive in your head as you are constructing. (JB).

When RN was asked whether she remembered an instance where her creativity has helped her overcome a problem, she explains how, when she feels unhappy, singing or listening to singing lifts her emotions and makes her feel happier. She emphasises the power of music to elevate one's spirit:

> Yes, well, singing certainly does. You know, dark thoughts are lessened really. So, yes I would if I am feeling down I'd sing a piece of chant or go over to the church and listen to it. Ehm [sic], so yes I think it's really when your emotions are affected really that you can dispel a certain darkness, you know and there's something very healing in singing or listening to it. Does not have to be singing yourself, you know. That's why music is so powerful; it just has that power to take you onto another level. (RN).

3.1.2.6. Creativity Provides Meaning

As with spirituality, meaning was implicated strongly within the participants' answers as to their creativity. KS, who believes that creativity is a gift from God, gives a beautiful account of why exactly she perceives creativity as meaningful. She said:

> It has been given to us to use to broaden our being, you know, to bring us out and help us to flower. You know, we are a seed and we are growing and our creativity has been given to us to enable us to blossom. (KS).

The view of creativity being inherent in human nature is incorporated into her quote, along with the idea of self-actualisation [24]. In other words, KS believes that the meaning of creativity is to enable people to be the best they can be.

The participants shared the view that life without creativity would be less meaningful. In ML's case, the immense significance that creativity has in her life, came across strongly in the interview where she talked about how it is one of her worst nightmares to be in a situation where she would not be able to pursue her art. The anxiety and horror of even just imagining such circumstances were obvious in her voice and facial expression during the discussion of this point: "It's having nothing to work with creatively, you know. When I think of that worst scenario, I always think 'What could I do?'" (LM).

JB thought along the same lines, although not with the same urgency by far. He believed that life would be very dull without being able to express himself creatively. However, I might mention at this point again, that he was also very spiritual and stated that his spirituality was more important to him than his creativity. "No, it certainly wouldn't be very exciting, you know, to have ideas and not be able to pursue them." (JB).

In contrast, LM saw herself as not spiritual (although she demonstrated that she believed in and observed some important spiritual values, e.g., respect for oneself, others and nature) and did, therefore, not resort to spirituality, but resorted to creativity as a much valued coping strategy.

3.1.2.7. Creativity Provides Self-Esteem

Self-esteem emerged as another subtheme to creative expression. It describes feelings of self-worth and pride resulting from having created something unique, as KS explains: "I love writing and to be able to take something and turn it into your own interpretation and to feel good about the work you have done." (KS).

SC, who started writing poetry after he came out of hospital 20 years ago following a mental breakdown, quietly, but proudly said: "I have some 68 published." (SC).

And LO captures the effects of self-esteem when he suggests that looking back on his creative achievements made him feel good about himself when he was going through more difficult times: "Well, I found if you are having a difficult time you look back on your achievements, and your achievements can be creative." (LO).

4. Discussion

The aim of the present study was to establish whether, and if so, to what extent individuals use their creativity as well as their spirituality in coping throughout their lifespan, how they are helped by resorting to them, and how important they are to them. The study critically examined the TTC and associated TCM-R from a qualitative perspective. Ten interviews were conducted among Northern Irish and Irish artists, contemplative prayer group members, and mental health service users. Data were analysed using IPA.

The participants provided an abundance of rich and complex data and have been very forthcoming not only in their answers to the interview questions but also in elaborations beyond that, thus providing an intimate picture of what the application of both creativity and spirituality meant for them and how important it was in their lives.

Eight out of ten participants saw themselves as creative and believed that creativity was in their nature (JB, LM, RN, LO, SC, PT, KS, MR). A further participant, although not actively creative, said he passively enjoyed others' creativity by watching films and listening to music in order to relax (HN). Another participant did not report resorting to creativity as a coping strategy either, yet seemed very familiar with poetry and proceeded to recite a poem ad-hoc during the interview (TC).

Out of the eight actively creative interviewees, six believed that their creativity had been nurtured in childhood (JB, LM, RN, LO, KS, MR), two did not (SC, PT). Four respondents have resorted to creativity in order to cope with illness (JB, LM, RN, MR). All eight have resorted to creativity in order to cope with stressful situations and with daily hassles; seven (all but PT) had resorted to it in difficult times and all eight had employed creativity to overcome a problem. None of them could imagine their life without being creative as they saw it as an intrinsic part of their lives. "It's a great source of help to me. I don't think I could survive without it." (MR)

Equally, most respondents (JB, RN, LO, SC, KS, TC, MR) saw themselves as spiritual and believed that spirituality was in their nature. Only three of them were also religious (KS, TC, MR), with the remaining four describing themselves as spiritual only (JB, RN, LO, SC). Three participants (LM, HN, PT) described themselves as not spiritual. Two of them (LM, PT) were creative, however. HN saw himself as neither actively creative nor spiritual. The distinction of spirituality from religion was an important one for four of the participants (JB, RN, LO, and SC). Out of the seven, six believed that their spirituality had been nurtured in childhood (all but JB). Four respondents had resorted to spirituality in order to cope with illness (JB, LO, SC, KC). All seven have resorted to spirituality in order to cope with stressful situations, daily hassles, and difficult times; and six had employed spirituality to overcome a problem (all but TC). None of the seven could imagine their life without being spiritual as they saw it as an intrinsic part of their lives, and, indeed, as part of their identity. "It's my essence, I think, yeah." (RN). "I would say that definitely God is a very central part of my life." (MR).

Overall, these findings indicate that both creativity and spirituality were important aspects in the participants' lives. Most of the interviewees applied either creativity or spirituality as a coping strategy on a regular basis in order to cope with stressful events and situations, with six out of ten applying a combination of both, effectively employing *transformative coping*. It is interesting to note that these six participants were equally distributed across the three groups, *i.e.*, they were two artists (JB and RN), two mental health group members (SC and LO), and two prayer group members (KS and MR). In line with the literature findings (e.g., [4,5,8,37,38]) creativity was found to be an aspect of spirituality. As JB put it: "My spirituality flows through my art, without a doubt."

The super-ordinate theme was identified as "Positive transformation" which contained the main theme of "Coping through creative expression", with the subthemes of "creativity is an aspect of spirituality", "creativity alleviates anxiety", "creativity facilitates sharing & connecting", "creativity provides focus", "creativity gives joy", "creativity provides meaning", and "creativity provides self-esteem"; and the main theme of "Coping through a spiritual attitude/way of life", with the subthemes of "Spirituality is distinct from religion", "spirituality fosters connectedness to God, self, and others", "Spirituality helps combat depression and addiction", "spirituality gives perspective", "spirituality gives hope", "spirituality provides meaning", and "spirituality provides guidance and protection". "Connecting with others" and "meaning" have emerged as shared benefits of creativity and spirituality (see Figure 2).

There were clear individual differences with regard to theme endorsement. In other words, certain themes were of particular importance to certain individuals. For example, MR's main benefits were joy and focus; TC's and JB's core benefit transpired as perspective; LM's and PT's main benefit was reduced anxiety; to LO and MR hope was an important theme, and for KS guidance had the greatest significance. This shows that, within the umbrella of a shared and collective understanding of the benefits of creativity and spirituality in coping, the participants attained personal meaning and its resulting benefits from transformative coping.

The TCM-R (see [6] for the original version) is supported by the findings of this study. In line with the model's premise, the theme of "creativity is an aspect of spirituality" emerged from the participant-driven analysis. Rather than focusing on their problems, the majority of the participants had chosen to enhance their psycho-spiritual wellbeing actively through the sustained application of a combination of creativity and spirituality and felt that this was a very important and integral part of their lives. They believed that they would not cope as well without it and could not imagine their lives without it (see Table 1). Transformation, a benefit derived from both creativity and spirituality [39,40] can be said to be of crucial importance to the participants. The replacing of negative emotions with positive ones and the consequent perceived improvement in mental health and well-being is central to this positive and proactive approach to coping in the interviewees' lives.

The findings indicated that the participants perceived creativity and spirituality to be associated and, more specifically, believed creativity to be an aspect of spirituality, providing support for the proposed link between creativity and spirituality (see [1–3,11,13,14,40,41]).

In support of the TCM-R the combined application of creativity and spirituality facilitated emotional expression and enabled the interviewees to increase their self-awareness, personal resources and growth. In line with Moritz, Kelly, Angen, Quan, Toews, and Rickhi's [28] findings, perspective was a shared benefit. The benefits of creative expression as a positive focus and perceiving God as a friend were reported as meaningful outcomes. Thus, the active and conscious application of creativity and spirituality combined in an effort to essentially manage emotions was shown to be of immense importance to six out of ten participants who felt that it was an integral part of their lives and that they would not cope as well without it. It can be said that the commitment to resort to the associated coping resources of creativity and spirituality constitutes transformative coping and is a consciously chosen way of life. As such the study supported previous research which reported on the mental health benefits of creativity (e.g., [41,42]) and spirituality (e.g., [43,44]) respectively, while adding a new dimension, namely that of the association between spirituality and creativity and their role in coping.

A somewhat unexpected finding was the extent to which they were united in having experienced adverse life events, and ongoing stressful situations in their lives and, in some cases, trauma. Six participants reported traumatic or stressful experiences, with a further two alluding to difficult situations. For example, loss of loved ones, loss of employment, loneliness, conflict (including the Northern Ireland "troubles") and separation. The traumas or stressful situations appeared to be directly implicated in the mental health history in each life story. Only three out of ten participants reported physical illness (such as food allergies, hernia, obesity, and a suspected heart attack). These findings lend support to Lazarus [15] who posits that hardship is inherent in human life, creating trauma and leading to negative emotions, resulting in psychological stress. Individuals who are deficient in coping resources are particularly vulnerable to suffer from mental ill-health. Ineffective coping with stress as a prelude to mental ill-health is emphasised by the World Health Organization [44]. The results are also in line with Holmes and Rahe's [45] observations that major changes in life (e.g., health, employment, moving, finances) precede the development of disease.

The majority of the interviewees had suffered some form of mental ill-health (see Table 1), albeit not all had been formally diagnosed and treated. Seven out of ten participants had been diagnosed with and treated for a mental illness in the past, with a further two respondents repeatedly referring to anxiety throughout the interview. In addition, two interviewees had contemplated suicide in the past.

Contrary to intentions, nine out of ten interviewees were Catholic and one was non-denominational. Further studies with a wider spread of religious denominations, in order to establish potential differences in transformative coping, are recommended. The findings demonstrated that all participants believed their creativity and spirituality were a result of both nature and nurture. This can be said to support a systemic view of the concepts (see e.g., [46]), placing them in a personal, cultural and historical context. It would be interesting and worthwhile to further qualitatively investigate the extent to which nurture and culture have a direct impact on creative and spiritual coping.

5. Practical Applications

Pending further studies testing the TTC and TCM-R with diverse populations, it is hoped that the TCM-R could be incorporated into therapy, mental health promotion and programs for recovery from mental illness and addiction, in order to enable individuals to resort to their inherent positive resources of creativity and spirituality by way of transformative coping, throughout the lifespan. Individuals may benefit greatly from connecting with their innate spirituality and creativity; from arriving at a mature understanding of the concepts, and from consequently harnessing their combined and mutually nurturing benefits. As a result they would have a more powerful and effective tool to transform negative emotions (e.g., anger, sadness, despair, hate, disappointment, guilt, fear, *etc.*) into positive ones (e.g., acceptance, understanding, forgiveness, hope, meaning, joy, love, optimism, self-esteem, *etc.*), in line with the conceptual framework for transformative coping (TCM-R). It may be that they would be able to appraise future traumas or stressful events from a position of improved inner strength and decreased vulnerability. Consequently, they may be more resilient and less likely to suffer from mental ill-health.

6. Conclusions

The rich data collated within this study have extended current theoretical knowledge in the areas of coping, creativity, spirituality and mental health. They substantiate and give meaning to the lived experience of transformative coping. The findings showed that there are differences in the extent to which individuals apply transformative coping. Therefore, the integration of creative and spiritual resources into client-centred counselling and psychotherapy is proposed, offering clients a positive, respectful and individualistic choice, enabling them to address coping difficulties throughout the lifespan. In order to aid the prevention of mental-ill health, promote mental health and build people's strengths and capacities, the principles of the TCM-R could be taught in educational settings and promoted by health centres, mental health charities, practitioners in primary care, and other health professionals in order to reach the wider population. To facilitate this, practitioners could be trained in how to apply the TTC and TCM-R in practice in order to be able to offer their clients a personalised coping strategy.

Author Contributions: Dr Dagmar A. S. Corry designed and performed the research, analysed the data, and wrote the paper. Dr Tracey assisted with the interpretation of results. Professor Christopher Alan Lewis helped to write the paper. All authors read and approved the final manuscript.

Conflicts of Interest: The authors declare no conflict of interest.

References

1. Wassily Kandinsky. *Concerning the Spiritual in Art*. Mineola: Courier Dover Publications, 2012.
2. Leo Tolstoy. *What is Art?* Translated by Richard Pevear, and Larissa Volokhonsky. London: Penguin Books Ltd., 1995.
3. Earle J. Coleman. *Creativity and Spirituality: Bonds between Art and Religion*. Albany: SUNY Press, 1998.
4. Christopher G. Edwards. "Creative writing as a spiritual practice: Two paths." In *Creativity, Spirituality and Transcendence: Paths to Integrity and Wisdom in the Mature Self*. Edited by Melvin E. Miller and Susanne R. Cook-Greuter. Stamford: Ablex Publishing Corporation, 2000, pp. 3–23.
5. Kelley Raab Mayo. *Creativity, Spirituality, and Mental Health: Exploring Connections*. Farnham: Ashgate Publishing, Ltd., 2013.
6. Dagmar A.S. Corry, Christopher A. Lewis, and John Mallett. "Harnessing the mental health benefits of the creativity—Spirituality construct: Introducing the Theory of Transformative Coping." *Journal of Spirituality in Mental Health* 16 (2014): 89–110.
7. Anthony D. Ong, Lisa M. Edwards, and Cindy S. Bergeman. "Hope as a source of resilience in later adulthood." *Personality and Individual Differences* 41 (2006): 1263–73.
8. Stanley Jacobs. "Creativity, science, and spirituality." *Perspectives*. 15 September 1996. Available online: http://metapsychology.mentalhelp.net/poc/view_doc.php?type=de&id=295 (accessed on 6 May 2009).
9. Peter Bray. "A broader framework for exploring the influence of spiritual experience in the wake of stressful life events: Examining connections between posttraumatic growth and psycho-spiritual transformation." *Mental Health, Religion & Culture* 13 (2010): 293–308.
10. John E. Roberts, Anne M. Shapiro, and Stephanie A. Gamble. "Level and perceived stability of self-esteem prospectively predict depressive symptoms during psychoeducational group treatment." *British Journal of Clinical Psychology* 38 (1999): 425–29.
11. Melvin E. Miller, and Susanne R. Cook-Greuter. *Creativity, Spirituality, and Transcendence: Paths to Integrity and Wisdom in the Mature Self*. Edited by Melvin E. Miller and Susanne R. Cook-Greuter. Santa Barbara: Greenwood Publishing Group, 2000.
12. Frances Reynolds, Kee H. Lim, and Sarah Prior. "Images of resistance: A qualitative enquiry into the meanings of personal artwork for women living with cancer." *Creativity Research Journal* 20 (2008): 211–20.
13. Kenneth I. Pargament. *Spiritually Integrated Psychotherapy: Understanding and Addressing the Sacred*. New York: Guilford Press, 2011.
14. Dana Zohar, and Ian Marshall. *Spiritual Intelligence: The Ultimate Intelligence*. London: Bloomsbury, 2000.
15. Richard S. Lazarus. "Hope: An emotion and a vital coping resource against despair." *Social Research* 66 (1999): 653–78.
16. Barbara L. Fredrickson. "The broaden-and-build theory of positive emotions." *Philosophical Transactions-Royal Society of London Series B Biological Sciences* 359 (2004): 1367–78.
17. Richard S. Lazarus, and Susan Folkman. *Stress, Appraisal, and Coping*. Berlin and Heidelberg: Springer Publishing Company, 1984.
18. Michelle Palmer, Michael Larkin, Richard de Visser, and Gráinne Fadden. "Developing an interpretative phenomenological approach to focus group data." *Qualitative Research in Psychology* 7 (2010): 99–121.
19. Richard C. Snyder. "Hope theory: Rainbows in the mind." *Psychological Inquiry* 13 (2002): 249–75.
20. Judith Lee. "Melancholy, the muse and mental health promotion—An analysis of the complex relationship between mood disorder and creativity, developing a specific model of mental health promotion: Six key themes." *International Journal of Mental Health Promotion* 9 (2007): 4–16.
21. Michael F. Valle, E. Scott Huebner, and Shannon M. Suldo. "An analysis of hope as a psychological strength." *Journal of School Psychology* 44 (2006): 393–406.
22. Vanessa Juth, Joshua M. Smyth, and Alecia M. Santuzzi. "How do you feel? Self-esteem predicts affect, stress, social interaction, and symptom severity during daily life in patients with chronic illness." *Journal of Health Psychology* 13 (2008): 884–94.
23. Joaquim J.F. Soares, and Giorgio Grossi. "The relationship between levels of self-esteem, clinical variables, anxiety/depression and coping among patients with musculoskeletal pain." *Scandinavian Journal of Occupational Therapy* 7 (2000): 87–95.

24. Abraham Maslow. "The creative attitude." In *Explorations in Creativity*. Edited by Ross L. Mooney and Taher A. Razik. New York: Harper & Row, 1967, pp. 43–57.
25. Viktor E. Frankl. *Man's Search for Meaning*. Boston: Beacon Press, 1959.
26. Mindy Greenstein, and William Breitbart. "Cancer and the experience of meaning: A group psychotherapy program for people with cancer." *American Journal of Psychotherapy* 54 (2000): 486–500.
27. Man Yee Ho, Fanny M. Cheung, and Shu Fai Cheung. "The role of meaning in life and optimism in promoting well-being." *Personality and Individual Differences* 48 (2010): 658–63.
28. Christopher Madden, and Taryn Bloom. "Creativity, health and arts advocacy." *International Journal of Cultural Policy* 10 (2004): 133–56.
29. Diarmuid Ó'Murchú. *Reclaiming Spirituality: A New Spiritual Framework for Today's World*. New York: The Crossroad Publishing Co., 1998.
30. Michael F. Steger, Shigehiro Oishi, and Todd B. Kashdan. "Meaning in life across the life span: Levels and correlates of meaning in life from emerging adulthood to older adulthood." *The Journal of Positive Psychology* 4 (2009): 43–52.
31. David J. Wilde, and Craig D. Murray. "The evolving self: Finding meaning in near-death experiences using Interpretative Phenomenological Analysis." *Mental Health, Religion & Culture* 12 (2009): 223–39.
32. Sheryl Zika, and Kerry Chamberlain. "On the relation between meaning in life and psychological well-being." *British Journal of Psychology* 83 (1992): 133–45.
33. Jonathan A. Smith. "Beyond the divide between cognition and discourse: Using interpretative phenomenological analysis in health psychology." *Psychology and Health* 11 (1996): 261–71.
34. Jonathan A. Smith, and Mike Osborn. "Interpretative phenomenological analysis." In *Qualitative Psychology: A Practical Guide to Research Methods*. Edited by Jonathan A. Smith. Thousand Oaks: Sage Publications Ltd., 2003, pp. 51–80.
35. Jonathan A. Smith, Maria Jarman, and Mike Osborn. "Doing interpretative phenomenological analysis." *Qualitative Health Psychology*, 1999, 218–39.
36. QSR International. "About QSR: Our History." Available online: http://www.qsrinternational.com/about-qsr_history.aspx (accessed on 2 April 2011).
37. Mahmoud Awara, and Christopher Fasey. "Is spirituality worth exploring in psychiatric out-patient clinics?" *Journal of Mental Health* 17 (2008): 183–91.
38. Co-Shi C. Chao, Chen Ching-Huey, and Yen Miaofen. "The essence of spirituality of terminally ill patients." *Journal of Nursing Research* 10 (2002): 237–45.
39. Deirdre Heenan. "Art as therapy: An effective way of promoting positive mental health?" *Disability & Society* 21 (2006): 179–91.
40. Sabine Moritz, Mary Kelly, Maureen Angen, Hude Quan, John Toews, and Badri Rickhi. "The impact of a home-based spirituality teaching programme: Qualitative exploration of participants' experiences." *Spirituality and Health International* 8 (2007): 192–205.
41. Shaun McNiff. *Art Heals*. Boston: Shambhala Publications, 2004.
42. Michal M. Mann, Clemens M.H. Hosman, Herman P. Schaalma, and Nanne K. de Vries. "Self-esteem in a broad-spectrum approach for mental health promotion." *Health Education Research* 19 (2004): 357–72.
43. Sean Fleming, and David S. Evans. "The concept of spirituality: Its role within health promotion practice in the Republic of Ireland." *Spirituality and Health International* 9 (2008): 79–89.
44. World Health Organization. *The World Health Report 2001. Mental Health: New Understanding, New Hope*. Geneva: World Health Organization, 2001.
45. Thomas H. Holmes, and Richard H. Rahe. "The Social Readjustment Rating Scale." *Journal of Psychosomatic Research* 11 (1967): 213–18.
46. Mihaly Csikszentmihalyi, and Judith LeFevre. "Optimal experience in work and leisure." *Journal of Personality and Social Psychology* 56 (1989): 815–22.

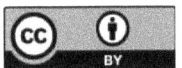

Chapter 2
Spirituality in Physical and Mental Disease

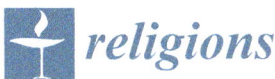

Article

Association between Health Behaviours and Religion in Austrian High School Pupils—A Cross-Sectional Survey

Gabriele Gäbler [1,*], Deborah Lycett [2] and René Hefti [3,4]

[1] Center for Medical Statistics, Informatics, and Intelligent Systems, Section for Outcomes Research, Medical University of Vienna, 1090 Vienna, Austria

[2] Faculty of Health and Life Sciences, Coventry University, Coventry CV15 FB, UK; deborah.lycett@coventry.ac.uk

[3] Medical Faculty, University of Bern, 3000 Bern, Switzerland

[4] Research Institute for Spirituality and Health and Clinic SGM for Psychosomatic Medicine, 4900 Langenthal, Switzerland; rene.hefti@rish.ch

* Correspondence: gabriele.gaebler@meduniwien.ac.at; Tel.: +43-664-473-4040

Received: 14 August 2017; Accepted: 25 September 2017; Published: 28 September 2017

Abstract: The prevalence of risk factors for chronic diseases such as smoking, alcohol abuse, low fruit and vegetable consumption, and lack of physical activity is high among young adults. Health behaviours are influenced by many factors and also by religious orientation, as American studies show. The aim of the present study was to explore whether a similar association with religion exists in Austria (Europe). A cross-sectional survey was carried out in seven randomly selected high schools, whereby a total of 225 11th-grade pupils (64% girls, 36% boys; average age 16.4 years) were surveyed by means of an online questionnaire. The study reveals a positive association between religion and healthy food choices as well as meal patterns. Smoking (number of cigarettes smoked daily) and alcohol consumption (getting drunk) was negatively associated with religion. These negative associations remained after adjusting for confounding factors using logistic regression analysis. Thus, the study showed that religion is associated with a reduction in these risky health behaviours in Austrian high school pupils. However, due to the limitations of the study design, causality cannot be inferred.

Keywords: health behaviours; adolescents; religion

---

1. Introduction

There is evidence that many chronic diseases, such as cardiovascular disease, cancer, diabetes mellitus, obesity and lung disease are largely influenced by lifestyle factors such as smoking, physical inactivity, alcohol use and an unhealthy diet (9; 26; 1). Ford et al. (2009) found that never smoking, having a body mass index lower than 30, performing 3.5 h or more physical activity per week and eating a healthy diet reduces the risk of developing a chronic disease by 78%. In a longitudinal study across several European countries (Belgium, Denmark, France, The Netherlands, Switzerland), Knoops (2004) showed that adherence to a Mediterranean diet and healthy lifestyle is associated with more than a 50% lower rate of all-cause and cause-specific (coronary heart disease, cardiovascular diseases, and cancer) mortality. This positive impact of a healthy lifestyle on mortality was also found by Khaw et al. (2008) in the EPIC-Norfolk prospective population study, which showed that four health behaviours combined (not smoking, being physically active, having a moderate alcohol intake and a fruit and vegetable intake of at least five servings a day) predict a 4-fold difference in total mortality, with an estimated impact equivalent to 14 years of life saved as a result of these health behaviours.

Health behaviours developed during adolescence often persist into adulthood (40; 34). Furthermore, the prevalence of certain risk factors such as smoking, alcohol abuse, low fruit and vegetable consumption, and lack of physical activity is high among young people in Europe (36; 8). These lifestyle factors influence one another and are further affected by social and environmental factors (36; 28). Causal pathways on health are depicted by Dahlgren and Whitehead (41) in their rainbow model of the main determinates of health which shows that health status results from a wide variety of factors, both directly and indirectly. These are firstly age, gender and genetic factors, secondly individual lifestyle factors such as smoking, alcohol use and diet, thirdly social and community networks such as family and friends, fourthly living and working conditions such as access to drinkable water, fast food and transport and fifthly socio-economic status, cultural and environmental factors such as climate, and political situation. Therefore, it is necessary to focus on improving health holistically and not focus simply on a single risk factor. Thus, youth care needs integrated health promotion (31).

Considering lifestyle as a whole also includes religious aspects. Religiosity/spirituality has been shown to be associated with an 18% reduced risk of mortality in healthy populations suggesting a protective effect of religious and spiritual involvement on longevity (7). Koenig et al. (2001, 2011) present a scientific model showing causal pathways from religion to physical health. Religion is conceptualized as individual's belief in, relationship with, and attachment to God or a higher power. Koenig illustrates that health can be directly and indirectly influenced by religious beliefs. Positive religious coping is associated with a reduction in stress and therefore with better physical and mental wellbeing. This may lead to improved health behaviours and reduced reliance on maladaptive coping strategies such as disordered eating, excessive alcohol consumption and smoking. Furthermore, low social acceptability of smoking and drinking alcohol in religious communities may result in lower prevalence of these unhealthy behaviours.

There is a growing body of evidence supporting this model (20, 2011). Furthermore, studies that examine the relationship between religion and health behaviours during adolescence, when independent lifestyle choices are often made are increasing in recent years. Wallace and Forman (1998) investigated a sample of 5000 high school students. They found a positive association between religion (measured religious importance, attendance and denominational affiliation) and a healthy diet (how often students have breakfast, green vegetables, and fruit). Similar results have been published by Bowen-Reid and Smalls (2004) and also by Callaghan (2006). Nagel and Sgoutas-Emch (2007) identified a significant positive association between religious involvement (spiritual experience, praying and church attendance) and physical activity in adolescents as well as a negative correlation with alcohol consumption. The protective influence of religiosity on alcohol use is in line with many other studies (35; 33; 10; 5). However, there are reported differences between ethnic groups, for example religious service attendance predicts alcohol use in black adolescents, while religious fundamentalism is the most predictive factor in white adolescents (4). No dose-response associations have been found (37). Furthermore, Wallace and Forman (1998) as well as Dunn (10) show results concerning the positive impact of religion on cigarette smoking. This is in line with Brown et al. (2001b). They analysed nationally representative data collected from 22 consecutive cohorts of high school seniors from 1976 to 1997. The authors investigated the associations between risk and protective factors for substance use. They found that religion (measured by religious attendance and importance) is negatively associated with smoking. Additionally, they indicate that religion is the strongest predictor determining cigarette use.

Most of these studies in adolescents have been carried out in the United States (US). Europe is generally lacking studies on religion and health behaviours although Bosnia and Germany have been involved in a study that investigating adolescent religiosity and psychosocial functioning (38). However, there are significant differences in the religious characteristics of European populations compared to those in the United States (US) which warrants investigation of the associations between religion and health within Europe. The US is predominantly protestant (2; 39) whereas Austria is predominantly Roman Catholic (2; 13). However, this landscape is changing, in 2001 3/4 of the Austrian population was Roman Catholic but in 2016, this had fallen to 2/3 with rising secularization. Seventeen percent of the Austrian population were estimated to be non-religious in 2016, compared to only 12% in 2001. Additionally, religious diversity has increased. For example, the number of Orthodox Catholics has more than doubled from 2% to 5%, and the number of Muslims has doubled from 4% to 8% between 2001 and 2016 (13).

The aim of the present study was to explore the association between religion and health behaviours in an Austrian sample of adolescents, contributing to the lack of European studies.

2. Methods

2.1. Design and Sample

A cross-sectional survey including seven randomly sampled high schools out of 23 in the province of Carinthia in Austria was conducted. Random sampling was carried out using the Microsoft Excel for Mac 2011 RAND function. All 11th-grade classes of the chosen schools were included in the study. Thus, the sample contained 13 classes and 225 11th-grade pupils in total, who were surveyed by an online questionnaire.

The study was approved by the ethic commission of the Medical University of Graz and the school inspectors for Carinthia. Parental approval was also obtained by teachers of the classes. The pupils were provided with information about the study and written instructions. Furthermore, a declaration of consent prior to the survey was obtained. The participation was voluntary and anonymous. Parents and pupils were informed that not participating would not have disadvantages. The online questionnaire lasting 10–15 min was completed during a school lesson.

2.2. Data Collection

The online questionnaire was implemented with assistance of SoSci Survey (25) and comprised 60 items in total. Measures of health status, health behaviours and religiosity were collected using validated instruments where possible or questions based on well-established questionnaires within the adolescent population as described below. Permission was obtained for the use of each questionnaire. The survey was piloted on a convenience sample of eight young people (17–22 years) of one city of Carinthia and found to be easy to complete.

Eating behaviour: Firstly, using the food frequency questionnaire of the well-established World Health Organization collaborative cross-national Health Behaviour in School-aged Children Survey (WHO-HBSC-Survey) (42; 28), the following questions were asked: "How many times a week do you usually drink fruit juice or eat fruit, vegetables/salad, cereal products, brown/whole-grain bread, white bread, French fries, red meat, sausages, chicken/turkey, fast-food, fish, crisps/chips/salt sticks, sweets/chocolates, sweetened soft drinks/energy drinks, ice tea and soft drinks without sugar? Answers were based on a 6-point Likert-type scale ranging from 1 = never to less than once a week, 2 = once a week, 3 = 2–4 days a week, 4 = 5–6 days a week, 5 = once a day/every day and 6 = more than once a day. For correlational analysis, a 'healthy eating' food frequency score was generated putting together positive items (fruit/vegetable/salad, brown bread/whole grain bread) and negative items (French fries, fast food, chips, soft drinks/energy drinks and ice tea) with reversed scoring (Cronbach's Alpha > 0.79). The possible range was 0 to 48. For logistic regression analyses responses were combined into binary outcomes. High Fruit and Vegetable Consumption means consuming at least one serving of fruit or vegetables a day, while low says neither fruit nor vegetable a day.

Secondly, the frequency of eating main meals (more than only a glass of beverages, an apple, a hamburger or other snacks) was assessed with six questions based on the WHO-HBSC-Survey 2002 (28). These were: On how many weekdays (0–5) do you usually eat breakfast (question 1), dinner (question 2) supper (question 3)? And on how many weekend days (0–2) do you usually eat breakfast (question 4), dinner (question 5) supper (question 6)? A meal frequency score with a possible range from 0 to 21 was calculated, for analysis of correlations. In terms of binary outcomes for logistic regression analyses high Main Meal Frequency refers to at least two a day main meals, while low refers to less than two main meals a day.

Disordered Eating: To assess indication of an eating disorder, a German version (15) of the SCOFF-Questionnaire (27; 30) was used. It is a brief tool (five items) designed to screen for eating disorders and has been shown to have excellent validity and reliability (27). Two or more positive answers to the five questions were suggestive of disordered eating.

Physical activity: Questions about physical activity were based on the well-established German Health Interview and Examination Survey for Children and Adolescents (KiGGS) (24). Two questions were asked to gauge the extent of physical activity. These were firstly "How often are you physically active in your leisure time, so much that you get out of breath or sweat?" Responses were based on a 6-point Likert-type scale ranging from 1 = never, 2 = 1–2 times per month, 3 = 1–2 times per week, 4 = 3–5 times per week, 5 = once a day and 6 = more than once a day. The second question asked: "How many hours per week are you usually [this] physically active?"

Cigarette smoking habits: The questions about cigarette smoking habits were also based on the KiGGS Survey (23). The following questions were asked: "Are you currently smoking?" (Yes/No) And: "If yes, how often do you smoke?" Response possibilities were 1 = no [I don't smoke], 2 = less than once a week, 3 = once a week, 4 = several times a week, 5 = once a day and 6 = more than once a day. An additional question was "If yes, how many cigarettes do you smoke a day, a week, a month? Answers were calculated on a fractional basis to calculate the daily number of cigarettes smoked. In terms of binary outcomes for logistic regression analyses high Number of cigarettes smoked daily refers to two or more cigarettes daily, while low refers to less than two cigarettes daily.

Alcohol drinking behaviour: Based on the WHO-HBSC-Survey 2002 (28). The questions were: "Have you ever had so much alcohol that you were really drunk?" Response options were: No, once, 2–3 times, 4–10 times, 11–20 times, more than 20 times. A previous study has suggested that the frequency of drunkenness has a better prediction power of problematic behaviour than the frequency of alcohol consumption per se (28). In terms of binary outcomes for logistic regression analyses high Drunkenness Frequency refer to being drunk more than once in their lifetime, while low refers to no drunken episodes.

Religiosity: Religiosity was assessed using the Centrality of Religiosity Scale (CRS) which consists of 10 items (CRS-10) (17; 16). It measures five dimensions of religion: public practice, private practice, religious experience, ideology and intellectual interest (two questions for each). Therefore, the CRS measures intrinsic religiosity as well as extrinsic religious involvement and is suitable for interreligious studies (17). Answers are scored from 1 to 5 based on perceived level or importance and frequency of engagement. In the calculation of the CRS-Score, the total score is divided by the number of items resulting in a range of the CRS-Score between 1.0 and 5.0. (17). The total score (CRS-Score) was used for correlation and regression analysis, additionally scores of each dimension were used for correlation analysis.

Other variables: A stress-score was used as a confounding variable. This stress-score included two questions assessing perceived stress frequency, "How often do you feel stress?" with eight response options, and perceived stress intensity, "How intensely do you feel this pressure?" with response options from 0 to 10.

Demographic questions included gender, age (years), and religious affiliation (10 options: Roman Catholic; Lutheran; old Catholic; Evangelical Free Churches; Jewish; Jehovah witness; Seventh-day Adventist; Islam; other denomination and no denomination).

2.3. Statistical Analyses

Descriptive statistics were conducted to present sample characteristics. Gender differences between health behaviours for dichotomous categories were estimated with Chi-squared (presented with p values).

Associations between health behaviours and religiosity were calculated using Spearman correlations with scores and Likert-type scales as described above. Multiple logistic (due to lack of linearity and data not being normal distributed) regression models were used to determine the magnitude of association between religiosity and health behaviours. For each of these analyses responses regarding each health behaviour were combined into binary outcomes. Four separate models with binary/dichotomous health behaviour variables (High/Low Fruit and Vegetable Consumption, High/Low Main Meal Frequency, High/Low Drunkenness Frequency and High/Low Cigarette Smoking Number as described above) as the outcome variable and the CRS-Score as the independent variable were performed. These were adjusted for gender and stress. In a further step, all health behaviour variables that were correlated with the outcome variable were entered into the model. Significance for regression models were set at 0.01 level according to Bonferroni correction ($\alpha = 0.05/4$). Statistical analyses were conducted using SPSS 20.

The sample size has been calculated a priori using G*Power (11) which showed that 55 individuals were needed to achieve 80% power to significantly identify an effect size of 0.35, using an α error probability of 0.01 and 4 predictor variables in the regression analyses.

3. Results

3.1. Sample Characteristics

From the 225 pupils recruited, 5 (2.2%) dropped out or did not complete the questionnaire seriously. As this drop-out rate was low, analysis was conducted on the 220 pupils who completed the questionnaire appropriately. The mean age of these pupils was 16, most were female and affiliated to the Roman Catholic denomination (Table 1).

Table 1. Sample characteristics (gender, religion, mean age with standard deviation) by schools.

School	Total		Gender		Religion						Age	
			Female	Male	rk	lu	efc	is	or	no	Years	
	n	%	*n*				*n*				m	SD
1	26	11.8	21	5	20	1	1	0	0	4	16.2	0.43
2	38	17.3	29	9	23	2	1	0	2	10	16.6	0.64
3	18	8.2	18	0	16	1	0	0	0	1	16.5	0.62
4	61	27.7	35	26	43	9	2	3	1	3	16.3	0.55
5	35	15.9	16	19	26	4	1	0	3	1	16.4	0.60
6	18	8.2	6	12	11	6	0	0	0	1	17.4	0.50
7	24	10.9	15	9	19	0	0	0	1	4	16.2	0.51
total	220		140	80	158	23	5	3	7	24	16.4	0.64

rk = Roman Catholic; lu = Lutherian; efc = Evangelical Free Church; is = Islam; or = Other religion (Greek orthodox, Buddhism); no = No religion.

3.2. Health Related Variables and Religiosity Scores of the Total Sample and by Gender

The sample had a mean CRS-Score of 1.41 (possible range 1–5) which was significantly lower in males than females with a mean difference and 95% CI of 0.26 [0.04–0.48]. While the stress score and also the healthy eating score were significantly higher in females than in males, the main meal frequency score was significantly lower in this subgroup.

A higher proportion of the total sample fell into the higher risk categories for episodes of drunkenness and levels of physical activity. Responses differed significantly by gender, proportionally more males were drunk more often and proportionally more females had lower levels of physical activity. For fruit and vegetable consumption, meal frequency, smoking status, and disordered eating the majority of the sample fell into the lower risk categories. While proportionally more males eating meals more often and exhibiting less disordered eating than females, proportionally more females ate greater amounts of fruit and vegetables than males (Table 2).

Table 2. Percentage frequency of transposed dichotomous health related variables of total sample and by gender.

	Total sample N = 220	Females N = 140	Males N = 80	Difference between Males and Females
	n (%)	*n* (%)	*n* (%)	*p* Value **
Fruit and Vegetable Consumption				
0 (High) = at least once a day	113 (51.4)	83 (59.3)	30 (37.5)	0.002
1 (Low) = none a day	107 (48.6)	57 (40.7)	50 (62.5)	
Main Meal Frequency				
0 = (High) at least 2 a day	154 (70)	91 (65.0)	63 (78.8)	0.032
1 = (Low) less than 2 a day	66 (30)	49 (35.0)	17 (21.2)	
Eating Disorder (Scoff-Score)				
0 = not suggestive of Eating disorder	165 (75)	93 (66.4)	72 (90.0)	<0.001
1 = suggestive of Eating disorder	55 (25)	47 (33.6)	8 (3.6)	
Cigarette Smoker				
0 = non-smoker	153 (69.5)	97 (69.3)	56 (70.0)	>0.5
1 = smoker	67 (30.5)	43 (30.7)	24 (30.0)	
Number of cigarettes smoked daily *				
0 = (Low) less than 2 Cigarettes daily	30 (44.8)	23 (53.5)	7 (29.2)	0.55
1 = (High) 2 or more Cigarettes daily	37 (55.2)	20 (46.5)	17 (70.8)	
Drunkenness Frequency				
0 = (Low) never or only once in lifetime	88 (40)	65 (46.4)	23 (28.8)	0.01
1 = (High) more than once in lifetime	132 (60)	75 (33.6)	57 (71.3)	
Physical Activity Frequency				
0 = at least 3 times a week	101 (45.9)	55 (39.3)	46 (57.5)	0.009
1 = less than 3 times a week	119 (54.1)	85 (60.7)	34 (42.5)	

* *n* = 67 only smokers (female *n* = 43, male *n* = 24); ** *p*-values calculated with Chi-square, tested 2-tailed.

3.3. Association between Health, Health Behaviours and Religion

There were significant weakly positive correlations between CRS-Score and Healthy Eating Score as well as Main Meal Frequency Score. There were significant weak to moderate negative correlations between CRS-Score and the Cigarette Smoking Number and Drunkenness Frequency (Table 3). Thus, for these behaviours a logistic (data not normally distributed) regression model was performed following the transformation into binary outcomes (Table 2).

Table 3. Spearman Correlation Coefficients for health behaviours and domains of religiosity.

	CRS-Score	Intellect	Ideology	Private	Experience	Public
Healthy Eating-Score	**0.141 ***	0.08	0.03	0.179 **	0.02	0.138 *
Main Meal Frequency-Score	**0.135 ***	0.140 *	0.08	0.07	0.135 *	0.09
Scoff-Score	0.12	0.01	0.55	0.203 **	0.06	0.12
Cigarette Smoking Frequency	−0.12	−0.03	−0.09	−0.13	−0.11	−0.08
Cigarette Smoking Number	**−0.480 ****	−0.13	−0.298 *	−0.459 **	−0.403 **	−0.461 **
Drunkenness Frequency	**−0.285 ****	−0.10	−0.195 **	−0.296 **	−0.231 **	−0.195 **
Physical Activity Frequency	0.03	0.03	−0.02	−0.03	0.09	0.05
Physical Activity Duration	0.04	0.03	−0.04	0.02	0.07	0.12

Note: Bold numbers show significant correlations between the total Centrality of Religiosity Scale-Score (CRS-Score) and health behaviour (* *p* < 0.05; ** *p* < 0.01.).

3.4. Strength of Association between Health, Health Behaviour and Religiosity

The results of the adjusted binary logistic regression analyses indicate that the CRS-Score was significantly associated with cigarette smoking and frequency of drunkenness. For every unit increase in religiosity (meaning having a higher religiosity by one point on the CRS-Score), the likelihood of getting drunk (never or only once in life compared to more than once) was reduced by 5% (Table 4).

For every unit increase in religiosity, the likelihood of smoking two or more cigarettes daily is reduced by 10% (Table 4).

Table 4. Logistic regression models for the association between religiosity and health behaviours.

		OR	95% CI		Sig
Drunkenness (High/Low)	CRS-Score (adjusted for gender and stress)	0.95	0.92	0.99	0.006
	CRS-Score (adjusted for gender, stress and other health behaviours)	0.95	0.91	0.99	0.010
Fruit and Vegetable Consumption (High/Low)	CRS-Score (adjusted for gender and stress)	1.00	0.97	1.04	n.s.
Main meal frequency (High/Low)	CRS-Score (adjusted for gender and stress)	0.97	0.94	1.01	n.s.
Number of Cigarettes smoked * (High/Low)	CRS-Score (adjusted for gender and stress)	0.89	0.82	0.96	0.002
	CRS-Score (adjusted for gender, stress and other health behaviours)	0.90	0.83	0.97	0.005

Note: CRS-Score = Centrality of Religiosity Scale-Score; * in smokers only $n = 67$.

Furthermore, the results of the binary logistic regression models show that fruit and vegetable consumption and main meal frequency is not significantly associated with the CRS-Score (Table 4).

4. Discussion

4.1. Main Findings

The aim of this study was to evaluate associations between health and risk behaviours with religion in adolescents in Carinthia, an Austrian province. Logistic regression analyses in our study confirmed that religiosity (CRS-Score) was significantly associated with the number of cigarettes smoked daily and of problem drinking (drunkenness). After controlling for gender, stress perception (stress-score) and other related health behaviours, this relationship remained significant. After adjustment of confounders, we found no significant association between religiosity and eating behaviours, neither for healthy eating nor for frequency of main meal consumption. This suggests that the association we found between eating behaviours and religiosity was explained by our confounding variables of gender, stress.

4.2. Consistency of Findings

We found that among smokers, those with higher CRS-Score smoked less cigarettes daily. However, frequency of smoking in our study was not associated with religiosity. Nagel and Sgoutas-Emch (2007) and Marsiglia et al. (2011) did not find any association with smoking amongst pupils from a Roman-Catholic background and suggested this could be due to the low prevalence of smokers in this population in general. Dunn (2005) found those who considered religion as important were significantly less likely to be a current smoker (OR = 1.47; 1.40). This was in an American 86.9% white population with data from the Monitoring the Future survey, a continuing study of American youth. Brown et al. (2001b) also found that religion (measured by religious attendance and importance) is negatively associated with smoking and the strongest predictor determining cigarette use. Nonnemaker et al. (2003) indicate that both public and private religiosity are protective factors against cigarettes and alcohol use. Concerning alcohol use, this is in line with Nagel and Sgoutas-Emch (2007). They found a lower prevalence in those who felt religion was important. The authors investigated the association with frequency of alcohol use. Our result showed no reduction of frequency of alcohol use with religiosity, however, there were fewer episodes of drunkenness in those with higher religiosity scores.

After adjusting for confounding variables, we found no association between religiosity and eating behaviours. Wallace and Forman (1998) found a positive association between religion and a healthy diet (how often students have breakfast, green vegetables, and fruit). Methodically, there are several similarities in comparison with our study, for example the use of self-administered questionnaires during a normal class period and the measure of religion by means of a multidimensional construct. However, there are several differences. Wallace and Forman use a less diverse measure (religious importance one question: How important is religion in your life?), attendance (one question: How often do you attend religious services?), and denominational affiliation (questions about religious preference). In contrast, our measure of religion included 5 dimension within the CRS-Score. Furthermore, our sample of 220 11th-grade pupils may not have been large enough to detect subtle associations. In contrast, Wallace and Forman's study was conducted in a national representative sample of 5000 high school students. Additionally, we may not have had a sufficient spread of religiosity within our sample to detect differences. In Wallace and Forman's study, religion was unimportant for 14.4% of their sample, but 37% of our sample were not religious, 32.1% considered religion very important in their study but in our study only 6 pupils (2.7%) have described themselves as "highly-religious". It might be that in our study, the association of religion and eating behaviour could not be found due to the small number of highly religious participants.

In this regard, it is important to discuss the religious demographics in Austria. We assumed differences in religiosity between Austria and the US. The US population is characterized by more protestant Christians and higher levels of religiosity (17; 2; 39). However, we did not expect such a low religiosity score. Namely, 37% of the Carinthia 11th-grade high school pupils described themselves as not-religious according categorization of the CRS-Score (17). This implies a mean CRS-Score of 1.41 in our sample. In contrast, the validation study of the CRS-Score in Austria shows a mean score of 2.93 (17). The validation study scores were derived from the Religion Monitor Project in 2008, which compared religiosity across 21 countries (2). In that investigation, a representative sample of Austrian population were surveyed. However, our sample was less diverse than the wider Austrian population and its homogeneity in terms of age, school attendance and religion. This fact may have been the reason for the low religiosity we found. Adolescents in particular are less religious than the rest of the population. The Religion Monitor Project describes 20% of the overall population of Austria as highly religious and 52% as somewhat religious, while the corresponding figures for young adults are only 5% and 53% respectively. Thirty-nine percent of young people are nonreligious, compared with only 25% of the whole population. These results are in line with an Austrian-wide youth survey (14 to 29 year old sample) conducted in 2011 (14). Where, questions on religiosity were based on a scale with 10 categories ranging from not religious to very religious. The results show that 72% of the young people scored themselves as low on religiosity (scale range between 1–5) and 28% as more religious (scale range between 6–10). Taking a closer look at the extreme values, 22% of these young people stated that they are not-religious and similar to our findings only 3% identified themselves as very religious.

Another fact that should be considered is the low effects of significant association we found. This might be because of the multi-factorial determinants of health behaviour of which religiosity is only one. We did not consider many other psychosocial determinants of health in our study. In Austria, a positive family situation (with a loving and affirming atmosphere), and a positive school environment (school satisfaction, good relationships with others, low levels of school pressure and high school performance) is positively associated with health in general, healthier eating behaviours and less substance use (36). Callaghan (2006) also investigated factors influencing adolescent's healthy behaviours. For example, he found significant relationships between the quality of social relationships, income of parents, religious involvement and healthy behaviours.

4.3. Strengths and Limitations

This study contained a representative sample of Austrian high school adolescents from the province of Carinthia. Random sampling of the high schools was performed to reduce the risk of a regional selection bias. Self-selection bias was also low with only five of the selected pupils (2.2%) not completing the questionnaire. The high response rate may be explained by the time set aside within school lessons to complete the questionnaire. Attention was given to clear and easily understandable written information for teachers and students to reduce the risk of information bias. However, it has to be mentioned due to the fact that we focused only on 11th grade high school pupils, the student population was quite homogenous in terms of the education as well as religious affiliation with a high percentage of pupils belonging to the Roman-Catholic church. Therefore, it cannot be generalised to those belonging to other religious groups. Nor can the findings be generalised to those adolescents who are not engaged with or attending high school. Kuntz and Lampert (2011) show that health behaviours (smoking, inactivity, alcohol consumption, excessive electronic media usage, and fruit and vegetable consumption) are associated with educational level, therefore it is unsurprising that in our well-educated sample, there was also lower smoking rates than in their large Austrian HBSC study which contained a more representative sample of all adolescents of Austria (n = 6496). This more representative sample included a variety of school types as well as those who had dropped out of school. However, in terms of alcohol consumption, physical activity and disordered eating, we did not find healthier behaviours in our high school pupils. Instead we found the prevalence of health and risk factors in our study comparable to others. Our results regarding excessive alcohol use are in line with results of the Carinthia survey, namely more young men had been drunk four times or more in their lives than young women (14%). Our results for physical activity are similar in both frequency and duration to the German survey (24) which found in the 11 to 17-year-old sample 64.7% of boys and 43.7% of girls who are physically active three times or more often weekly. In the 14 to 17-year-old adolescents group, physical activity was for a duration of 7.8 h per week in males and 4.2 h in females. Rates of physical activity declined with age in both our study and this German survey. We found 25% of young people showed signs of disordered eating (33.6% in girls and 10.0% in boys). These findings are comparable to 30.1% girls and 12.8% boys (n = 6634) in the German survey which also used the SCOFF-Questionnaire that we used (15).

This study was limited by our self-reported questionnaires which may have been influenced by social desirability bias. This may be particularly more evident in a school situation where students are usually required in their school work to choose the 'correct answer'. Whether this was more likely for those who were more religious or not is unknown—if it is more likely through a desire to please for those who are more religious, then this could have explained our findings. However, if it is less likely and those who are more religious are more reflective of their honesty, then our effect size might have been underestimated.

Additionally, we were unable to measure and adjust for all potential confounding factors, as described above, for example psychosocial factors, social-economic status, home and school environment, and peer or social support. If those who were more religious were also of higher social-economic status then this may have explained the relationship. Or such confounders may have mediated the relationship we found, for example, social support from a religious community could explain why more religious adolescents also have healthier behaviours.

Our study is also limited by its cross-sectional design. A lack of temporality means that we cannot prove causality, as we cannot determine the direction of this association. We do not know whether becoming more religious leads to healthier behaviours or whether those who already have healthier behaviours seek out spiritual health through religious engagement, for example.

A larger study would increase the confidence in our results as our study was limited by a relatively small sample size. The a priori power calculation was based on conducting linear regression analysis assuming a normal distribution of variables. However, not all variables were normally distributed therefore we finally conducted a logistic regression analysis. So, our study may have been underpowered to detect small effect sizes. Nonetheless the narrow confidence intervals of our results suggest these are reasonably precise.

5. Conclusions

There is growing evidence for an interaction between religion and health behaviour. Many studies show positive associations with health, health behaviour and even reduced mortality, if a religious lifestyle is practiced in "healthy years" before a disease is developed.

However, there are few studies in adolescents which investigated the associated between religion and health behaviour in Europe. Our study showed that religiosity was associated with less smoking and drunkenness, however it is limited by its cross-sectional design and unmeasured confounding variables. It provides evidence that the relationship between religiosity and health behaviours among adolescents should be explored further. To this end it would be prudent for national surveys, for example the WHO-HBSC-Survey, to include questions on religion and spirituality.

Acknowledgments: We would like to thank the pupils and their teachers for participating in this survey.

Author Contributions: All authors contributed to the design of this study and to the manuscript. G.G. collected and analysed the data with supervision of R.H. and wrote the manuscript with supervision of D.L.

Conflicts of Interest: The authors declare no conflict of interest.

References

1. Albers, Torsten. 2012. Lebensstilfaktoren und Krebs. *Public Health Forum* 20: 21.e1–21.e3. [CrossRef]
2. Bertelsmann Stiftung. 2009. *What the World Believes: Analyses and Commentary on the Religion Monitor 2008*. Gütersloh: Verlag Bertelsmann Stiftung.
3. Bowen-Reid, Terra L., and Ciara Smalls. 2004. Stress, spirituality and health promoting behaviors among African American college students. *Western Journal of Black Studies* 28: 283–91.
4. Brown, Tamara L., Gregory S. Parks, Rick S. Zimmerman, and Clarenda M. Phillips. 2001a. The role of religion in predicting adolescent alcohol use and problem drinking. *Journal of Studies on Alcohol* 62: 696–705. [CrossRef]
5. Brown, Tony N., John Schulenberg, Jerald G. Bachman, Patrick M. O'Malley, and Lloyd D. Johnston. 2001b. Are Risk and Protective Factors for Substance Use Consistent across Historical Time?: National Data from the High School Classes of 1976 through 1997. *Prevention Science* 2: 29–43. [CrossRef]
6. Callaghan, Donna. 2006. Basic Conditioning Factors' Influences on Adolescents' Healthy Behaviors, Self-Efficacy, and Self-Care. *Issues in Comprehensive Pediatric Nursing* 29: 191–204. [CrossRef] [PubMed]
7. Chida, Yoichi, Andrew Steptoe, and Lynda H. Powell. 2009. Religiosity/Spirituality and Mortality. *Psychotherapy and Psychosomatics* 78: 81–90. [CrossRef] [PubMed]
8. Currie, Candace. 2012. *Social Determinants of Health and Well-Being among Young People: Health Behaviour in School-Aged Children (HBSC) Study: International Report from the 2009/2010 Survey*. Copenhagen: World Health Organization, Regional Office for Europe.
9. Danaei, Goodarz, Eric L. Ding, Dariush Mozaffarian, Ben Taylor, Jürgen Rehm, Christopher J. L. Murray, and Majid Ezzati. 2009. The Preventable Causes of Death in the United States: Comparative Risk Assessment of Dietary, Lifestyle, and Metabolic Risk Factors. *PLoS Medicine* 6: e1000058. [CrossRef] [PubMed]
10. Dunn, Michael S. 2005. The Relationship between Religiosity, Employment, and Political Beliefs on Substance Use among High School Seniors. *Journal of Alcohol and Drug Education* 49: 73.
11. Faul, Franz, Axel Buchner, Edgar Erdfelder, and Albert-Georg Lang. 2011. G*Power (version 3.1.3) (software). Available online: http://www.psycho.uni-duesseldorf.de/abteilungen/aap/gpower3/download-and-register/Dokumente/GPower_3 (accessed on 20 September 2011).
12. Ford, Earl S., Manuela M. Bergmann, Janine Kroger, Anja Schienkiewitz, Cornlia Weikert, and Heiner Boeing. 2009. Healthy living is the best revenge: Findings from the European Prospective Investigation Into Cancer and Nutrition-Potsdam study. *Archives of Internal Medicine* 169: 1355–62. [CrossRef] [PubMed]
13. Goujon, Anne, Sandra Jurasszovich, and Michaela Potančoková. 2017. *Religious Denominations in Vienna & Austria: Baseline Study for 2016-Scenarios until 2046*. Vienna: Vienna Institute of Demography, Austrian Academy of Sciences.
14. Heinzlmaier, Bernhard, and Phillipp Ikrath. 2012. *Bericht zur Jugend-Wertestudie 2011*. Vienna: Institut für Jugendkulturforschung, Wien.

15. Hölling, Heike, and Robert Schlack. 2007. Eating disorders in children and adolescents. First results of the German Health Interview and Examination Survey for Children and Adolescents (KiGGS). *Bundesgesundheitsblatt, Gesundheitsforschung, Gesundheitsschutz* 50: 794–99. [CrossRef] [PubMed]

16. Huber, Stefan. 2004. Zentralität und multidimensionale Struktur der Religiosität: Eine Synthese der theoretischen Ansätze von Allport und Glock zur Messung der Religiosität. In *Religiosität: Messverfahren und Studien zu Gesundheit und Lebensbewältigung: Neue Beiträge zur Religionspsychologie*. Edited by Christian Zwingmann and Helfried Moosbrugger. Münster: Waxmann.

17. Huber, Stefan, and Odilo W. Huber. 2012. The Centrality of Religiosity Scale (CRS). *Religions* 3: 710–24. [CrossRef]

18. Khaw, Kay-Tee, Nicholas Wareham, Sheila Bingham, Ailsa Welch, Robert Luben, and Nicholas Day. 2008. Combined Impact of Health Behaviours and Mortality in Men and Women: The EPIC-Norfolk Prospective Population Study. *PLoS Medicine* 5: e12. [CrossRef] [PubMed]

19. Knoops, Kim T. B. 2004. Mediterranean Diet, Lifestyle Factors, and 10-Year Mortality in Elderly European Men and Women: The HALE Project. *JAMA: The Journal of the American Medical Association* 292: 1433–39. [CrossRef] [PubMed]

20. Koenig, Harold, Michael E. McCullough, and David B. Larson. 2001. *Handbook of Religion and Health.* Oxford: Oxford University Press.

21. Koenig, Harold G., Dana E. King, and Verna Benner Carson. 2011. *Handbook of Religion and Health.* Oxford and New York: Oxford University Press.

22. Kuntz, Benjamin, and Thomas Lampert. 2011. Potenzielle Bildungsaufsteiger leben gesünder. *Prävention und Gesundheitsförderung* 6: 11–18. [CrossRef]

23. Lampert, Thomas, and Michael Thamm. 2007. Consumption of tobacco, alcohol and drugs among adolescents in Germany. Results of the German Health Interview and Examination Survey for Children and Adolescents (KiGGS). *Bundesgesundheitsblatt, Gesundheitsforschung, Gesundheitsschutz* 50: 600–8. [CrossRef] [PubMed]

24. Lampert, Thomas, Gert B. Mensink, Natalie Romahn, and Alexander Woll. 2007. Physical activity among children and adolescents in Germany. Results of the German Health Interview and Examination Survey for Children and Adolescents (KiGGS). *Bundesgesundheitsblatt, Gesundheitsforschung, Gesundheitsschutz* 50: 634–42. [CrossRef] [PubMed]

25. Leiner, Dominik J. 2012. *SoSci Survey* (version 2.0) (computer software). Available online: https://www.soscisurvey.de/ (accessed on 24 October 2012).

26. Lopez, Alan D. 2006. *Global Burden of Disease and Risk Factors.* New York: Oxford University Press, Washington: World Bank.

27. Luck, Amy J., John F. MorganLuck, Fiona Reid, Aileen O'Brien, Joan Brunton, Clare Price, Lin Perry, and J. Hubert Lacey. 2002. The SCOFF questionnaire and clinical interview for eating disorders in general practice: Comparative study. *BMJ* 325: 755–56. [CrossRef] [PubMed]

28. Ludwig Boltzmann Institut (LBI). 2006. *Kinder und Jugend Gesundheitsbericht Kärnten.* Klagenfurt: Amt der Kärntner Landesregierung.

29. Marsiglia, Flavio Francisco, Stephanie L. Ayers, and Steven Hoffman. 2011. Religiosity and Adolescent Substance Use in Central Mexico: Exploring the Influence of Internal and External Religiosity on Cigarette and Alcohol Use. *American Journal of Community Psychology* 49: 87–97. [CrossRef] [PubMed]

30. Morgan, John Farnill, Fiona D. A. Reid, and Hubert John Lacey. 1999. The SCOFF questionnaire: assessment of a new screening tool for eating disorders. *BMJ (Clinical Research ed.)* 319: 1467–68. [CrossRef]

31. Mur, Ingrid, and Mariken Leurs. 2006. Developing youth care: The challenge of integrated school health promotion. *International Journal of Integrated Care* 6: e26. [CrossRef] [PubMed]

32. Nagel, Erik, and Sandra Sgoutas-Emch. 2007. The relationship between spirituality, health beliefs, and health behaviors in college students. *Journal of Religion and Health* 46: 141–54. [CrossRef]

33. Nonnemaker, James M., Clea A. McNeely, and Robert Wm Blum. 2003. Public and private domains of religiosity and adolescent health risk behaviors: Evidence from the National Longitudinal Study of Adolescent Health. *Social Science & Medicine* 57: 2049–54.

34. Paul, Seana L., Leigh Blizzard, George C. Patton, Terry Dwyer, and Alison Venn. 2008. Parental smoking and smoking experimentation in childhood increase the risk of being a smoker 20 years later: The Childhood Determinants of Adult Health Study. *Addiction* 103: 846–53. [CrossRef] [PubMed]

35. Porche, Michelle V., Lisa R. Fortuna, Amy Wachholtz, and Rosalie Torres Stone. 2015. Distal and Proximal Religiosity as Protective Factors for Adolescent and Emerging Adult Alcohol Use. *Religions (Basel)* 6: 365–84. [CrossRef] [PubMed]

36. Ramelow, Daniela, Robert Griebler, Felix Hofmann, Katrin Unterweger, Ursula Mager, Rosemarie Felder-Puig, and Wolfgang Dür. 2011. *Gesundheit und Gesundheitsverhalten von Österreichischen Schülerinnen und Schülern: Ergebnisse des WHO-HBSC-Survey 2010.* Wien: Bundesministerium für Gesundheit (BMG).

37. Steinman, Kenneth J., Amy K. Ferketich, and Timothy Sahr. 2008. The dose-response relationship of adolescent religious activity and substance use: Variation across demographic groups. *Health Education & Behavior* 35: 22–43.

38. Stolz, Heidi E., Joseph A. Olsen, Teri M. Henke, and Brian K. Barber. 2013. Adolescent religiosity and psychosocial functioning: Investigating the roles of religious tradition, national-ethnic group, and gender. *Child Development Research.* [CrossRef]

39. Wallace, John M., and Tyrone A. Forman. 1998. Religion's role in promoting health and reducing risk among American youth. *Health Education & Behavior* 25: 721–41.

40. Wang, Li Yan, David Chyen, Sarah Lee, and Richard Lowry. 2008. The Association Between Body Mass Index in Adolescence and Obesity in Adulthood. *Journal of Adolescent Health* 42: 512–18. [CrossRef] [PubMed]

41. Whitehead, Margaret, and Göran Dahlgren. 1991. What can be done about inequalities in health? *The Lancet* 338: 1059–63. [CrossRef]

42. World Health Organization (WHO). 2012. Health Behaviour in School-aged Children Survey. Available online: http://www.hbsc.org/about/index.html (accessed on 23 March 2017).

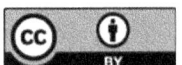

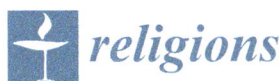

Article

Does the Spiritual Well-Being of Chronic Hemodialysis Patients Differ from that of Pre-Dialysis Chronic Kidney Disease Patients?

Areewan Cheawchanwattana [1,*], Darunee Chunlertrith [2], Warapond Saisunantararom [3] and Nutjaree Pratheepawanit Johns [4]

[1] Social and Administrative Pharmacy Department, Faculty of Pharmaceutical Sciences, Khon Kaen University, Khon Kaen, 40002, Thailand

[2] Renal Service Center, Srinagarind Hospital, Faculty of Medicine, Khon Kaen University, Khon Kaen 40002, Thailand; darchu@kku.ac.th

[3] Graduate School, Khon Kaen University, Khon Kaen 40002, Thailand; warapond@hotmail.com

[4] Clinical Pharmacy Department, Faculty of Pharmaceutical Sciences, Khon Kaen University, Khon Kaen 40002, Thailand; pnutja@kku.ac.th

* Author to whom correspondence should be addressed; areche@kku.ac.th; Tel. +66-4336-2090; Fax: +66-4336-2090.

Academic Editors: René Hefti, Stefan Rademacher and Arndt Büssing

Received: 30 October 2014; Accepted: 22 December 2014; Published: 29 December 2014

Abstract: Spiritual well-being is viewed as an essential component of health-related quality of life (HRQOL) in the modernized biopsychosocial-spiritual model of health. Understanding spiritual well-being should lead to better treatment plans from the patients' point of view, and improved patient adherence. There are numerous studies of traditional HRQOL, physical, mental, and social well-being; however, studies of spiritual well-being in chronic kidney disease (CKD) patients are limited. Thus, this study compared spiritual well-being of chronic hemodialysis patients and pre-dialysis CKD patients. A total of 31 chronic hemodialysis and 63 pre-dialysis CKD patients were asked for consent and then interviewed for spiritual well-being using the Functional Assessment of Chronic Illness Therapy–Spiritual Well-Being (FACIT-Sp). Analysis of covariance was applied to compare FACIT-Sp scores between pre-dialysis CKD and chronic hemodialysis groups that were adjusted by patient characteristics. The FACIT-Sp scores of pre-dialysis CKD patients were non-significantly greater than those of chronic hemodialysis patients after adjustment for gender, age, and marital status. However, all FACIT-Sp scores of males were significantly lower than those of females [FACIT Meaning -1.59 ($p = 0.024$), FACIT Peace -2.37 ($p = 0.004$), FACIT Faith -2.87 ($p = 0.001$), FACIT Total Score -6.83 ($p = 0.001$)]. The spiritual well-being did not significantly differ by stages of chronic kidney disease; however, patient gender was associated with spiritual well-being instead. To improve spiritual well-being, researchers should consider patient gender as a significant factor.

Keywords: spiritual well-being; quality of life (QOL); health-related quality of life (HRQOL); Functional Assessment of Chronic Illness Therapy – Spiritual Well-Being (FACIT-Sp); end-stage renal diseases (ESRD); chronic kidney disease (CKD); hemodialysis; pre-dialysis

---

1. Introduction

Since 1948, when the World Health Organization [1] defined *'health'* as *"a state of complete physical, mental, and social well-being and not merely the absence of disease infirmity"*, quality of life (QOL) and health related QOL (HRQOL), the more specific term, have been important issues in healthcare practice and research [2]. HRQOL is based on physical, mental, and social domains of health as perceived by the individual person [2]. There is evidence suggesting that spiritual and religious experiences also contribute to HRQOL, and are important for coping with illness [3]. The more traditional HRQOL domains, physical, mental, social well-being, have been expanded to cover spiritual well-being as another essential component, and this is the so called the biopsychosocial-spiritual model of health [4]. This model should help healthcare professionals concerning patients' spiritual well-being, especially those who are suffering from serious illnesses.

The definition of spirituality is still a debatable issue in that the term has no single and widely-agreed definitions [5,6]. Spirituality is considered to be a more wide-ranging and inclusive concept than religion, though their concept relationships are quite complex [6]. Based on an earlier literature review, the key components of spirituality were 'meaning', 'hope', 'relatedness/connectedness', and 'beliefs/beliefs systems' [5]. Büssing and Koenig also suggested the important of caring for spiritual, existential, and psychological needs of patients who are suffer from long-term chronic illnesses until the end of their lives [7]. They proposed the spiritual needs quantification model that included 'connection' (social dimension), 'peace' (emotional dimension), 'meaning/purpose' (existential dimension), and 'transcendence' (religious dimension) [7].

Chronic kidney disease (CKD) is defined as 'kidney damage or glomerular filtration rate (GFR) lower than 60 mL/min/1.73 m^2 for three months or longer. The worldwide prevalence of CKD is estimated to be within the range of 8–16% [8]. CKD patients experience life disturbances in many HRQOL areas including physical, sexual, social dysfunction, and mental problems such as depression, anxiety, pain, and sleep disturbance [9]. When patients reach a GFR of less than 15%, they are classified into the end-stage renal disease (ESRD) group. Most ESRD patients are treated with chronic dialysis leading to a dependency on healthcare professionals and dialysis machines. Moreover, they lose their normal lifestyle because of limitations of food, beverage intake, and normal activities [10–12]. HRQOL decline in CKD patients has long been recognized, and the deterioration is more pronounced with the progression of disease. Numerous studies have reported the better HRQOL of pre-dialysis CKD patients when compared with dialysis ESRD patients [13]. The associations of HRQOL and morbidity and mortality in dialysis patients are well-established, and this had led to the recommendation of routine HRQOL assessment in dialysis patients [9].

Research on the spirituality of CKD patients is however limited. Davison and Jhangri studied 253 CKD and dialysis patients and reported the prevalence of spiritual/existential needs in the range of 35–53%, with the highest need in 'finding hope' [14]. Their later study found that spirituality independently provided unique variances in HRQOL, and also associated with psychological adjustment to illness [15]. Spiritual care experiences of 10 nephrology nurses revealed that giving spiritual care led to a closer relationship between patients and nurse, nurses sensed the pain of patient spiritual distress, and giving spiritual care was much deeper than psychological [16]. A recent qualitative study of Thai CKD patients who lived in the United Stated showed that religion helped patients to cope with emotional stress [17]. Despite its importance, previous studies explored spirituality in western or Christian culture. This area has never been investigated in CKD patients in the Thai context.

A number of measures for spiritual well-being have been developed. The Functional Assessment of Chronic Illness Therapy-Spiritual Well-Being Scale (FACIT-Sp) is commonly used and has been validated in a large sample of patients with serious illnesses (N = 1,617) [18]. It covers domains specified as important for spiritual well-being in chronic patients [18]. The strength is not only its rigorous validity and reliability tests, but also its applicability to a wide range of spiritual and religious traditions [4]. Recent study on spiritual well-being for Thai-Buddhist has defined three components involving 'having hope and sense of connectedness', 'understanding self and nature of life', and 'being happy' [19]. The measure is being developed but is still in its infancy. The majority of Thai people are Buddhist, and their spiritual well-being has been influenced by Thai-Buddhist beliefs which involve Kamma, merit making and reincarnation. Especially in a Thai context, however, their way of life and beliefs have also been associated with supernatural power, ghosts and spirits of Brahmist influence [19]. Therefore, a measure of spiritual well-being with wider coverage should be more applicable to the Thai population.

Religions **2015**, *6*, 14–23

The objective of this present study was to compare the spiritual well-being of chronic hemodialysis patients and pre-dialysis CKD patients. As previous reports have suggested that disease progression leads to HRQOL deterioration, the study aim was to determine whether spiritual well-being would be different at different stages of disease progression. Such information should enhance the understanding of healthcare professionals and leading to a comprehensive and holistic care in this patient group.

2. Methods

This was a cross-sectional study using the structured questionnaire. The study sites were a community hospital and a medical school hospital in the northeast of Thailand. The protocol of study was approved by the Khon Kaen University Ethics Committee for Human Research.

Eligible patients were recruited between July 1, 2013 and December 31, 2013. Inclusion criteria for the pre-dialysis CKD were patients with GFR less than 15 mL/min/1.73 m^2 for three months or longer who visited the nephrology out-patient clinic at one of the study hospitals. Eligibility for chronic hemodialysis patients were ESRD patients who were on chronic hemodialysis for three months or longer and were being treated at one of the study hospitals. The trained interviewers and research assistants invited each patient to participate in the study and written informed consent was obtained prior to data collection. Patients were interviewed in a private area of the nephrology out-patient clinic for pre-dialysis patients, and during the first two hours of a dialysis session for chronic hemodialysis patients. An interview method was used as it is more acceptable for the local people, many of whom were elderly, often unfamiliar with the reading, or uncomfortable to read due to limited education or poor eyesight. The trained interviewers administered the questionnaire by carefully reading the question and answer choices without interpretation, and then recorded the response to each question. Interview sessions lasted approximately 30 minutes.

The questionnaire consisted of patient demographic variables and the FACIT-Sp. The FACIT-Sp consists of 12 items that are classified into three factors: Meaning, Peace, and Faith [4]. The response choices for every item is a 5-point Likert-type scale (0 = Not at all; 1 = A little bit; 2 = Somewhat; 3 = Quite a bit; and 4 = Very much). The recall period of each question was seven days. The three domain scores and total scores were transformed according to the developer's guideline [4]. Scores were transformed into separate three domains: Meaning (FACIT Meaning), Peace (FACIT Peace), and Faith (FACIT Faith), and total scores (FACIT Total Scores). Higher scores reflect better spiritual well-being. The FACIT-Sp is a reliable and valid measure. The Cronbach's alpha of the FACIT-Sp was in range of 0.81 to 0.88. The validity of FACIT-Sp was examined by using concurrent spirituality measures, and moderate to strong correlation was found [4]. The Thai version of FACIT-Sp was translated and validated by Dr. Supalak Khemthong (with permission from Jason Bredle). The report of validity and reliability of FACIT-Sp Thai version has not been published. However, preliminary results indicated good validity and reliability (Cronbach's alpha = 0.80) [20].

Descriptive statistics were appropriately applied according to measurement levels and data distributions. To compare categorical variables between pre-dialysis CKD and chronic hemodialysis groups, chi-square test was applied; however, if the assumption of chi-square was not met, the Fisher's exact test was applied instead. For continuous numerical data, the independent t-test was used to compare between the two groups, if data were highly skewed, the Mann-Whitney U-test was used instead. Additionally, analysis of covariances (ANCOVA) were applied to compare the scores between the two groups that were adjusted by patient characteristics. The significance levels were set at 0.05 (2-sided tests) for all analyses.

3. Results

3.1. Patients' Characteristics

A total of 31 chronic hemodialysis and 63 pre-dialysis CKD patients were studied. Table 1 shows that the two patient groups significantly differed in all demographic factors. Almost four out of five pre-dialysis CKD patients were female (79.4%), while more than half of chronic hemodialysis patients were male (54.8%), and the gender difference between groups was significant ($p = 0.001$). Pre-dialysis CKD patients were significantly older than chronic hemodialysis patients (64.0 *versus* 54.5 years, $p < 0.001$). Almost all of the chronic hemodialysis patients were married (87.1%), while just over half of pre-dialysis CKD patients were married (58.7%), and the marital status of two groups was significantly different ($p = 0.006$).

Table 1. Demographic data of pre-dialysis chronic kidney diseases (CKD) and chronic hemodialysis patients (N = 94).

	Pre-dialysis CKD (n = 63)		Chronic hemodialysis (n = 31)		*p*-value
	n	(%)	n	(%)	
Gender					
Female	50	(79.4%)	14	(45.2%)	0.001 *
Male	13	(20.6%)	17	(54.8%)	
Age (years) [Mean±SD]	64.0	±9.1	54.5	±10.2	<0.001 **
Marital status					
Single/ widow/ divorced	26	(41.3%)	4	(12.9%)	0.006 *
Married	37	(58.7%)	27	(87.1%)	

Notes: SD = standard deviation; * Chi-square test; ** Independent t-test.

3.2. Comparisons of FACIT-Sp Scores When Classified by Patient Demographic Characteristics

All FACIT-Sp scores (FACIT Meaning, FACIT Peace, FACIT Faith, and FACIT Total Scores) were highly skewed towards high spirituality scores, thus Mann-Whitney U-tests were used. Female patients had significantly better spiritual well-being than male when comparing all FACIT-Sp scores ($p < 0.001$). When classified into age-groups, patients above 60 years (elderly) and 60 years or lower, elderly patients had greater spiritual well-being scores than the younger patients in total scores and in two out of three domains (except FACIT Peace). Married patients had lower spiritual scores than other marital status, but scores were not significantly different (Table 2).

Table 2. Functional Assessment of Chronic Illness Therapy–Spiritual Well-Being (FACIT) domains and total scores by patient demographic characteristics.

	n	FACIT Meaning *		FACIT Peace *		FACIT Faith *		FACIT Total Scores **	
		Mean	±SD	Mean	±SD	Mean	±SD	Mean	±SD
Gender									
Male	30	11.17	±2.68	10.73	±3.89	10.50	±3.99	32.40	±9.38
Female	64	13.28	±3.11	13.75	±3.22	13.97	±3.26	41.0	±8.52
p-value ***		<0.001		<0.001		<0.001		<0.001	
Age groups									
Age < 60 years	40	12.03	±2.89	12.08	±3.87	11.83	±4.17	35.93	±9.78
Age > 60 years	54	13.04	±3.25	13.31	±3.53	13.63	±3.42	39.98	±9.25
p-value ***		0.042		0.070		0.033		0.020	
Marital status									
Married	64	12.30	±3.05	12.42	±3.72	12.58	±3.94	37.30	±9.71
Single/widow/divorced	30	13.27	±3.27	13.57	±3.63	13.47	±3.63	40.30	±9.31
p-value ***		0.102		0.081		0.255		0.103	

Notes: SD = standard deviation; *score range 0–16; ** score range 0–48; *** Mann-Whitney U test.

3.3. Comparisons of FACIT-Sp Scores When Classified by Patient Treatment Groups: Results Adjusted by Patient Demographic Characteristics

All unadjusted FACIT-Sp scores of pre-dialysis CKD patients were significantly greater than those of chronic hemodialysis patients (Table 3). The pre-dialysis CKD patient group consisted of significantly more females, unmarried status and older patients than the chronic hemodialysis patient group. ANCOVA adjusting for gender, age, and marital status, was used to compare the scores of the pre-dialysis CKD and chronic hemodialysis groups. Based on unadjusted scores, the adjusted scores were slightly lower for pre-dialysis CKD patients, but slightly higher for chronic hemodialysis patients. All adjusted FACIT-Sp scores of pre-dialysis CKD patients were still greater than those of chronic hemodialysis patients, but they were not significant ($p > 0.05$). Controlling for covariate factors, gender was the only significant factor that affected all FACIT-Sp scores. The demographic variables, age and marital status, were non-significant in ANCOVA of all FACIT-Sp scores, however analysis of results revealed a similar trend as previously analyzed by using Mann-Whitney U-test. In conclusion, spiritual well-being FACIT-Sp scores of pre-dialysis CKD patients were not significantly greater than those of chronic hemodialysis patients after being adjusted for gender, age, and marital status. Among study demographic variables, gender was the most influential factor for spiritual well-being in the study patients.

Table 3. Analysis of covariances of Functional Assessment of Chronic Illness Therapy – Spiritual Well-Being (FACIT) domain and total scores as the dependent variables by patient treatment groups and covariates.

Dependent Variables	FACIT Meaning *	FACIT Peace *	FACIT Faith *	FACIT Total Scores **
Main Factor and Covariates				
Main factor				
Unadjusted mean (95% CI)				
Pre-dialysis CKD	13.25 (12.51, 14.00)	13.67 (12.80, 14.53)	13.68 (12.78, 14.58)	40.60 (38.41, 42.80)
Chronic hemodialysis	11.29 (10.16, 12.42)	11.00 (9.65, 12.35)	11.19 (9.77, 12.62)	33.48 (29.90, 37.07)
Adjusted mean (95% CI)				
Pre-dialysis CKD	12.95 (12.12, 13.73)	13.32 (12.14, 14.23)	13.15 (12.23, 14.08)	39.42 (37.12, 41.73)
Chronic hemodialysis	11.92 (10.73, 13.10)	11.70 (10.33, 13.07)	12.27 (10.88, 13.66)	35.88 (32.40, 39.36)
Pre-dialysis CKD versus chronic hemodialysis score differences (95% CI)	1.03 (−0.50, 2.56)	1.63 (−0.14, 3.39)	0.89 (−0.90, 2.68)	3.55 (−0.93, 8.02)
p-value	0.183	0.070	0.327	0.119
Covariates: Parameter estimates (95%CI)				
Age (years)	0.03 (−0.04, 0.09)	0.01 (−0.06, 0.09)	0.06 (−0.02, 0.14)	0.10 (−0.09, 0.29)
p-value	0.397	0.774	0.119	0.304
Male versus female score differences (95% CI)	−1.59 (−2.98, −0.21)	−2.37 (−3.96, −0.77)	−2.87 (−4.49, −1.25)	−6.83 (−10.87, −2.78)
p-value	0.024	0.004	0.001	0.001
Married versus other marital status score differences (95% CI)	−0.45 (−1.80, 0.91)	−0.45 (−2.01, 1.11)	−0.19 (−1.77, 1.40)	−1.09 (−5.05, 2.87)
p-value	0.513	0.566	0.814	0.587

Notes: 95% CI = 95% Confident Interval; CKD=chronic kidney disease; * score range 0–16; ** score range 0–48.

4. Discussion

This study was conducted to test whether spiritual well-being of patients with different disease stages would differ as previously reported in HRQOL. Spiritual well-being is considered to be an important part of QOL, but it is distinct from traditional HRQOL, physical, mental, and social well-being [4]. Thus, spiritual well-being may or may not be influenced by disease stages in the same way as QOL. Though unadjusted comparison analyses of spiritual well-being scores between pre-dialysis CKD and chronic hemodialysis patients revealed significant differences, these results may be due to influencing factors of different patient characteristics. Since gender and age of patients were also associated with spiritual well-being, and these factors significantly differed across the two treatment groups, analyses should therefore account for these differences. With ANCOVA analysis, gender was the only significant factor that was associated with all spiritual well-being FACIT-Sp scores, instead of treatment groups. Thus the effect of gender on spiritual well-being was more pronounced than that of disease stages in ESRD patients.

The association of gender and spirituality was also reported in the study of Kao *et al.* in Taiwanese hemodialysis patients. They found that the proportion of male patients with strong spiritual beliefs (34.6%) was significant smaller than those of male patients with none (52.8%) or weak (47.5%) spiritual beliefs ($p = 0.005$) [21]. Additionally, the study of Reig-Ferrer *et al.* in Spanish hemodialysis patients reported in the association of religiosity and gender that female hemodialysis patients tended to be more spiritual and religious than male hemodialysis patients (percentages of very religious; female 36.4% *vs.* male 6.6%, $p < 0.001$) [22]. The phenomenon of more religiousness and spirituality in women was reconfirmed in this study. Non-significant effect of disease stages on spirituality were revealed by this study, while previous evidence reported lower HRQOL in hemodialysis patients than CKD patients [13]. An explanation of this phenomenon might be that HRQOL measures aspects of daily living such that physical, mental, and social well-being, while spiritual well-being measures aspects of inner peace and beliefs. Since this was a cross-sectional study, it did not take into account patients' adaptations to the chronic disease situation. As the effect of disease stage on daily living distress occurs and is long lasting, a patient might learn to cope with the disease and spirituality by a number of methods [23], which may result in response shift on the spiritual well-being scores, or else, the disease might not even change their spiritual well-being.

This study added to the evidence of gender difference in spiritual well-being after controlling for age, marital status, and different stages of chronic renal diseases. However, the limitations of this study were the small number of patients. There is an imbalance of gender distribution with more male in the chronic hemodialysis group, and more female in the pre-dialysis CKD group. Nevertheless, the gender difference was expected in our setting. The Renal Replacement Therapy Registry of Thailand Year 2011 reported 52.6% male in chronic hemodialysis patients [24] which is similar to 54.8% reported in this study. The gender distribution of pre-dialysis CKD patients also reflects population in the setting, and as women generally take better care of themselves, it is common to have more females in this early stage of disease. Nevertheless, the interpretation of the results should take into consideration the skewed gender distribution in pre-dialysis CKD patients. In addition, study variables were limited to only a few demographic characteristics, and thus other important variables such as laboratory measures, HRQOL, and social support should be considered in future research. It should be noted that Kao *et al.* found weak spiritual beliefs in less-educated hemodialysis patients [21].

Acknowledgments: The authors thank Supalak Khemthong for providing the FACIT-Sp Thai version to be applied in this study, and facilitating the permission of FACIT-Sp application. We also thank Jason Bredle for permission to use FACIT-Sp. We thank Jeff Johns for his hard work on English editing service. We thank Faculty of Pharmaceutical Sciences, Khon Kaen University for funding of this study. Finally, we thank the pre-dialysis CKD-V and chronic hemodialysis patients that made this study possible through their participation.

Author Contributions: AC is PI of the study, designed the study and developed the proposal for approval by the ethic committee, analyzed the data using statistical methods, and drafted the manuscript. DC and WS interviewed patients, and helped draft the manuscript. NPJ contributed on revising the final draft manuscript. The final manuscript was approved by all authors.

Abbreviations

QOL	quality of life
HRQOL	health-related quality of life
FACIT-Sp	Functional Assessment of Chronic Illness Therapy – Spiritual Well-Being
GFR	glomerular filtration rate
ESRD	end-stage renal disease
CKD	chronic kidney disease
ANCOVA	analysis of covariance

Conflicts of Interest: The authors declare no conflict of interest.

References

1. World Health Organization. "WHO definition of Health." Available online: http://www.who.int/about/definition/en/print.html (accessed on 23 October 2014).
2. Marcia A. Testa, and Donald C. Simonson. "Assessment of quality-of-life outcomes." *NEJM* 334 (1996): 835–40.
3. WHOQOL SRPB Group. "A cross-cultural study of spirituality, religion, and personal beliefs as components of quality of life." *Social Science & Medicine* 62 (2006): 1486–97.
4. Jason M. Bredle, John M. Salsman, Scott M. Debb, Benjamin J. Arnold, and David Cella. "Spiritual well-being as a component of health-related quality of life: the Functional Assessment of Chronic Illness Therapy-Spiritual Well-Being Scale (FACIT-Sp)." *Religions* 2 (2011): 77–94.
5. Jane Dyson, Mark Cobb, and Dawn Forman. "The meaning of spirituality: A literature review." *Journal of Advanced Nursing* 26 (1997): 1183–88.
6. Mélanie Vachon, Lise Fillion, and Marie Achille. "A conceptual analysis of spirituality at the end of life." *Journal of Palliative Medicine* 12 (2009): 53–59.
7. Arndt Büssing, and Harold G. Koenig. "Spiritual needs of patients with chronic diseases." *Religions* 1 (2010): 18–27.
8. Vivekanand Jha, Guillermo Garcia-Garcia, Kunitoshi Iseki, Zuo Li, Saraladevi Naicker, Brett Plattner, Rajiv Saran, Angela Yee-Moon Wang, and Chih-Wei Yang. "Chronic kidney disease: Global dimension and perspectives." *Lancet* 382 (2013): 260–72.
9. Fredric O. Finkelstein, Diane Wuerth, and Susan H. Finkelstein. "Health related quality of life and the CKD patient: Challenges for the nephrology community." *Kidney International* 76 (2009): 946–52.
10. Natale Gaspare De Santo, Alessandra Perna, Aziz El Matri, Rosa Maria De Santo, and Massimo Cirillo. "Survival is not enough." *Journal of Renal Nutrition* 22 (2012): 211–19.
11. Kai-Uwe Eckardt, Josef Coresh, Olivier Devuyst, Richard J. Johnson, Anna Köttgen, Andrew S. Levey, and Adeera Levin. "Evolving importance of kidney disease: From subspecialty to global health burden." *Lancet* 382 (2013): 158–69.
12. Anjay Rastogia, and Allen R. Nissenson. "The future of renal replacement therapy." *Advances in Chronic Kidney Disease* 14 (2007): 249–55.
13. Marina Avramovic, and Vladisav Stefanovic. "Health-related quality of life in different stages of renal failure." *Artificial Organs* 36 (2012): 581–89.
14. Sara N. Davison, and Gian S. Jhangri. "Existential and supportive care needs among patients with chronic kidney disease." *Journal of Pain and Symptom Management* 40 (2010): 838–43.
15. Sara N. Davison, and Gian S. Jhangri. "The relationship between spirituality, psychological adjustment to illness, and health-related quality of life in patients with advanced chronic kidney disease." *Journal of Pain and Symptom Management* 45 (2013): 170–78.
16. Belinda Deal, and Jane S. Grassley. "The lived experience of giving spiritual care: A phenomenological study of nephrology nurses working in acute and chronic hemodialysis settings." *Nephrology Nursing Journal* 39 (2012): 471–96.
17. Chutikarn Chatrung, Siroj Sorajjakool, and Kwanjai Amnatsatsue. "Wellness and religious coping among Thai individuals living with chronic kidney disease in Southern California." *Journal of Religion and Health*. 10 October 2014. Available online: http://link.springer.com/article/10.1007%2Fs10943-014-9958-4 (accessed on 29 October 2014). [CrossRef]

18. Stéfanie Monod, Mark Brennan, Etienne Rochat, Estelle Martin, Stéphane Rochat, and Christophe J. Büla. "Instruments measuring spirituality in clinical research: A systematic review." *Journal of General Internal Medicine* 26 (2011): 1345–57.

19. Saengduean Promkaewngam, Linchong Pothiban, Wichit Srisuphan, and Khanokporn Sucamvang. "Development of the spiritual well-being scale for Thai Buddhist adults with chronic illness." *Pacific Rim International Journal of Nursing Research* 18 (2014): 320–32.

20. Supalak Khemthong. Personal communication with the authors. 14 November 2014.

21. Tze-Wah Kao, Pau-Chung Chen, Chia-Jung Hsieh, Hong-Wei Chiang, Lap-Yuen Tsang, Ing-Fang Yang, Tun-Jun Tsai, and Wan-Yu Chen. "Correlation between spiritual beliefs and health-related quality of life of chronic hemodialysis patients in Taiwan." *Artificial Organs* 33 (2009): 576–79.

22. Abilio Reig-Ferrer, M. Dolores Arenas, Rosario Ferrer-Cascales, Dolores Fernández-Pascual, Natalia Albaladejo-Blázquez, M. Teresa Gil, and Vanesa de la Fuente. "Evaluation of spiritual well-being in haemodialysis patients." *Nefrología* 32 (2012): 731–42.

23. Jeremy P. Cummingsa, and Kenneth I. Pargament. "Medicine for the spirit: Religious coping in individuals with medical conditions." *Religions* 2 (2010): 28–53.

24. The Nephrology Society of Thailand. "Thailand Renal Replacement Therapy Year 2011." Available online: http://www.nephrothai.org/nephrothai_boffice/images_upload/news/391/files/trt2011.pdf (accessed on 30 November 2014).

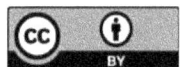

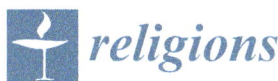

Article

Associations among Spirituality, Health-Related Quality of Life, and Depression in Pre-Dialysis Chronic Kidney Disease Patients: An Exploratory Analysis in Thai Buddhist Patients

Waraporn Saisunantararom [1], Areewan Cheawchanwattana [2,*], Talerngsak Kanjanabuch [3], Maliwan Buranapatana [4] and Kornkaew Chanthapasa [2]

[1]   Graduate School, Khon Kaen University, Khon Kaen 40002, Thailand; warapond@hotmail.com
[2]   Social and Administrative Pharmacy Department, Faculty of Pharmaceutical Sciences,
      Khon Kaen University, Khon Kaen 40002, Thailand; dedar13@yahoo.com
[3]   Division of Nephrology, Department of Internal Medicine and Kidney & Metabolic Disorders Research Unit,
      Faculty of Medicine, Chulalongkorn University, Bangkok 10330, Thailand; golfnephro@hotmail.com
[4]   Thai Language Department, Faculty of Humanities and Social Sciences, Khon Kaen University,
      Khon Kaen 40002, Thailand; toysuda@hotmail.com
*   Author to whom correspondence should be addressed; areche@kku.ac.th; Tel./Fax: +6-643-362-090.

Academic Editor: Arndt Büssing
Received: 2 August 2015; Accepted: 19 October 2015; Published: 22 October 2015

Abstract: There are numerous studies of quality of life (QOL) in chronic kidney disease (CKD) patients; however, there are a few studies of spirituality and its association with QOL. Previous studies were done focusing on Western cultures; thus, the study of CKD patients in Eastern cultures would reveal interesting insights. This study was conducted to explore the spirituality, QOL, and depression of Thai CKD patients, and the associations between spirituality, QOL, and depression. This cross-sectional descriptive study using structured questionnaires was approved by the Khon Kaen University Ethics Committee in Human Research, Thailand. A total of 63 pre-dialysis CKD stage V patients who visited the kidney diseases clinic as appointed at the outpatient department in a community hospital in northeastern Thailand were recruited. The patients were asked for consent and then interviewed. Spirituality was assessed by using the WHOQOL Spirituality, Religiousness and Personal Beliefs (WHOQOL-SRPB) and the Functional Assessment of Chronic Illness Therapy-Spiritual Well-Being Scale (FACIT-Sp). The 9-item Thai Health Status Assessment Instrument (9-THAI) was used to assess QOL. The Beck Depression Inventory-II (BDI-II) was used to evaluate the depression. The study patients had high WHOQOL-SRPB and FACIT-Sp spirituality scores (median = 18.0, and 44.0, respectively). The 9-THAI QOL scores were within the normal range of the Thai general, healthy population (physical health score [PHS]; median = 48.0, mental health score [MHS]; median = 32.0). Based on BDI-II scores, most patients were in the minimal depression group (63.5%). The Spearman rho correlation coefficients (rs) of PHS and WHOQOL-SRPB and FACIT-Sp were moderate with 0.34 for both spirituality measures. Similarly, also the mental health scores (MHS) correlated moderately with WHOQOL-SRPB (rs = 0.46) and FACIT-Sp (rs = 0.37). Depressive symptoms (BDI-II) strongly negatively correlated with WHOQOL-SRPB (rs = −0.58) and FACIT-Sp (rs = −0.55). Overall results were consistent with previous studies in Western contexts. Understanding spirituality would lead to the better management of depression and improving patient survival. These significant associations suggest that further research is needed on how provider knowledge of patient spirituality could affect the outcomes for patients both in terms of depression and patient survival.

Keywords: spirituality; quality of life; depression; chronic kidney disease

1. Introduction

Chronic kidney disease (CKD) is a significant chronic disease as it leads to patient morbidity and mortality [1]. Based on the third National Health Examination Survey (NHES III), a national representative survey of the Thai population, the prevalence of age-adjusted CKD stage III-V in the year 2004 was 8.9%, and the prevalence of CKD stage V was 0.2% [2]. The report also showed the highest prevalence of CKD in the northeastern region of Thailand (10.8%). Thus, CKD is a chronic disease of concern for hospitals in the northeastern region of Thailand.

Advanced medical technologies prolong patient lives, thus healthcare outcomes have become broader than patient survival. According to the definition of *"health"*, as physical, mental, and social well-being, stated by the World Health Organization (WHO) [3], quality of life (QOL) has become an important outcome of healthcare services. The specific term, health-related quality of life (HRQOL), has been recommended as a frame of reference for QOL in healthcare research [4,5]. Based on recommendations resulting from a focus group of lay people of 18 participating countries, including Thailand, a spirituality domain was included as a part of the QOL measure developed by WHO (WHOQOL) [6]. Both QOL and spirituality are ill-defined terms, thus consensus on their definitions still has not been reached [5,7,8]. The definition of spirituality is also a debatable issue [9,10], and both QOL and spirituality definitions vary according to the frameworks defined by the measures' developers [4,9,10]. Numerous QOL questionnaires have been developed to measure QOL [11], and considerable numbers of spirituality measures have been developed [12]. However, experts seemingly agree that HRQOL should be composed of physical, mental, and social well-being components [4,5], while spirituality should address meaning, purpose, and hope [13].

The burdens imposed by the multiple symptoms of CKD from disease and treatment experienced by patients are well recognized [14]. Patient function limitations and QOL declination with disease progression are also well known [15,16]. Apart from QOL deterioration, depression is common in CKD as well, since a recent meta-analysis study reported the prevalence of depression in CKD ranged from 21.4%–39.3% varying by stages of disease and assessment methods [17]. Both QOL and depression significantly predicted morbidity and mortality in CKD patients [18–23]. There are numerous studies of QOL in CKD patients; however, spirituality studies in this patient group are limited [24,25]. Studies on the relationship of QOL, depression and spirituality in CKD patients [25–27] reported a positive relationship between QOL and spirituality/religiosity, while the relationship between depression and spirituality/religiosity was negative. Spirituality and beliefs are important elements for helping patients cope with their illness [28,29], thus understanding spirituality and its relationship with QOL and depression might lead to better care in this patient group.

There has been some research on QOL measures in Thai CKD patients [30–34], and most of the measures were developed in Western countries except for a measure called the 9-item Thai Health status Assessment Instrument (9-THAI) [33,34]. The 9-THAI was developed to be a culturally specific health status (or so-called HRQOL) measure for the Thai population. It was thoroughly psychometrically examined, and results showed that it is a valid, reliable and responsive measure in both the Thai general population and end stage renal disease patients [33,34]. Since the validity property of measures should clearly link with score interpretation as suggested by theory [35], the norm-based scoring system of the 9-THAI is considered to be a major advantage [34]. The norm-based scores of 9-THAI are the standardized T scores that are calculated by using the averages and standard deviations (SDs) of the general healthy Thai population data of the National Health and Welfare Survey Year 2003, and thus the scores provide meaningful interpretation by comparison with the general healthy Thai population. Apart from QOL research, there is limited amount of research that is concerned with depression or spirituality in Thai renal disease patients. One study reported a 6.7% prevalence of depression in Thai dialysis patients [36], and a qualitative research reported that spiritual experience was valuable in Thai CKD patients [37]. In addition, the authors recently reported that spiritual well-being, as measured by FACIT-Sp, of pre-dialysis CKD and chronic hemodialysis patients was not significantly different between the two groups [38].

The association of QOL, spirituality, and depression has been previously studied in Western culture [25–27]. The concept of spirituality varied according to different societies, cultures, beliefs, philosophies of living, and particular religions [39]. Most Thai people are Buddhists, and the way of life and spirituality has been influenced by Buddhist doctrine and Buddha's teachings. Spirituality in a Thai context has also been influenced by Brahmanism and other supernatural beliefs such as ghosts, spirits, magical amulets, and magical incantations, *etc.* Since the study of QOL, spirituality, and depression associations in Thai CKD patients is still limited, this study was conducted to examine the associations.

2. Methods

2.1. Materials and Methods

The present study was a cross-sectional descriptive study using structured questionnaires. The protocol of study was approved by the Khon Kaen University Ethics Committee for Human Research, Thailand. Eligible patients were recruited between 1 July 2013 and 30 September 2013. Inclusion criteria for pre-dialysis CKD were patients with a glomerular filtration rate less than 15 mL/min/1.73 m^2 for three months or longer who visited the kidney diseases clinic, outpatient department, in a community hospital located in northeastern Thailand. A trained interviewer invited all eligible patients to participate in the study, and written informed consents were obtained prior to data collection. Patients were excluded if they were unable to communicate such as unconsciousness, confusion, speaking or hearing loss. Patients who refused to participate in the study were also excluded. Since people in northeastern Thailand are classified in the low socioeconomic group, most CKD patients in this hospital had the limitation of literacy, and the interview mode of questionnaire administration was considered to be the most appropriate method. Each patient was interviewed in a private area of the kidney diseases clinic during a regular visit to the clinic as appointed during the study time frame. To prevent bias from interviews, the trained interviewer only read questions and response choices without interpretation. The interviewer then carefully recorded the answer according to patients' responses to each question. Interview sessions lasted approximately one hour.

2.2. Measurement

The questionnaires used in this study were the World Health Organization Quality of Life-Spirituality, Religiousness and Personal Beliefs (WHOQOL-SRPB) [40], the Functional Assessment of Chronic Illness Therapy-Spiritual Well-Being Scale (FACIT-Sp) [41], the Beck Depression Inventory-II (BDI-II) [42], and the 9-THAI [34]. The spirituality was measured by using the WHOQOL-SRPB and the FACIT-Sp. The validation study of WHQOL-SRPB was based on the largest and most diverse population [12], and Thailand was one of the 18 study countries [40]. The FACIT-Sp was validated in the largest patient sample [12]. The HRQOL was measured by the 9-THAI as previously explained, with meaningful score interpretation based on the norm-based scoring system [34]. The depression was measured by BDI-II, since BDI-II is commonly applied in research on CKD patients [24]. The Thai versions of these four questionnaires were available.

The WHOQOL-SRPB is composed of 32 questions that are divided into eight facets: spiritual connection, meaning and purpose in life, experiences of awe and wonder, wholeness and integration, spiritual strength, inner peace, hope and optimism and faith. Scores were coded and calculated as indicated in the manual [43]. Scores range from 0–20 with higher scores indicating greater spiritual well-being. The authors have previously reported the psychometric properties of WHOQOL-SRPB Thai version based on these study CKD patients [44]. The WHOQOL-SRPB Thai version was valid and reliable. The convergent validity was assessed by using FACIT-Sp and Spearman Rho correlation of total scores of WHOQOL-SRPB and FACIT-Sp was 0.73. A high value of Cronbach's alpha (0.94; 95% CI 0.91–0.96) of the overall WHOQOL-SRPB 32 items indicated a high reliability.

The FACIT-Sp (Version 4) Thai Version consists of 12 items that are divided into three subscales: meaning, peace, and faith. Scores were coded and calculated according to the manual [42] with higher scores indicating higher spiritual well-being. The FACIT-Sp total scores range from 0–48, and the three subscales scores range from 0–16. The FACIT-Sp is a reliable and valid measure. The Cronbach's alpha of the FACIT-Sp was in range of 0.81–0.88. The validity of FACIT-Sp was examined by using concurrent spirituality measures, and moderate to strong correlation was found [41]. The Thai version of FACIT-Sp was translated and validated by Dr. Supalak Khemthong (with permission from Jason Bredle). The preliminary results indicated good validity and reliability (Cronbach's alpha = 0.80) [45].

The 9-THAI [33,34] was used to evaluate QOL. The 9-THAI is composed of seven domains and two global health ratings. The seven domains enable subjects to rate their experience with health problems during the last month, It includes four domains (mobility, self-care, usual activities, illness/discomfort) that measure physical constructs, and three domains (anxiety/depressed, cognition, social functions) that measure mental constructs. The scores of all items are coded such that higher scores reflect better health status. The 9-THAI was transformed into two scale scores, physical and mental health scores (PHS, MHS). The PHS and MHS are the standardized T scores that are based on the averages and SDs of gender (male, female) and age-groups (15–19, 20–29, 30–39, 40–49, 50–59, $\geq$60 years) of the Thai general healthy population. Based on the National Health and Welfare Survey Year 2003 of Thailand, data of Thai general healthy population (defined as self-reported with no any chronic diseases, no history of illness during the past month, and no history of hospitalization during the past year) were used to calculate the averages and SDs. To comprehensibly interpret the scores based on the normal distribution, the score range of 20 to 80 ($\pm$3SDs) indicate the possible distribution of Thai general healthy population scores. If 9-THAI PHS or MHS of patients are above 20, they are justified to be equal to the Thai general healthy population. The 9-THAI is a valid and reliable QOL measure in Thai renal replacement therapy patients. In brief, the validity was shown in terms of convergent and divergent validity using SF-36 as a concurrent measure, and the concurrent validity was also assessed by using clinical variables as concurrent measures. The test-retest reliability of 9-THAI was satisfactory as the intraclass correlation coefficients were 0.78 (mental) and 0.79 (physical).

The Beck Depression Inventory-II (BDI-II) Thai Version was used to evaluate the severity of depression. The BDI-II contains of 21 questions, and scores were coded and calculated as indicated in the manual [42]. Scores range from 0–63 and higher total scores indicate more severe depression. Scores were also used to classify patients into groups as follows: 0–13 = minimal, 14–19 = mild, 20–28 = moderate, 29–63 = severe depression.

2.3. Statistics

Descriptive statistics were used to analyze the demographic variables. Due to skewed distributions of scores, Spearman Rho correlation was applied for assessing correlation of spirituality, QOL, and depression. Analyses were done using IBM SPSS v 19.0, and the significance level was set at 0.05.

3. Results

The 63 study patients were all eligible CKD stage V patients who registered in the hospital's CKD clinic during the study period. Since the study hospital is a small 30-bed hospital that is responsible for healthcare services of 20,394 people in the area, these 63 patients constituted all CKD stage V patients in the area, indicating a 0.3% prevalence of CKD stage V, a little greater than the 0.2% prevalence given in the national report [2]. The patients were invited to participate in the study, and all of them gave informed consent and agreed to participate. The patients' socio-demographic characteristics are presented in Table 1. Most of the patients were female (79.4%) with the average age of 64 years. All patients were Buddhist (100%). Most of them (90.5%) had a limited literacy with the highest education level of primary school (Grade 6). More than half of them were married (58.7%) and unemployed

(58.7%). The most common co-morbidities of study patients were diabetes mellitus (77.8%) and hypertension (63.5%), respectively.

Table 1. Socio-demographic characteristics of the study patients (*N* = 63).

Variables	*n*	%
Gender		
Female	50	79.4
Male	13	20.6
Age (years) mean±SD	64	±9.1
min-max	31	79
Religion		
Buddhist	63	100
Educational level		
Uneducated	2	3.2
Primary school	57	90.5
Secondary school or higher level	4	6.3
Marital status		
Married	37	58.7
Widowed	22	34.9
Single	4	6.4
Occupation		
Unemployed or retired	37	58.7
Agriculture	16	25.4
House-work	9	14.3
Own business	1	1.6
Co-morbidity		
Diabetes mellitus	49	77.8
Hypertension	40	63.5
Dyslipidemia	25	39.7
Kidney stones	10	15.9
Gout	5	7.9
Heart diseases	3	4.8
Other diseases	9	14.3

In terms of QOL, depression and spirituality, most of study patients had good QOL, low depression and high spirituality. The median of the WHOQOL-SRPB total scores was 18.0 (interquartile range; IQR = 2.9, range 8.63–20.0), and the median of FACIT-Sp total scores was 44.0 (IQR = 10.0, range 11.0–48.0). The spirituality scores of both measures indicated the high spirituality of these patients. On average, the WHOQOL-SRPB scores of the study patients were greater than those of hemodialysis patients in Brazil [46], and schizophrenia patients in India [47]. Based on the FACIT-Sp scores, the spirituality of the study patients was higher than those of hospitalized elderly patients in Switzerland [48], aortic stenosis patients in USA [49], psychiatric inpatients in Brazil [50], and cancer patients in Iran [51]. On average, 9-THAI PHS and MHS of these patients were within the range of the Thai general healthy population (PHS: median = 48.0, IQR = 20.5, range −18.3–59.1, MHS: median = 32.0, IQR = 38.8, range −13.3–58.5). In terms of depression status as measured by BDI-II, the percentages of patients with minimal, mild, moderate, severe depression were 63.5%, 19%, 14.3%, and 3.2%, respectively.

Table 2 shows the Spearman rho correlation coefficients (*rs*) of spirituality, QOL, and depression. Spirituality as measured by WHOQOL-SRPB and FACIT-Sp showed greater associated with mental health and depression than physical health. The *rs* of BDI-II depression scores and spirituality were −0.55 (FACIT-Sp) and −0.58 (WHOQOL-SRPB), this showed significant moderate negative associations between depression and spirituality. The associations conformed to the associations of spirituality and mental health as measured by 9-THAI MHS, since the correlations were 0.37 (FACIT-Sp) and 0.46 (WHOQOL-SRPB). However, the associations of physical health as measured by 9-THAI PHS and spirituality showed a lesser degree of relationship with spirituality in that both correlation coefficients were 0.34.

The associations of mental health and spirituality domains of WHOQOL-SRPB and FACIT-Sp were further examined. A noteworthy association between depression and peaceful spirituality was revealed. The *rs* of the "Peace" domain of FACIT-Sp with BDI-II scores was −0.62, and this was the highest negative correlation among the three domains of FACIT-Sp and BDI-II scores. Additionally, the *rs* of the "Peace" domain of FACIT-Sp and 9-THAI MHS was also the highest (0.42) among the three domains of FACIT-Sp and 9-THAI MHS. In terms of WHOQOL-SRPB "Inner Peace" domain, the *rs* with 9-THAI MHS (0.44), and BDI-II scores (−0.59) were also high. The correlations between questions of the questionnaires were then further analyzed (details not shown). The highest negative correlation (*rs* = −0.43) was found between question no. 5 of 9-THAI ("*During the past 1 month, have you felt depressed, blue, or anxious, or not? If so, to what level?*") and question no. 4 of the "Peace" domain of FACIT-Sp ("*I have trouble feeling peace of mind*"). The *rs* were also high between question no. 5 of 9-THAI and another two questions of the "Peace" domain of FACIT-Sp ("*I am able to reach down deep into myself for comfort*": 0.40, and "*I feel peaceful*": 0.37). The further examination of the correlations between questions no. 5 of 9-THAI and the questions of WHOQOL-SRPB revealed the three highest *rs* with three questions of the "Inner Peace" domain ("*To what extent do you feel peaceful within yourself?*": 0.49, "*How much are you able to feel peaceful when you need to?*": 0.43, and "*To what extent do you have inner peace?*": 0.42). These results indicated the considerable association between depression and peace. It may be difficult for patients to have a peaceful state of mind, when they feel anxious or depressed.

Table 2. Spearman rho correlation coefficients of spirituality, quality of life, and depression of the study patients (*N* = 63).

Spirituality	Quality of Life: 9-THAI[1]		Depression: BDI-II[2]
	Physical health [PHS]	**Mental health [MHS]**	
WHOQOL-SRPB[3]			
Spiritual Connection	0.27	0.39	−0.52
Meaning and Purpose In Life	0.19 *	0.20 *	−0.30
Experiences of Awe and Wonder	0.25 *	0.24 *	−0.36
Wholeness and Integration	0.42	0.48	−0.59
Spiritual Strength	0.23 *	0.35	−0.50
Inner Peace	0.30	0.44	−0.59
Hope and Optimism	0.28	0.42	−0.42
Faith	0.25	0.42	−0.47
Total score	0.34	0.46	−0.58
FACIT-Sp[4]			
Meaning	0.42	0.39	−0.54
Peace	0.36	0.42	−0.62
Faith	0.12 *	0.18 *	−0.31
Total score	0.34	0.37	−0.55

Notes: All values in the Table are Spearman rho correlations. Values were significant (*p* < 0.05) except for * *p* ≥ 0.05; (1) 9-item Thai Health status Assessment Instrument; (2) Beck Depression Inventory II; (3) World Health Organization Quality of Life-Spirituality, Religiousness and Personal Beliefs; (4) Functional Assessment of Chronic Illness Therapy-Spiritual Well-Being Scale.

The *rs* of the "Meaning" domain of FACIT-Sp with QOL and depression were also considerable (PHS: 0.42, MHS: 0.39, and BDI-II: −0.54). Details of correlations between questions of the questionnaires were further analyzed. The highest *rs* (0.44) was found between that of question no.1 of 9-THAI PHS ("*During the past 1 month, have you had difficulty with the mobility of your hand, limb, torso or the whole body or not? If so, to what level?*") and question no. 2 of FACIT-Sp ("*I have a reason for living*"). Problems with physical mobility might lead to desperation and questioning of the reasons for living. Moreover, the association between the anxiety/depression question and the meaning/purpose question was considerable. The *rs* of question no. 5 of 9-THAI and question no. 8 of FACIT-Sp ("*My *life lacks meaning and purpose"*) was 0.44. In addition, the *rs* of question no. 8 of FACIT-Sp and BDI-II scores was −0.49. When patients feel depressed, they may be desperate and think that their lives have no meaning. The associations of "Meaning and Purpose In Life" domain of WHOQOL-SRPB with QOL and depression (PHS: 0.19, MHS: 0.20, and BDI-II: −0.30) were less than those of the "Meaning" domain of FACIT-Sp with QOL and depression. The weaker relationships resulted from the very low correlations of the "Purpose In Life" item with QOL/depression, since the *rs* of the question *"To what extent do you feel your life has a purpose?"* (WHOQOL-SRPB) and 9-THAI PHS, MHS, BDI-II were 0.03, −0.03, and −0.05, respectively. The belief of lack of control of one's life, the inheritance of the last life into the present life, and the expectation of many future lives make the question of "the purpose of life" less relevant for Buddhists. Western culture focuses on maximizing one's achievements in a single present life, particularly for Christians, so "purpose of life" has great importance. The ultimate reality paradigm of Buddhism leads to realistic hope and living goals [39], and thus the purpose of life is less relevant for Thai Buddhists.

The relationship of the 'Wholeness and Integration' domain of WHOQOL-SRPB and QOL (PHS: 0.42, MHS: 0.48, and BDI-II: −0.59) was further examined. The relationship of the question *"To what extent do you feel the way you live is consistent with what you feel and think?"* of WHOQOL-SRPB and all four questions of 9-THAI PHS were noteworthy (9-THAI questions no. 1–4; *rs* = 0.41, 0.43, 0.48, 0.32, respectively). The four questions assessed the problems of mobility, self-care, usual works, and illness/discomfort; thus, these problems might lead to patients having undesirable lives. In terms of mental health and depression, the two questions of the "Wholeness and Integration" domain of WHOQOL-SRPB, *"How satisfied are you that you have a balance between mind, body and soul?"* and *"To what extent do you feel any connection between your mind, body and soul?"*, significantly associated with anxiety and depression question of 9-THAI (question no. 5) (*rs* = 0.37, 0.33, respectively) and BDI-II scores (*rs* = −0.50, −0.44, respectively). The depression condition may lead to imbalance of mind, body, and soul.

4. Discussion

This is the first quantitative study of spirituality in Thai CKD patients, where all study patients are Buddhists. Most spiritual studies in CKD patients were conducted in Western cultures, and patients were mainly Christian. The spirituality and beliefs of Thai people are influenced by the Dhamma of the Buddha and other supernatural beliefs. This study was conducted to firstly explore spirituality and its associations with QOL/depression, and to answer whether the associations would be similar to those previously observed in Western countries. The results of this study revealed consistent evidence as shown in previous studies [26,27]. The results were as expected that spirituality was positively associated with QOL, and negatively associated with depression. Moreover, the associations of QOL and spirituality were explored in detail, and a greater association between spirituality and mental health was found when comparing with the association between spirituality and physical elements. The greater association between mental and spiritual elements was consistent with previous studies [40]. Depression was closely related with lack of peacefulness and meaning of life, and imbalance of mind, body, and soul. This information is potentially useful for healthcare professionals since understanding spirituality might lead to better management of depression in CKD patients if future research can demonstrate that provider knowledge of patient spirituality leads to better outcomes. However, the results should be cautiously applied, since study patients were limited to only CKD patients in one healthcare center. Still, this study opens the door to further research on Thai dialysis patients, associations between spirituality and survival, spirituality intervention, *etc.*

5. Conclusions

In summary, spirituality was found to be positively associated with QOL, and negatively associated with depression. Spirituality was more associated with mental health than physical health and depression played an important role in the association. Healthcare professionals should be concerned with the spirituality of CKD patients, since understanding spirituality might lead to less depression and prolonging of patient lives.

Acknowledgments: The authors wish to thank the competent staff of the United Nations in Thailand, the FACIT organization, Jason Bredle, Supalak Khemthong, Artchara Mungpanich, Nutjaree Pratheepawanit Johns, Supattra Porasuphatana, and all participating pre-dialysis CKD patients. We thank Jeff Johns for providing English editing services.

Author Contributions: Waraporn Saisunantararom and Areewan Cheawchanwattana are principal investigators of the study. We designed the study and developed the proposal for approval by the ethics committee, analyzed the data using statistical methods, and drafted the manuscript. Waraporn Saisunantararom interviewed patients. Talerngsak Kanjanabuch and Maliwan Buranapatana contributed in the processes of proposal finalization and WHOQOL-SRPB translation. Kornkaew Chanthapasa contributed to the draft manuscript. The final manuscript was approved by all authors.

Conflicts of Interest: The authors declare no conflicts of interest.

Abbreviations

QOL	quality of life
CKD	chronic kidney disease
FACIT-Sp	Functional Assessment of Chronic Illness Therapy—Spiritual Well-Being
WHOQOL-SRPB	WHOQOL Spirituality, Religiousness and Personal Beliefs
BDI-II	Beck Depression Inventory-II
9-THAI	9-item Thai Health status Assessment Instrument
rs	Spearman rho correlation coefficient

References

1. Marcello Tonelli, Natasha Wiebe, Bruce Culleton, Andrew House, Chris Rabbat, Mei Fok, Finlay McAlister, and Amit X. Garg. "Chronic kidney disease and mortality risk: A systematic review." *Journal of the American Society of Nephrology* 17 (2006): 2034–47. [CrossRef] [PubMed]
2. Leena Ong-ajyooth, Kriengsak Vareesangthip, Panrasri Khonputsa, and Wichai Aekplakorn. "Prevalence of chronic kidney disease in Thai adults: a national health survey." *BMC Nephrology* 10 (2009): 35. [PubMed]
3. World Health Organization. "WHO definition of Health." Available online: http://www.who.int/about/definition/en/print.html (accessed on 30 June 2015).
4. Marcia A. Testa, and Donald C. Simonson. "Assessment of quality-of-life outcomes." *New England Journal of Medicine* 334 (1996): 835–40. [PubMed]
5. Sharon Wood-Dauphinee. "Assessing quality of life in clinical research: From where have we come and where are we going? " *Journal of Clinical Epidemiology* 52 (1999): 355–63. [CrossRef]
6. Marcelo P. Fleck, and Suzanne Skevington. "Explaining r the meaning of the WHOQOL-SRPB." *Revista de Psiquiatria Clínica* 34 (2007): 67–69.
7. Peter M. Fayers, and David Machin. *Quality of life: Assessment, Analysis, and Interpretation.* West Sussex: John Wiley & Sons Ltd., 2000.
8. Ann Bowling. *Measuring Health: A Review of Quality of Life Measurement Scales*, 3rd ed. Glasgow: Bell & Bain Ltd., 2005.
9. Michael B. King, and Harold G. Koenig. "Conceptualising spirituality for medical research and health service provision." *BMC Health Services Research* 9 (2009): 116. [CrossRef] [PubMed]
10. Mélanie Vachon, Lise Fillion, and Marie Achille. "A conceptual analysis of spirituality at the end of life." *Journal of Palliative Medicine* 12 (2009): 53–59. [CrossRef] [PubMed]
11. Andrew Garratt, Louise Schmidt, Anne Mackintosh, and Ray Fitzpatrick. "Quality of life measurement: Bibliographic study of patient assessed health outcome measures." *British Medical Journal* 324 (2002): 1417–21. [CrossRef] [PubMed]
12. Stéfanie Monod, Mark Brennan, Etienne Rochat Theologian, Estelle Martin, Stéphane Rochat, and Christophe J. Büla. "Instruments measuring spirituality in clinical research: A systematic review." *Journal of General Internal Medicine* 26 (2011): 1345–57. [CrossRef] [PubMed]

13. Arndt Büssing, Klaus Baumann, Niels Christian Hvidt, Harold G. Koenig, Christina M. Pulchalski, and John Swinton. "Spirituality and Health." *Evidence-Based Complementary and Alternative Medicine (eCam).* 2014 (2014): 1–2, Article 682817. [CrossRef] [PubMed]

14. Hayfa Almutary, Ann Bonner, and Clint Douglas. "Symptom burden in chronic kidney disease: A review of recent literature." *Renal Care* 39 (2013): 140–50. [CrossRef] [PubMed]

15. Natale Gaspare De Santo, Alessandra Perna, Aziz El Matri, Rosa Maria De Santo, and Massimo Cirillo. "Survival is not enough." *Journal of Renal Nutrition* 22 (2012): 211–19. [CrossRef] [PubMed]

16. Marina Avramovic, and Vladisav Stefanovic. "Health-related quality of life in different stages of renal failure." *Artificial Organs* 36 (2012): 581–89. [CrossRef] [PubMed]

17. Suetonia Palmer, Mariacristina Vecchio, Jonathan C. Craig, Marcello Tonelli, David W. Johnson, Antonio Nicolucci, Fabio Pellegrini, Valeria Saglimbene, Giancarlo Logroscino, Steven Fishbane, and *et al.* "Prevalence of depression in chronic kidney disease: Systematic review and meta-analysis of observational studies." *Kidney International* 84 (2013): 179–91. [CrossRef] [PubMed]

18. Edmund G. Lowrie, Roberta Braun Curtin, Nancy LePain, and Dorian Schatell. "Medical Outcomes Study Short Form-36: A consistent and powerful predictor of morbidity and mortality in dialysis patients." *American Journal of Kidney Diseases* 41 (2003): 1286–92. [CrossRef]

19. Donna L. Mapes, Antonio Alberto Lopes, Sudtida Satayathum, Keith P. McCullough, David A. Goodkin, Francesco Locatelli, Shunichi Fukuhara, Eric W. Young, Kiyoshi Kurokawa, Akira Saito, and *et al.* "Health-related quality of life as a predictor of mortality and hospitalization: The Dialysis Outcomes and Practice Patterns Study (DOPPS)." *Kidney International* 64 (2003): 339–49. [CrossRef] [PubMed]

20. Yi-Chun Tsai, Chi-Chih Hung, Shang-Jyh Hwang, Shu-Li Wang, Shih-Ming Hsiao, Ming-Yen Lin, Lan-Fang Kung, Pei-Ni Hsiao, and Hung-Chun Chen. "Quality of life predicts risks of end-stage renal disease and mortality in patients with chronic kidney disease." *Nephrology Dialysis Transplantation* 25 (2010): 1621–26. [CrossRef] [PubMed]

21. Fabiane Rossi dos Santos Grincenkov, Natália Fernandes, Beatriz dos Santos Pereira, Kleyton Bastos, Antônio Alberto Lopes, Fredric O. Finkelstein, Roberto Pecoits-Filho, Abdul Rashid Qureshi, José Carolino Divino-Filho, and Marcus Gomes Bastos. "Impact of baseline health-related quality of life scores on survival of incident patients on peritoneal dialysis: A cohort study." *Nephron* 129 (2015): 97–103. [CrossRef] [PubMed]

22. Paul L. Kimmel, Rolf A. Peterson, Karen L. Weihs, Samuel J. Simmens, Sylvan Alleyne, Illuminado Cruz, and Judith H. Veis. "Multiple measurements of depression predict mortality in a longitudinal study of chronic hemodialysis outpatients." *Kidney International* 57 (2000): 2093–98. [CrossRef] [PubMed]

23. Antonio Alberto Lopes, Jennifer Bragg, Eric Young, David Goodkin, Donna Mapes, Christian Combe, Luis Piera, Phillip Held, Brenda Gillespie, Friedrich K. Port, and Dialysis Outcomes and Practice Patterns Study (DOPPS). "Depression as a predictor of mortality and hospitalization among hemodialysis patients in the United States and Europe." *Kidney International* 62 (2002): 199–207. [CrossRef] [PubMed]

24. Veena D. Joshi. "Quality of life in end stage renal disease patients." *World Journal of Nephrology* 3 (2014): 308–16. [CrossRef] [PubMed]

25. Fredric O. Finkelstein, William West, Jaya Gobin, Susan H. Finkelstein, and Diane Wuerth. "Spirituality, quality of life, and the dialysis patient." *Nephrology Dialysis Transplantation* 22 (2007): 2432–34. [CrossRef] [PubMed]

26. Sara N. Davison, and Gian S. Jhangi. "The relationship between spirituality, psychosocial adjustment to illness, and health-related quality of life in patients with advanced chronic kidney disease." *Journal of Pain and Symptom Management* 45 (2013): 170–8. [CrossRef] [PubMed]

27. Samir S. Patel, Viral S. Shah, Rolf A. Peterson, and Paul L. Kimmel. "Psychosocial variables, quality of life, and religious beliefs in ESRD patients treated with hemodialysis." *American Journal of Kidney Diseased* 40 (2002): 1013–22. [CrossRef] [PubMed]

28. Christina M. Puchalski. "The role of spirituality in health care." *Baylor University Medical Center Proceedings* 14 (2001): 352–57. [PubMed]

29. Arndt Büssing, and Harold G. Koenig. "Spiritual needs of patients with chronic diseases." *Religions* 1 (2010): 18–27. [CrossRef]

30. Nipa Aiyasanon, Nalinee Premasathian, Akarin Nimmannit, Pantip Jetanavanich, and Suchai Sritippayawan. "Validity and reliability of CHOICE Health Experience Questionnaire: Thai version." *Journal of Medical Association of Thailand* 92 (2009): 1159–66.

31. Phantipa Sakthong, and Vijj Kasemsup. "Health-related quality of life in Thai peritoneal dialysis patients." *Asian Biomedicine* 5 (2011): 799–805.

32. Tanita Thaweethamcharoen, W. Srimongkol, P. Noparatayaporn, Paweena Jariyayothin, N. Sukthinthai, Nipa Aiyasanon, Panupong Kitisriworapan, K. Jantarakana, and Somkiat Vasuvattakul. "Patient-reported outcomes (PRO) or quality of life (QOL) studies: Validity and reliability of KDQOL-36 in Thai kidney disease patient." *Value in Health Regional Issue* 2 (2013): 98–102. [CrossRef]

33. Areewan Cheawchanwattana, Chulaporn Limwattananon, Cynthia Gross, Supon Limwattananon, Viroj Tangcharoensathien, Cholatip Pongskul, and Dhavee Siriwongs. "The validity of a new practical quality of life measure in patients on renal replacement therapy." *Journal of Medical Association of Thailand* 89 (2006): S207–17.

34. Areewan Cheawchanwattana. "The psychometric property of a new generic health status measure: The 9-item Thai Health status Assessment Instrument (9-THAI)." Ph.D. dissertation, Khon Kaen University, 23 July 2007.

35. David A. Cook, and Thomas J. Beckman. "Current concepts in validity and reliability for psychometric instruments: Theory and application." *The American Journal of Medicine* 119 (2006): 166.e7–166.e16. [CrossRef] [PubMed]

36. Pasiri Sithinamsuwan, Suchada Niyasom, Samart Nidhinandana, and Ouppatham Supasyndh. "Dementia and depression in end stage renal disease: Comparison between hemodialysis and continuous ambulatory peritoneal dialysis." *Journal of Medical Association of Thailand* 88 (2005): S141–47.

37. Supin Prekbunjun. "Spiritual experience of patients with end stage of renal failure." Master degree thesis, Chulalongkorn University, 14 July 2004.

38. Areewan Cheawchanwattana, Darunee Chunlertrith, Warapond Saisunantararom, and Nutjaree Pratheepawanit Johns. "Does the Spiritual Well-Being of Chronic Hemodialysis Patients Differ from that of Pre-dialysis Chronic Kidney Disease." *Religions* 6 (2015): 14–23. [CrossRef]

39. Saengduean Promkaewngam, Linchong Pothiban, Wichit Srisuphan, and Khanokporn Sucamvang. "Development of the spiritual well-being scale for Thai Buddhist adults with chronic illness." *Pacific Rim International Journal of Nursing Research* 18 (2014): 320–32.

40. WHOQOL SRPB Group. "A cross-cultural study of spirituality, religion, and personal belief as components of quality of life." *Social Science & Medicine* 62 (2006): 1486–97.

41. Jason M. Bredle, John M. Salsman, Scott M. Debb, Benjamin J. Arnold, and David Cella. "Spiritual well-being as a component of health-related quality of life: The Functional Assessment of Chronic Illness Therapy-Spiritual Well-Being Scale (FACIT-Sp)." *Religions* 2 (2011): 77–94. [CrossRef]

42. Aaron T. Beck, Roberts A. Steer, and Gregory K. Brown. *BDI-II Beck Depression Inventory—Second Edition Manual*. San Antonio: Pearson, 1996.

43. World Health Organization. *WHOQOL-SRPB Users Manual Scoring and Coding for the WHOQOL SRPB Field-Test Instrument*. Geneva: World Health Organization, 2002, pp. 2–4.

44. Waraporn Saisunantararom, Areewan Cheawchanwattana, Talerngsak Kanjanabuch, and Maliwan Burapatana. "The psychometric property of WHOQOL-SRPB Thai version in chronic kidney diseases stage V patients." In Paper presented at European Conference on Religion, Spirituality and Health (EC RSH14), University of Malta/Mater Dei Hospital, Malta, 22–24 May 2014.

45. Supalak Khemthong. Personal communication with the authors, 14 November 2014.

46. Suzana Gabriela Rusa, Gabriele Ibanhes Peripato, Sofia Cristina Iost Pavarini, Keika Inouye, Marisa Silvana Zazzetta, and Fabiana de Souza Orlandi. "Quality of life/spirituality, religion and personal beliefs of adult and elderly chronic kidney patients under hemodialysis." *Revista Latino-Americana de Enfermagem* 22 (2014): 911–17. [CrossRef] [PubMed]

47. Ruchita Shah, Parmanand Kulhara, Sandeep Grover, Suresh Kumar, Rama Malhotra, and Shikha Tyagi. "Relationship between spirituality/religiousness and coping in patients with residual schizophrenia." *Quality of Life Research* 20 (2011): 1053–60. [CrossRef] [PubMed]

48. Stéfanie Monod, Estelle Lécureux, Etienne Rochat, Brenda Spencer, Laurence Seematter-Bagnoud, Anne-Sylvie Martin-Durussel, and Christophe Büla. "Validity of the FACIT-Sp to Assess Spiritual Well-Being in Elderly Patients." *Psychology* 6 (2015): 1311–22. [CrossRef]

49. Kristin E. Sandau, Charlene Boisjolie, and James S. Hodges. "Use of The Minnesota Living With Heart Failure Questionnaire among elderly patients with aortic stenosis: Results from a pilot study." *Journal of Cardiovascular Nursing* 29 (2014): 185–97. [CrossRef] [PubMed]

50. Giancarlo Lucchetti, Alessendra Lamas Granero Lucchetti, Juliane Piasseschi de Bernardin Gonçalves, and Homero P. Vallada. "Validation of the Portuguess Version of the Functional Assessment of Chronic illness Therapy-Spiritual Well-Being Scale (FACIT-Sp12) among Brazilian Psychiatric Inpatients." *Journal of Religion and Health* 54 (2015): 112–21. [CrossRef] [PubMed]

51. Najmeh Jafari, Ahmadreza Zamani, Mark Lazenby, Ziba Farajzadegan, Hamid Emami, and Amir Loghmani. "Translation and validation of the Persian version of the functional assessment of chronic illness therapy-Spiritual well-being scale (FACIT-Sp) among Muslim Iranians in treatment for cancer." *Palliative and Supportive Care* 11 (2013): 29–35. [CrossRef] [PubMed]

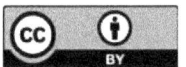

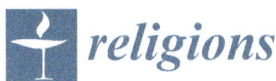

Article

Interpretation of Illness in Patients with Chronic Diseases from Poland and Their Associations with Spirituality, Life Satisfaction, and Escape from Illness—Results from a Cross Sectional Study

Arndt Büssing [1,†,*] and Janusz Surzykiewicz [2,3,†]

[1] Quality of Life, Spirituality and Coping, Institute for Integrative Medicine, Witten/Herdecke University, 58313 Herdecke, Germany; arndt.buessing@uni-wh.de
[2] Faculty for Religious Education, Catholic University Eichstätt-Ingolstadt, 85072 Eichstätt, Germany; janusz.surzykiewicz@ku-eichstaett.de
[3] Faculty of Paedagogy, Cardinal Wyszynski University, 01-815 Warsaw, Poland
* Author to whom correspondence should be addressed; arndt.buessing@uni-wh.de; Tel.: +49-2330-623-246; Fax: +49-2330-623-810.
† These authors contributed equally to this work.

Academic Editor: Peter Iver Kaufman
Received: 28 April 2015; Accepted: 5 June 2015; Published: 25 June 2015

Abstract: To analyse how patients with chronic diseases would interpret their illness, and how these interpretations were related to spirituality/religiosity, life satisfaction, and escape from illness, we performed a cross-sectional survey among patients with chronic diseases from Poland (n = 275) using standardized questionnaires. Illness was interpreted mostly as an Adverse Interruption of life (61%), Threat/Enemy (50%), Challenge (42%), and rarely as a Punishment (8%). Regression analyses revealed that escape from illness was the best predictor of negative disease perceptions and also strategy associated disease perceptions, and a negative predictor of illness as something of Value, while Value was predicted best by specific spiritual issues. Patients' religious Trust and partner status were among the significant contributors to their life satisfaction. Data show that specific dimensions of spirituality are important predictors for patients' interpretation of illness. Particularly the fatalistic negative perceptions could be indicators that patients may require further psychological assistance to cope with their burden.

Keywords: interpretation of illness; chronic disease; coping; life satisfaction; spirituality; Poland

1. Background

Based on the assumptions of Leventhal's Self-Regulation Theory [1], the individual being is an active problem solver that consciously activates efforts to modulate his thoughts, emotions and behaviours—particularly when facing illness or health affections. An important aspect for dealing with illness in terms of coping and illness interpretation are individual representations of disease. Relying on Diefenbach and Leventhal [2,3], there are two main types of representations, *i.e.*, cognitive and emotional processes. With respect to the "Transactional Model of Stress and Coping" of Park and Folkman [4], the ability to cope with stress (including illness) requires that people can find meaning in it and recognize it as important. Taylor [5] argued that patients with breast cancer adapted psychologically when they were able to find positive meanings in their illness.

Patients' religiosity was found to be an important factor for individual coping strategies [6]. Moreover, spirituality/religiosity can be seen also a resource of hope [7–9] and transformation [10,11]. Wiechman and Magyar-Russell [12] have shown that trauma survivors who use religious coping strategies show signs of posttraumatic growth' with "greater appreciation of life and changed priorities; warmer, more intimate relations with others; a greater sense of personal strength, recognition of new possibilities, and spiritual development".

The findings of previous studies that patients' spirituality was related particularly with positive interpretations of illness (*i.e.*, illness as something of value to grown on, or as a challenge) [13] would indicate that spirituality may influence cognitive processes related to meaning finding, and utilization of strategies to find hope despite of illness. These interpretations may be co-influenced by patients' positive or negative emotions to God (or other transcendent resources).

The psychiatrist Lipowski [14] described eight categories of how persons may interpret their illness (*i.e.*, Challenge, Value, Enemy, Punishment, Weakness, Loss, Relief, and Strategy) which may have influence on patients' choice of coping strategies. With respect to these categories, Challenge was rated most often by British [15], Canadian [16], Swedish [17] and German [13] cancer patients, and also by British patients with chronic renal diseases [18]. In contrast, German patients with chronic pain diseases rated their disease most often as an Adverse Interruption of life [19]; also predominantly a-religious patients with chronic diseases (60% cancer) from Shanghai rated their disease as an Adverse Interruption or as a Threat / Enemy, but also as a Challenge [20].

With respect to the findings described above, it is clear that a person's spirituality/religiosity may have an influence on how her/she may see illness [13,21], and this may have an influence on life satisfaction, too. Yet, the underlying dimensions of spirituality/religiosity which may be related are so far unclear.

We assume that different qualities of spirituality (*i.e.*, religious trust in God, existential search for meaning, ethical sensitivity, harmony, positive/negative emotions towards God) may be associated with different interpretations of illness, either positive or negative (*i.e.*, illness as a value, as a chance, as a punishment *etc.*), and that these variables may have an influence on patients' life satisfaction on the one hand or their (depressive) intention to escape from illness on the other hand.

Therefore we intended to analyse how patients with chronic diseases from Catholic Poland would interpret their illness, and how these specific interpretations were related to their religiosity/spirituality, their life satisfaction, and an intention to escape from illness. We hypothesize that both, the negative perceptions of illness (*i.e.*, threat, interruption of life, punishment, failure) and also strategy associated disease perceptions (*i.e.*, relieving break, call for help) are strongly influenced by patients' attitudes to escape from illness rather than reframing reflective strategies, while positive disease perceptions are associated primarily with patients' religiosity/spirituality and reflexive processes. Moreover, we assume that emotions towards God, either positive or negative, may be associated with their view of illness and also their life satisfaction, assuming that particularly negative emotions or disinterest in God would decrease life satisfaction.

2. Methods

Participants

This is the last part of a larger study among patients with chronic diseases from Poland [22,23]. All individuals were informed of the purpose of the study, were assured of confidentiality, and gave informed consent to participate. The patients were recruited consecutively by a psychologist and educators in Oncology Hospital in Wieliszew and in Department of Social Welfare in the province of Warsaw. Demographic information of these patients is presented in Table 1.

Individuals provided informed consent to participate by returning a completed questionnaire which did not ask for names, initials, addresses, or clinical details (with the exception of a diagnosis). The internal review boards in the persons of the Directorate Institutions and psychologists working in these institutions approved the survey. The study did not provide financial incentives to patients. All completed the questionnaires by themselves.

Table 1. Characteristics of 275 Patients.

Variables	Mean/%
Gender, %	
Women	74
Men	26
Age, years (Mean, standard deviation)	56 ± 16
Family status, %	
Married	54
Divorced	26
Widowed	20
Educational level, %	
basic	12
professional	20
medium	42
higher	25
Religious Denomination, %	
Christian (Catholic)	100
Spiritual/religious self-categorization, %	
R + S +	78
R + S –	7
R – S +	2
R – S –	13
Underlying diseases, %	
Cancer	35
Chronic pain diseases	10
Diabetes mellitus	16
Other chronic conditions	40
(incl. Asthma bronchiale, Multiple sclerosis, *etc.*	

3. Measures

All instruments were provided in their Polish language version.

3.1. Interpretation of Illness

The interpretation of illness was measured with 8 items according to Lipowski's "Meaning of Illness" [14] which were validated as a scale in patients with chronic diseases [13]. This Interpretation of Illness Scale (IIS; Cronbach's alpha = 0.73) includes positive interpretations (*i.e.*, challenge, value), strategy-associated interpretations (*i.e.*, relieving break of life, call for help), but also guilt-associated interpretations (*i.e.*, punishment, weakness/failure), and fatalistic negative interpretations (*i.e.*, threat/enemy, interruption of life). The items were scored on a 5-point scale from disagreement to agreement (0, does not apply at all; 1, does not truly apply; 2, don't know (neither yes nor no); 3, applies quite a bit; 4, applies very much).

3.2. Escape from Illness

The 3-item scale Escape from Illness is an indicator of a depressive/fearful escape-avoidance strategy to deal with illness (*i.e.*, "fear what illness will bring", "would like to run away from illness", "when I wake up, I don't know how to face the day") [24]. In patients with depressive and addictive diseases, the Escape scale correlates strongly positive with depressive symptoms (BDI; $r = 0.57$) [25] and strongly negative with various disease acceptance styles (Büssing *et al.*, 2010a), while in patients with cancer Escape correlated moderately positive with anxiety (HADS, $r = 0.47$) and depression (HADS; $r = 0.34$), and negatively with SF-12's mental health component ($r = -0.38$) [13].

The items were scored on a 5-point scale from disagreement to agreement (0, does not apply at all; (1) does not truly apply; (2) don't know (neither yes nor no); (3) applies quite a bit; (4) applies very much). Scores > 50% indicate an intention to escape from illness.

3.3. Life Satisfaction

Life satisfaction was measured with the Brief Multidimensional Life Satisfaction Scale (BMLSS) [26] which refers to Huebner's "Brief Multidimensional Students" Life Satisfaction Scale' [27,28]. The items of the BMLSS address intrinsic (Myself, Life in general), social (Friendships, Family life), external (Work situation, Where I live), and prospective dimensions (Financial situation, Future prospects). The internal consistency of the instrument was good (Cronbach's alpha = 0.87) [26]. Here we included two further items addressing patients' health situation and their abilities to deal with daily life concerns. Each item was introduced by the phrase "I would describe my level of satisfaction as … ", and scored on a 7-point scale from dissatisfaction to satisfaction (0, terrible; 1, unhappy; 2, mostly dissatisfied; 3, mixed (about equally satisfied and dissatisfied); 4, mostly satisfied; 5, pleased; 6, delighted). The BMLSS-10 sum score refers to a 100% level ("delighted"). Scores > 50% indicate higher life satisfaction, while scores < 50% indicate dissatisfaction.

3.4. Self-Description Questionnaire of Spirituality

The Self-description Questionnaire of Spirituality (SQS) is an instrument tested first in Polish individuals [29], and was used as an external measure sensitive for spiritual activities of Polish individuals. The scale uses originally 20 items and differentiates 3 factors, *i.e.*

- Religious Attitudes (*i.e.*, faith allows me to survive difficult periods in my life". "while making decisions, I rely on my religious beliefs", *etc.*)
- Ethical Sensitivity (*i.e.*, "react when someone is being hurt", "care about other people's situations", *etc.*)
- Harmony (*i.e.*, "I am part of the world", "while thinking about my life I experience peace and happiness", *etc.*)

However, when testing this scale in our sample, explorative factor analysis indicated four main factors and some items which loaded weakly on the respective factors (< 0.5). These items were thus eliminated. The resulting 17-item version of the instrument (SQS-17) with its 2 main scales Religious Attitudes and Ethical Sensitivity, and the third scale Peace/Harmony with two sub-constructs, has a very good reliability coefficient (Cronbach's alpha = 0.90) and explains 68% of variance. For this analysis, we used the SQS-17 version. The SQS-17 scores on a 5-point Likert scale ranging from "not at all" to "very much". The sum of the subscales indicates overall spirituality.

3.5. Spirituality/Religiosity and a Resource

The contextual SpREUK-15 questionnaire (SpREUK; which is an acronym of the German translation of "Spiritual and Religious Attitudes in Dealing with Illness") measures spirituality/religiosity attitudes and convictions of patients dealing with chronic diseases [30,31]. Referring to 15 items, it differentiates three factors, *i.e.*, Search, Trust and Reflection (Büssing, 2010). Confirmatory factor analysis confirmed the already established three subscales also in SpREUK's Polish version with good internal consistency coefficients ranging from alpha 0.74 to 0.91, yet with 10 items (SpREUK-Polish) [22]:

- Search scale, or search (for support/access to spirituality/religiosity), deals with patients' intention to find access to a spiritual or religious resource, which may be beneficial for coping with illness, and with their interest in spiritual or religious issues (insight and renewed interest).
- Trust scale, or trust (in higher guidance/source), is a measure of intrinsic religiosity; the factor deals with patients' conviction that they want to be connected with a higher source, and with

their desire to be sheltered and guided by that source, whatever may happen to them, conviction that death is not an end.

- Reflection scale, deals with a patient's cognitive reappraisal of his or her life because of illness and subsequent attempts to change or see illness differently (*i.e.*, change aspects of life or behavior, see illness as a chance for individual development, believing that the illness has meaning).

- The items scored on a 5-point scale from disagreement to agreement (0, does not apply at all; 1, does not truly apply; 2, don't know (neither yes nor no); 3, applies quite a bit; 4, applies very much). The scores were referred to a 100% level (transformed scale score). Scores > 50% indicate higher agreement (positive attitude), while scores < 50% indicate disagreement (negative attitude).

3.6. Positive Emotions (Associated with God)

To measure positive or negative emotions associated with God, we used a 12-item scale which was not yet validated for the Polish population. The instrument addresses positive emotions with 6 items (*i.e.*, Happiness/Joy, Love, Affection, Security, Shelter, Confidence/Trust), negative emotions with 5 items (*i.e.*, Guilt, Punishment, Failure, Fear, Anger/Rage), while 1 item addresses a person's disinterest in God. Within this sample, the sub-scale measuring positive emotions has a very good internal reliability (alpha = 0.95), and the sub-scale measuring negative perceptions a good internal reliability (alpha = 0.85).

These items were scored on a 5-point scale from disagreement to agreement (0, does not apply at all; 1, does not truly apply; 2, don't know (neither yes nor no); 3, applies quite a bit; 4, applies very much). The score was referred to a 100% level (transformed scale score).

3.7. Statistical Analysis

The research team performed descriptive data analyses, cross tabulation (Pearson Chi2), analyses of variance (ANOVA), correlation (Spearman rho), stepwise regression and linear regression analyses with SPSS 22.0.

The team judged $p < 0.05$ as significant. With respect to the correlation analyses, we regarded r > 0.5 as a strong correlation, an r between 0.3 and 0.5 as a moderate correlation, an r between 0.2 and 0.3 as a weak correlation, and r < 0.2 as no or a negligible correlation.

4. Results

4.1. Participants

As shown in table 1, patients' mean age was 56 ± 16 years; 74% were women and 26% men. Most were married and had a medium educational level. All had chronic diseases, predominantly cancer (35%), diabetes mellitus (16%), chronic pain diseases (10%), and other chronic conditions.

Polish patients were 100% Catholics; 78% regarded themselves as religious and spiritual (R + S +), 7% as religious but not spiritual (R + S −), 2% as not religious but spiritual (R − S +), and 13% as neither religious nor spiritual (R − S −).

4.2. Patients' Interpretations of Illness

As shown in Table 2, most regarded their disease as an Adverse Interruption of life (61%) or as a Threat/Enemy (50%), but also as a Challenge (42%). Several may see their illness as a Call for help (22%), as an own Weakness/Failure (20%), or as something of Value to grow (18%), and only a few as a Relieving Break from the demands of life (12%) or as a Punishment (8%).

Table 2. Interpretations of Illness (multiple answers).

	NO (%)	Undecided (%)	YES (%)	Non-responder (%)
Threat/Enemy	26	24	50	< 1
Adverse interruption of life	21	19	61	0
Punishment	70	22	8	< 1
Own Failure	53	27	20	1
Relieving break from the demands of life	68	20	12	0
Call for help	58	21	22	< 1
Something of value to grow	52	30	18	1
Challenge	35	23	42	< 1

Data are % of responders for each of these 8 items (no = scores 0 and 1; undecided = score 2; yes = scores 3 and 4).

Because patients had multiple options to assess their illness, there might be also combinations. We focused on the most often cited disease perception, and found that 71% of those who see their illness as an Adverse Interruption may see it also as a Threat/Enemy, while 41% can see it also as a Challenge (Table 3).

Table 3. Interpretations of Illness with respect to adverse interruption (cross tabulation).

		Adverse interruption of life		*p*-value (Chi^2)
		Disagreement/undecided (%)	Agreement (%)	
Threat/Enemy	No/undecided	83	29	< 0.0001
	Agreement	17	71	
Punishment	No/undecided	96	89	
	Agreement	4	11	0.018
Own Failure	No/undecided	87	76	
	Agreement	13	24	0.022
Relieving break from the demands of life	No/undecided	90	86	n.s.
	Agreement	10	14	
Call for help	No/undecided	89	72	< 0.0001
	Agreement	11	28	
Something of value to grow	No/undecided	71	89	< 0.0001
	Agreement	29	11	
Challenge	No/undecided	56	59	n.s.
	Agreement	44	41	

Results are % of *adverse interruption* statements as either no/undecided or agreement.

We next intended to analyse the influence of socio-demographic data, and found that the view of illness as something of Value was significantly lower in male patients than in women, while the view of illness as a Threat/Enemy was higher in men (Table 4). Patients with cancer had significantly higher perceptions of illness as a Threat/Enemy than those with other (primarily non-fatal) diseases, while all other interpretations did not significantly differ between both subgroups (Table 4). Of interest, patients who would regard themselves as R-S- had significantly higher scores for Adverse Interruption and Punishment and had lower scores for Value than their religious/spiritual counterparts. Age, educational level and family status had no significant influence on the disease interpretations (data not shown), with the exception of Call for Help, which was highest in elderly (F = 4.5; *p* = 0.001) and widowed persons (F = 4.6, *p* = 0.11), and also in those with a lower educational level (F = 3.2; *p* = 0.024).

Table 4. Interpretations of illness and socio-demographic variables.

		Threat/Enemy	Adverse Interruption	Punishment	Weakness/ Failure	Relieving Break	Call for Help	Value	Challenge
All patients	Mean	2.37	2.61	1.01	1.47	1.16	1.47	1.50	2.01
	SD	1.22	1.20	1.04	1.19	1.13	1.23	1.12	1.28
Gender									
Women (74%)	Mean	2.25	2.57	0.99	1.42	1.16	1.47	1.63	1.94
	SD	1.27	1.21	1.04	1.19	1.10	1.19	1.14	1.27
Men (26%)	Mean	2.68	2.74	1.08	1.64	1.17	1.47	1.13	2.24
	SD	1.05	1.16	1.04	1.19	1.22	1.34	0.95	1.27
F value		6.6	1.1	0.4	1.9	0.0	0.0	11.2	3.0
P value		0.011	n.s.	n.s.	n.s.	n.s.	n.s.	0.001	0.087
Disease									
Chronic diseases (65%)	Mean	2.22	2.52	0.97	1.49	1.14	1.38	1.49	2.01
	SD	1.18	1.19	1.03	1.21	1.06	1.22	1.12	1.24
Cancer (35%)	Mean	2.64	2.78	1.10	1.44	1.21	1.63	1.52	2.02
	SD	1.26	1.18	1.07	1.16	1.26	1.24	1.12	1.35
F value		7.3	3.2	1.1	0.1	0.2	2.6	0.0	0.0
P value		0.007	0.077	n.s.	n.s.	n.s.	n.s.	n.s.	n.s.
Religious orientation (R-S- *vs.* R/S)									
No (15%)	Mean	2.59	3.10	1.37	1.73	1.27	1.41	0.83	1.98
	SD	0.97	0.83	1.11	1.16	1.32	1.26	0.83	1.27
Yes (85%)	Mean	2.32	2.52	0.95	1.42	1.15	1.48	1.62	2.02
	SD	1.26	1.23	1.02	1.18	1.10	1.23	1.12	1.28
F value		1.6	8.4	5.7	2.5	0.4	0.1	18.4	0.0
P value		n.s.	0.004	0.018	n.s.	n.s.	n.s.	< 0.0001	n.s.

4.3. Interpretations of Illness and Their Association with External Measures

To clarify which specific interpretations of illness were associated with different aspects of spirituality on the one hand, and life satisfaction and escape from illness on the other hand, we performed first order correlation analyses.

In line with our hypothesis, particularly the positive interpretation Value was moderately to strongly related to patients' religiosity/spirituality (particularly with religious Trust and Reflection), while Challenge (which was only marginally related to Value) was weakly associated only with spiritual Search and Reflection (Table 5).

In line with our suggestion, the Escape scale was strongly correlated with fatalistic negative interpretations (*i.e.*, Threat/Enemy, Interruption) and moderately with Call for Help and Punishment (Table 5). Life satisfaction correlated best (and negative) with Call for help. Because Escape and life satisfaction are negatively correlated (r = −0.50), it is evident that the pattern of the aforementioned variables is inversely associated.

Table 5. Interpretations of illness and their correlations with life Satisfaction, escape from illness, and aspects of spirituality.

	Threat/Enemy	Adverse Interruption	Punishment	Weakness/ Failure	Relieving Break	Call for Help	Value	Challenge
Interpretations of Illness								
Threat/Enemy	1.000	0.650 **	0.312 **	0.177 **	0.120	0.366 **	−0.150	0.157 **
Adverse interruption		1.000	0.281 **	0.140	0.056	0.250 **	−0.266 **	−0.023
Punishment			1.000	0.387 **	0.223 **	0.386 **	−0.038	0.037
Failure				1.000	0.136	0.194 **	0.074	−0.051
Relieving break					1.000	0.455 **	0.207 **	0.140
Call for help						1.000	0.153	0.145
Something of value							1.000	0.206 **
Challenge								1.000
Spirituality (SQS and SpREUK Polish)								
Religious attitudes	−0.069	−0.161 **	−0.134	−0.104	0.034	0.168 **	0.356 **	0.045
Ethical Sensitivity	0.019	0.032	−0.094	−0.047	−0.018	0.120	0.313 **	0.062
Harmony	−0.168 **	−0.188 **	−0.143	−0.085	0.050	−0.044	0.230 **	0.166 **
Search	0.017	−0.108	−0.005	−0.034	0.029	0.217 **	0.369 **	0.215 **
Trust	−0.083	−0.163 **	−0.093	−0.021	0.010	0.136	0.511 **	0.174 **
Reflection	−0.173 **	−0.260 **	−0.160 **	−0.134	0.033	0.124	0.478 **	0.201**
Emotions towards God								
Positive	−0.191 **	−0.248 **	−0.111	−0.102	−0.035	0.059	0.310 **	0.055
Negative	0.211 **	0.208 **	0.222 **	0.067	0.175 **	0.203 **	−0.008	0.079
Life satisfaction								
Life Satisfaction	−0.277 **	−0.285 **	−0.287 **	−0.116	−0.125	−0.381 **	0.237 **	−0.031
Escape from Illness	0.589 **	0.546 **	0.363 **	0.119	0.175 **	0.482 **	−0.235 **	0.005

** $p < 0.01$ (Spearman rho); Moderate and strong correlations were highlighted (bold).

4.4. Predictors of Interpretations of Illness

To analyse which variables may be the best predictors of the specific perceptions of illness, particularly with respect to measures of spirituality, we performed stepwise regression analyses. Because the included variables predicted less than 15% of variance of the disease perceptions Weakness/Failure ($R^2 = 0.05$), Relieving Break ($R^2 = 0.04$), Punishment ($R^2 = 0.12$) and Challenge ($R^2 = 0.14$), the respective models were too weak to draw valid conclusion.

As shown in Table 6, Threat can be predicted best by Escape from Illness and male gender ($R^2 = 0.38$). Interruption of Life can be predicted best by Escape from Illness, with a further negative influence of Reflection, and a positive influence of Ethical Sensitivity ($R^2 = 0.36$). Also The strategy-associated interpretation Call for Help was explained best by Escape from Illness, with further influences of spiritual Search and Ethical Sensitivity, and a negative influence of life satisfaction ($R^2 = 0.35$). The positive interpretation Value was explained best by religious Trust, with further negative influences of Escape from Illness, living with partner, and positive influence of Reflection ($R^2 = 0.33$).

Table 6. Predictors of interpretations of illness (stepwise regression analyses).

		Beta	T	*p*	Collinearity Statistics *	
					Tolerance	VIF
	Threat					
	(constant)		0.739	0.461		
Model 2: R^2 = 0.38	Escape from Illness	0.595	12.359	0.000	1.000	1.000
	Male gender	0.154	3.205	0.002	1.000	1.000
	Interruption					
	(constant)		1.723	0.086		
Model 3: R^2 = 0.36	Escape from Illness	0.515	10.326	0.000	0.961	1.041
	Reflection	−0.237	−4.380	0.000	0.819	1.221
	Ethical Sensitivity	0.158	2.987	0.003	0.850	1.177
	Call for Help					
	(constant)		0.785	0.433		
Model 4: R^2 = 0.35	Escape from Illness	0.368	6.550	0.000	0.775	1.290
	Search	0.188	3.448	0.001	0.819	1.222
	Life Satisfaction	−0.268	−4.671	0.000	0.741	1.349
	Ethical Sensitivity	0.135	2.419	0.016	0.781	1.280
	Value					
	(constant)		1.177	0.240		
Model 4: R^2 = 0.33	Trust	0.363	4.572	0.000	0.404	2.473
	Escape from Illness	−0.170	−3.314	0.001	0.963	1.039
	Reflection	0.171	2.149	0.033	0.399	2.506
	living with partner	−0.106	−2.079	0.039	0.983	1.017

Included variables were measures of spirituality (SpREUK-Polish, SQS. and Emotions towards God), life satisfaction (BMLSS), Escape from illness (Escape), gender, age, relation status (with/without partner), and disease (cancer *vs.* other). Only significant models were presented; * As the regression coefficients may be compromised by collinearity, we checked the Variance Inflation Factor (VIF) as an indicator for collinearity. VIF > 10 is indicative for high collinearity.

Thus, religious issues were of strong relevance particularly for Value, and also for Call for help, while fatalistic negative interpretations were predicted best by patients' intention to escape from illness with no significant influence of specific religious issues.

4.5. Predictors of Life Satisfaction and Escape from Illness

Now we intended to analyse the influence of specific disease interpretations (*i.e.*, Value, Call for Help, Threat/Enemy and Adverse interruption) and other variables (*i.e.*, emotions towards God, religious Trust, gender, age and living with or without a partner) on life satisfaction and Escape from Illness. To identify the best fitting predictors, we therefore applied linear regression models (Table 7). It is expected that the positive variable Value will have a positive influence on life satisfaction, while the negative disease perceptions will have a negative (promoting) influence on escape from illness.

In the first linear regression model with life satisfaction as dependent variable (Table 7), the illness interpretation Call for Help was the best (negative) predictor, with further promoting effects of Value, living with a partner, and religious Trust. These variables account of 29% of variance.

Table 7. Predictors of life satisfaction and escape from illness (stepwise regression analyses).

		Beta	T	*p*	Collinearity statistics *	
					tolerance	VIF
Dependent variable: Life satisfaction						
Model 4: $R^2 = 0.29$	(constant)		23.789	< 0.0001		
	Illness = Call for Help	−0.434	−8.183	< 0.0001	0.963	1.039
	Illness = Value	0.239	3.893	< 0.0001	0.719	1.390
	Living with partner	0.131	2.470	0.014	0.962	1.039
	Religious Trust	0.149	2.420	0.016	0.719	1.392
Dependent variable: Escape						
Model 5: $R^2 = 0.51$	(constant)		7.462	< 0.0001		
	Illness = Threat/Enemy	0.313	5.262	< 0.0001	0.535	1.869
	Illness = Call for Help	0.332	6.864	< 0.0001	0.814	1.229
	Illness = Value	−0.215	−4.589	< 0.0001	0.861	1.161
	Illness = Adverse Interruption	0.199	3.440	0.001	0.566	1.768
	Male gender	−0.106	−2.347	0.020	0.934	1.071

Included variables were measures of were gender, age, relation status (with/without partner), positive and negative emotions towards God, religious Trust, spiritual Search, Reflection, and specific disease interpretations (*i.e.*, Threat/Enemy, Adverse Interruption, Call for Help, Value). Only significant models were presented; * As the regression coefficients may be compromised by collinearity, we checked the Variance Inflation Factor (VIF) as an indicator for collinearity. VIF > 10 is indicative for high collinearity.

In the second linear regression model with Escape as dependent variable ($R^2 = 0.51$), both negative disease perceptions Call for Help and Threat/Enemy were the strongest predictors, with further promoting (aggravating) effect of Adverse Interruption, and negative (ameliorating) effects of Value and male gender.

Religious Trust explains only 5% of variance in life satisfaction, and positive emotions towards God 4% of variance; both variables were thus not of relevance in the prediction model. Religious Trust explains 3% of Escape's variance, and positive emotions towards God explains 4%, and were thus not of relevance in the respective prediction model.

5. Discussion

Most of the Catholic Polish patients investigated in this study exhibited fatalistic negative interpretations of their illness (*i.e.*, Adverse Interruption, Threat/Enemy), while a large fraction can nevertheless see it also as a Challenge. Interestingly, 41% of those who regard their illness as an Adverse Interruption would see it also as a Challenge.

In line with our primary hypothesis, the current data underline that the intention to escape from illness, as a depressive escape-avoidance strategy, is strongly related to fatalistic negative perceptions of disease but also with the perception of illness as Call for help or even a Punishment, but not with illness as a Challenge. Patients' ability to reflect their life concerns, to change attitudes and behaviour, and to see illness differently (SpREUK's Reflection subscale), was moderately associated only with Value. It is consistent with the underlying theory that having trust in God is related with the view that even illness can be something of value for an inner development or even "spiritual transformation", as observed also in persons with HIV [10,11], and/or a feeling of control in difficult situations [32]. Moreover, exclusively Value as an interpretation of illness was associated moderately with different dimensions of patients' spirituality and positive emotions towards God. This would confirm our second hypothesis that a positive disease interpretation is associated primarily with patients' religiosity/spirituality. However, while this is true for Value, the view of illness as a Challenge was only weakly associated with measures of spirituality. Challenge was neither related to life satisfaction, nor negatively to Escape from Illness, nor to positive or negative emotions towards God, and only weakly associated with a persons' ability to reflect life concerns (which is consistent with the underlying construct) on the one hand, and an attitude of Search for a spiritual source which might be helpful, and marginally with religious Trust. Yet, it was not significantly associated with Religious attitudes or Ethical Sensitivity. This would indicate that the view of illness as a Challenge is rather related to spirituality as a strategy to cope (state) than an intrinsic aspect of religiosity (trait).

The role of Polish patients' spirituality was investigated by Krok [33], too. In his study using the Self-description Questionnaire of Spirituality (which was used in this study, too), spirituality was an important buffer against stressful events to help people to cope with distress and difficulties in life. Interestingly, the underlying three spiritual dimensions (*i.e.*, Religious Attitudes, Ethical Sensitivity, and Harmony) have a different impact on particular coping styles depending. While Religious Attitudes were not significantly related to specific coping styles, Ethical Sensitivity was associated with Avoidance and Social Diversion coping, and the subscale Harmony was related to a Task-oriented coping, and negatively with Avoidance-oriented coping [33]. This means that people characterized by a high level of spirituality will try to solve problems through efforts aimed at solving the problem and seeking social support.

5.1. Interaction Model between Interpretations of Illness, Emotions towards God, Life Satisfaction and Escape from Illness

It is intuitive that having a positive view of the illness (*i.e.*, something of value to grow) would be of benefit to cope, and thus would increase patients' life satisfaction. Moreover, having or not a concrete partner to rely on in times of need would mean, patients have someone who is providing support and care on the one hand, or a positive relation towards God who is expected to help in times of need and thus providing hope and emotional comfort, would all contributing to higher life satisfaction, too. In contrast, when illness is interpreted as a Call for Help then patients are in strong need for external support, and thus their life satisfaction might be low. This Call for Help can, but must not necessarily have a religious connotation. In the respective regression model, it was patients' religious Trust on the one hand and living with a partner were among the significant contributors to life satisfaction. This means, having a reliable source of help (either a concrete partner or a helping God) will contribute to a persons' experienced life satisfaction. This is consistent with the theory and literature that loneliness is negatively related to life satisfaction [34], while partnership is positively related with life satisfaction [35,36].

In contrast, seeing illness as something negative was in fact the best predictor of patients' intention to escape from illness. Theoretically, negative emotions towards God (implying illness as a punishment) might be associated with higher intention to escape from illness and lower life satisfaction; yet, neither positive nor negative emotions were among the significant predictors in both models. However, in a small study enrolling patients with multiple sclerosis from Poland found a negative correlation between negative emotion and consequences of own illness, and SQS's Harmony scale [37]. In our study, we did not analyse the association of negative emotions with measures of spirituality, yet we can confirm that negative disease interpretations are related to negative interpretations. However, in our sample these negative interpretations were only marginally related with SQS's Harmony or other scales.

The main findings of this interaction model are summarized in Figure 1.

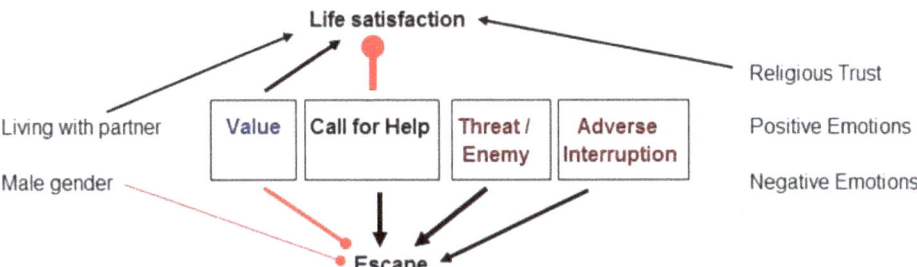

Figure 1. Interaction model with respect to the regression analyses. Positive influences on the dependent variables on life satisfaction or escape were indicated as arrow lines, while inhibitory influences were indicated as lines with thickened ends. The thickness of lines correspond with the T values of the regression models. Round ends indicate negative influences, while arrowed ends indicate positive influences.

5.2. Limitations

A limitation of this study is the cross-sectional design, which does not allow for causal interpretations. To substantiate the findings, longitudinal studies are needed. We also have no information about how many patients rejected to fill the questionnaire at all, and thus the sample should be regarded as a convenience sample Moreover, the data may not be representative for patients from whole Poland because the patients were recruited only in the city of Wieliszew and in the province of Warsaw; thus, a more diverse sample is highly encouraged.

6. Conclusions

The data show that specific dimensions of spirituality are important predictor for patients' distinct interpretation of illness. Particularly religious Trust was identified as the best predictor of Polish patients' interpretation of illness as something of Value, indicating potentially the chance for a "spiritual transformation". Yet, religious Trust has only a very weak influence on patients' depressive intention to escape from the current life situation; it is not a buffer against suffering, but might be a positive resource to cope and to find new perspectives—and thus a matter of hope. In fact, a study among Polish cancer patients by Wnuk *et al.*, [38] confirmed a positive relationship between frequency of spiritual experiences and strength of hope. Indeed, the ability to reflect life concerns and to change life or behaviour (Reflection scale), which was also related in this study to the disease interpretation Value, has clearly a religious connotation and is strongly associated with positive views of God, also the experience of gratitude and awe [22].

In this context, it is of importance to underline that negative interpretations were mainly related to the intention to escape from illness and reduced life satisfaction. Particularly when patients' state negative disease perceptions, psychologists, nurses and physicians should be aware that these may be indicators that patients may require further psychological and/or pastoral assistance to cope with their burden. These disease interpretations may help to understand how patients react towards their illness, which strategies they may use to cope, and how they can be supported to adapt to the complex process of chronic illness. When positive interpretations predominate they may indicate some kind of "inner transformation" with processes to change attitudes, priorities, and life style, while persisting negative interpretations indicate the need for specific psychological support. In fact, although the causality is unclear, in Canadian breast cancer patients their negative disease perceptions (*i.e.*, Enemy, Loss, or Punishment) were related to higher mental health affections and lower quality of life within a 3 year follow up than women who indicated a more positive meaning [16]. Moreover, also the view of illness as a call for help means that patients are searching for a helpful source because they feel that they cannot manage the implications of illness alone. These persons obviously require further support, either by chaplains, psychologists, social workers, nurses, physicians, or their relatives.

Acknowledgments: The authors would like to dedicate this manuscript to the memory of Kazimierz Franczak who started this study with us, but passed away during the process of data evaluation. We are grateful to Daniela Rodrigues Recchia for her support in statistical analyses.

Author Contributions: Arndt Büssing and Janusz Surzykiewicz initiated the project, Janusz Surzykiewicz organized recruitment of patients, and Arndt Büssing analyzed the data. Both authors interpreted the data, and contributed to write the manuscript. All authors have read and approved the final manuscript.

Conflicts of Interest: The authors declare no conflict of interest.

References

1. Howard Leventhal, Daniel Meyer, and David Nerenz. "The common sense representation of illness danger." In *Medical Psychology*. Edited by S. Rachman. New York: Pergamon Press, 1980, vol. 2, pp. 7–30.
2. Howard Leventhal, Michael Diefenbach, and Elaine A. Leventhal. "Illness Cognition: Using common sense to understand treatment adherence and affect cognition interactions." *Cognitive Therapy and Research* 16 (1992): 143–63. [CrossRef]
3. Michael A. Diefenbach, and Howard Leventhal. "The common-sense model of illness representation: Theoretical and practical considerations." *The Journal of Social Distress and the Homeless* 5 (1996): 11–38. [CrossRef]
4. Crystal L. Park, and Susan Folkman. "Meaning in the context of stress and coping." *Review of General Psychology* 1 (1997): 115–44. [CrossRef]
5. Elisabeth Johnston Taylor. "Transformation of tragedy among women surviving breast cancer." *Oncology Nursing Forum* 27 (2000): 781–88. [PubMed]
6. Kenneth I. Pargament. *The Psychology of Religion and Coping: Theory, Research, Practice.* New York: Guilford, 1997.
7. Wendy Greenstreet. "From spirituality to coping strategy: making sense of chronic illness." *British Journal of Nursing* 15 (2006): 938–42. [CrossRef] [PubMed]
8. Ingela C. Thuné-Boyle, Jan A. Stygall, Mohammed R. Keshtgar, and Stanton P. Newman. "Do religious/spiritual coping strategies affect illness adjustment in patients with cancer? A systematic review of the literature." *Social Science & Medicine* 63 (2006): 151–64.
9. Océane Agli, Nathalie Bailly, and Claude Ferrand. "Spirituality and religion in older adults with dementia: A systematic review." *International Psychogeriatrrics* 26 (2014): 1–11. [CrossRef] [PubMed]
10. Heidemarie Kremer, and Gail Ironson. "Longitudinal spiritual coping with trauma in people with HIV: implications for health care." *AIDS Patient Care STDS* 28 (2014): 144–54. [CrossRef] [PubMed]
11. Gail Ironson, and Heidemarie Kremer. "Spiritual transformation, psychological well-being, health, and survival in people with HIV." *International Journal of Psychiatry in Medicine* 39 (2009): 263–81. [CrossRef] [PubMed]
12. Shelley Wiechman Askay, and Gina Magyar-Russell. "Post-traumatic growth and spirituality in burn recovery." *International Review of Psychiatry* 21 (2009): 570–79. [CrossRef] [PubMed]
13. Arndt Büssing, and Julia Fischer. "Interpretation of illness in cancer survivors is associated with health-related variables and adaptive coping styles." *BMC Women's Health* 9 (2009): 2. [CrossRef] [PubMed]
14. Zbigniew J. Lipowski. "Physical illness, the individual and the coping processes." *Psychiatry in Medicine* 1 (1970): 91–102. [CrossRef] [PubMed]
15. Karen A. Luker, Kinta Beaver, Sam J. Leinster, and R. Glyn Owens. "Meaning of illness for women with breast cancer." *Journal of Advanced Nursing* 23 (1996): 1194–201. [CrossRef] [PubMed]
16. Lesley F. Degner, Thomas Hack, John O'Neil, and Linda J. Kristjanson. "A new approach to eliciting meaning in the context of breast cancer." *Cancer Nursing* 26 (2003): 169–78. [CrossRef] [PubMed]
17. Birgitta Wallberg, Helena Michelson, Marianne Nystedt, Christina Bolund, Lesley Degner, and Nils Wilking. "The meaning of breast cancer." *Acta Oncologica* 42 (2003): 30–35. [CrossRef] [PubMed]
18. Ann-Louise Caress, Karen A. Luker, and R. Glynn Owens. "A descriptive study of meaning of illness in chronic renal disease." *Journal of Advanced Nursing* 33 (2011): 716–27. [CrossRef]

19. Arndt Büssing, Thomas Ostermann, Edmund AM Neugebauer, and Peter Heusser. "Adaptive coping strategies in patients with chronic pain conditions and their interpretation of disease." *BMC Public Health* 10 (2010): 507. [CrossRef] [PubMed]

20. Arndt Büssing, Ariane von Bergh, Xiao-feng Zha, and Chang-quan Ling. "Interpretation of illness in patients with chronic diseases from Shanghai and their associations with life satisfaction, escape from illness, and ability to reflect the implications of illness." *Journal of Integrative Medicine* 12 (2014): 409–16. [CrossRef]

21. Arndt Büssing, and Götz Mundle. "Changes in Emotional Acceptance of Disease after Therapeutic Intervention in Patients with Addictions and Depressive Disorders." *Integrative Medicine: A Clinician's Journal* 9 (2010): 40–46.

22. Arndt Büssing, Kazimierz Franczak, and Janusz Surzykiewicz. "Spiritual and Religious Attitudes in Dealing with Illness in Polish Patients with Chronic Diseases: Validation of the Polish Version of the SpREUK Questionnaire." *Journal of Religion and Health*, 2014. Available online: http://link.springer.com/article/10.1007%2Fs10943-014-9967-3 (accessed on 26 October 2014).

23. Arndt Büssing, Iwona Pilchowska, and Janusz Surzykiewicz. "Spiritual Needs of Polish Patients with Chronic Diseases." *Journal of Religion and Health*. 2014. Available online: http://link.springer.com/article/10.1007%2Fs10943-014-9863-x#page-1 (accessed on 1 May 2014).

24. Arndt Büssing, Nadja Keller, Andreas Michalsen, Susanne Moebus, Gustav Dobos, Thomas Ostermann, and Peter F. Matthiessen. "Spirituality and adaptive coping styles in German patients with chronic diseases in a CAM health care setting." *Journal of Complementary and Integrative Medicine* 3 (2006): 4. [CrossRef]

25. Arndt Büssing, Peter F. Matthiessen, and Götz Mundle. "Emotional and rational disease acceptance in patients with depression and alcohol addiction." *Health and Quality of Life Outcomes* 6 (2008): 4. [CrossRef] [PubMed]

26. Arndt Büssing, Julia Fischer, Almut Haller, Thomas Ostermann, and Peter F. Matthiessen. "Validation of the Brief Multidimensional Life Satisfaction Scale in patients with chronic diseases." *European Journal of Medical Research* 14 (2009): 171–77. [CrossRef] [PubMed]

27. E. Scott Huebner, Shannon Suldo, Robert F. Valois, J. Wanzer Drane, and Keith Zullig. "Brief multidimensional students' life satisfaction scale, sex, race, and grade effects for a high school sample." *Psychological Reports* 94 (2004): 351–56. [CrossRef] [PubMed]

28. Keith J. Zullig, E. Scott Huebner, Rich Gilman, Jon M. Patton, and Karen A. Murray. "Validation of the brief multidimensional students' life satisfaction scale among college students." *American Journal of Health Behavior* 29 (2005): 206–14. [CrossRef] [PubMed]

29. Irena Heszen-Niejodek, Ewa Gruszczyńska, and A. Metlak. *Kwestionariusz Samoopisu (The Self-description Questionnaire)*; Katowice: Uniwersytet Slaski, 2003. Available online: http://www.ipri.pl/badania-naukowe/narzedzia-psychometryczne/duchowosc-2/kwestionariusz-samoopisu/ (accessed on 19 June 2015).

30. Arndt Büssing, Thomas Ostermann, and Peter F. Matthiessen. "Role of religion and spirituality in medical patients, Confirmatory results with the SpREUK questionnaire." *Health and Quality of Life Outcomes* 3 (2005): 10. [CrossRef] [PubMed]

31. Arndt Büssing. "Spirituality as a resource to rely on in chronic illness, The SpREUK questionnaire." *Religions* 1 (2010): 9–17. [CrossRef]

32. Fred Rothbaum, John R. Weisz, and Samuel S. Snyder. "Changing the world and changing the self: A two process model of perceived control." *Journal of Personality and Social Psychology* 42 (1982): 5–37. [CrossRef]

33. Dariusz Krok. "The role of spirituality in coping: Examining the relationships between spiritual dimensions and coping styles." *Mental Health, Religion & Culture* 11 (2008): 643–53.

34. Ana M. Fernández-Alonsoa, Martina Trabalón-Pastora, Carmen Varaa, Peter Chedrauib, Faustino R. Pérez-Lópezc, and MenopAuse Risk Assessment (MARIA) Research Group. "Life satisfaction, loneliness and related factors during female midlife." *Maturitas* 72 (2012): 88–92. [CrossRef] [PubMed]

35. Tanja Besier, Tim. G. Schmitz, and Lutz Goldbeck. "Life satisfaction of adolescents and adults with cystic fibrosis: Impact of partnership and gender." *Journal of Cystic Fibrosis* 8 (2009): 104–09. [CrossRef] [PubMed]

36. Markus H. Schafer, Sarah A. Mustillo, and Kenneth F. Ferraro. "Age and the tenses of life satisfaction." *Journals of Gerontology, Series B: Psychological Sciences and Social Sciences* 68 (2013): 571–79. [CrossRef] [PubMed]

37. Marta Lenkiewicz, Agata Silczak, Anna Szymańska, and Martyna Żyłkowska. "Reprezentacja własnej choroby i poczucie koherencji jako predykatory zdrowia u osób z sm (Self-perception of the disease and sense of coherence as health predictors in group of patients with sm)." *Pielęgniarstwo Polskie* 3 (2011): 175–80.
38. Marcin Wnuk, Jerzy Tadeusz Marcinkowski, Mateusz Hędzelek, and Sylwia Świstak-Sawa. "Religijno-duchowe korelaty siły nadziei oraz poczucia sensu życia pacjentów onkologicznych." *Psychonkologia* 1 (2010): 14–20.

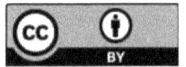

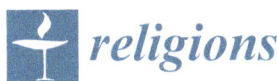

Review

Religious Beliefs and Their Relevance for Treatment Adherence in Mental Illness: A Review

Paweł Zagożdżon * and Magdalena Wrotkowska

Department of Hygiene and Epidemiology, Medical University of Gdansk, 80-211 Gdansk, Poland;
m.wrotka@gumed.edu.pl
* Correspondence: pzagoz@gumed.edu.pl; Tel.: +48-58-349-1928

Received: 6 July 2017; Accepted: 8 August 2017; Published: 14 August 2017

Abstract: Approximately 50% of patients do not adhere to medical therapy. Religious and spiritual factors may play an important role in determining medication compliance in mental illness. The aim of this paper is to review published evidence documenting a relationship between religion/spirituality (R/S) and treatment adherence in mental illness, in particular in schizophrenia, depression and substance abuse. This review summarizes, categorizes and defines the role of religious beliefs as a factor improving medication compliance in mental illness. Randomized controlled trials and observational studies were eligible for the review if they were published in December 2015 or earlier, analyzed the effects of religious beliefs or spirituality on medication compliance, or adherence to other therapeutic interventions in mental illness. The vast majority of published studies analyzed the effects of religion on medication compliance in schizophrenia and addiction. In schizophrenia patients, religious beliefs turned out to be a predictor of worse treatment adherence. However, spiritual orientation was shown to play an important role in the recovery from addiction, and to improve adherence in patients with this condition. Furthermore, better treatment adherence was observed in more religious patients diagnosed with depression. While religious beliefs and spirituality may represent an important source of hope and meaning, they often interfere with treatment adherence. Therefore, psychiatrists should consider religious and spiritual beliefs of their patients, and verify if and to what extent they improve their medication compliance.

Keywords: religion; treatment adherence; mental illness

1. Introduction

While lack of medication adherence may be observed in essentially all chronic conditions, it is particularly challenging in mental disorders. The latter are typically associated with social isolation, stigmatization, comorbid substance abuse, lack of insight, depression and cognitive impairment. Moreover, treatment adherence may be affected by both positive and negative symptoms of the mental illness itself.

The key therapeutic objectives in mental illness is to adequately control its symptoms and to ensure treatment adherence of the patient. Treatment adherence improves mental health and facilitates resolution of the underlying illness. Adherence is defined as the extent to which the patient's behaviors, such as medication taking, diet and lifestyle modification comply with doctor's recommendations (12). Religion beliefs may influence medication compliance in mental illness to a large extent. If a mental illness is supposed to result from or may be associated with spiritual problems, pharmacotherapy may not be enough. Some patients may believe that medication taking or medical advice seeking reflect the lack of their faith in God's ability to heal the disease without a medical intervention. However, if religious beliefs promote self-care for somatic and mental health as a manifestation of good overall status, they may also exert a beneficial effect on medication compliance (32). Some persons may consider treatment adherence as a disobedience to religious doctrines. Such opinions may be shared by patients, their relatives and/or members of local communities, influencing their attitude to prescribed treatment.

Published evidence suggests that lack of treatment adherence is a more serious issue in psychiatry than in general medicine. In a review paper analyzing treatment adherence in psychiatric and somatic disorders throughout a 20-year period between 1975 and 1996, medication compliance for antipsychotics, antidepressants and agents used in the therapy of physical ailments was estimated at 58%, 65% and 76%, respectively (7). Mean rate of medication non-compliance in schizophrenia identified in a systematic review of 39 studies was 41%. However, when the analysis was limited solely to five methodologically flawless studies, the proportion of patients who took less than 75% of prescribed medications had increased up to 50% (23). Lack of compliance with antipsychotic treatment results in exacerbation of symptoms, and is associated with worse prognosis and increased demand for inpatient and acute outpatient healthcare services (37; 24; 31).

Lack of treatment adherence was shown to be associated with a worse insight, negative attitude or subjective response to pharmacotherapy, past history of non-compliance, substance abuse, shorter duration of underlying illness, inadequate discharge planning or aftercare environment, and poor therapeutic alliance (34). Other predictors of non-adherence identified in some, albeit not all, studies dealing with the problem in question, were age, sex, ethnicity, marital status, education level, neurocognitive impairment, intensity of psychotic symptoms, medication type and route of its administration, severity of side-effects, use of drugs at higher antipsychotic doses, presence of mood symptoms, and family involvement. However, these are patients' beliefs about their illness and potential benefits of a given treatment, its subjectively assessed side-effects (among them extrapyramidal side-effects), as well as neuroleptic dysphoria, akathisia, sexual dysfunction and weight gain, which are particularly important for medication compliance (13). Also a good relationship with the physician in charge is considered an important determinant of treatment adherence (39).

There is no universal definition of religiosity and spirituality. Koenig et al. (2012) define spirituality as distinguished from humanism, values, morals, and mental health, by its connection to which is sacred, the transcendent' and that religion 'involves beliefs, practices, and rituals related to the transcendent, where the transcendent is God'. Huguelet in his book *Religion and Spirituality in Psychiatry* used the term *religion* to indicate specific behavioral, social, doctrinal, and denominational characteristics (14). Religious and spiritual factors may play an important role in determining medication compliance in mental illness. However, systematic assessment of available evidence in this matter is needed. The aim of this paper is to review published evidence documenting a relationship between religion/spirituality (R/S) and treatment adherence in mental illness, in particular in schizophrenia, depression, and substance abuse. We summarized, categorized and defined the role of religious beliefs as a factor improving medication compliance in these major psychiatric conditions.

2. Methods

This study is a systematic review of published evidence regarding the influence of R/S on treatment adherence in mental illness following PRISMA (Preferred Reporting Items for Systematic reviews and Meta-Analyses) guidelines for search strategy and data collection process. The study was conducted between January 2016 and May 2016, and then its results were updated in April 2017.

2.1. Eligibility Criteria

Published observational and experimental studies were eligible for the review if they explored the association between R/S and outcomes in three mental illnesses: depression, anxiety and addiction. R/S were defined as a non-medical process or message aimed at improvement of patient's status and framed by the themes of spiritual relevance.

The search was limited to articles in English published till April 2017 and searched during period specified above.

2.2. Search Strategies

Original research papers and review articles identified using PubMed.

The search included the following medical subject headings: *religion, spirituality* combined with *medication adherence, compliance/noncompliance* and *schizophrenia, depression, psychosis, anxiety, phobia, dissociative disorders, addiction.*

Two researchers (PZ and MW) reviewed titles and abstracts of all identified articles independently, to exclude those in which R/S were not analyzed in the context of treatment adherence in mental illness, as well as to eliminate off-topic and duplicate papers.

Publications were identified as eligible for the review if based on their abstract they could be classified as (1) observational studies, addressing spirituality or religion as the determinants of treatment adherence, or (2) non-randomized or randomized studies testing the effect(s) of a given intervention on the adherence, or (3) qualitative articles, such as editorials or review papers.

Separate search strategy was used to identify other potential sources of evidence, such as textbooks and systematic reviews analyzing treatment adherence or spirituality in mental illness (21; 27; 33; 11; 17).

2.3. Data Items

The lists of items extracted from each eligible publication included (1) clinical diagnosis, (2) sample size, (3) type of intervention or exposure, (4) outcome measures, and (5) results of the intervention. The results were analyzed as a qualitative variable, i.e., improvement of adherence or lack thereof.

2.4. Risk of Bias

Due to the nature of the R/S intervention and influencing variable adopted, the risk of selection bias in our review is high. A known threat to the validity of meta-analysis is publication bias, which occurs when studies with statistically significant or clinically favourable results are more likely to be published than studies with non-significant or unfavourable results. There has also been the suggestion that the potential for publication bias is greater for observational studies. Reviewer selection bias could also occur when reviewers search for studies based on specific exposure variable from a subset of existing studies through secondary search and selection takes place with knowledge of individual study results. Caution should be exercised when combining and reporting systematic reviews of observational and experimental studies. It is commonly accepted that observational studies are prone to greater degree of bias than experimental studies. There were few non-randomised studies in our review that used any method of adjustment. Some authors questions whether meta-analytic techniques can be applied to epidemiological studies at all. We did not use any methods that detect publication bias as we were unable to extract any common measure of treatment effect (adherence summary measures). Additionally within specific therapeutic area there were singular studies found (depression and anxiety). Therefore some PRISMA items requiring study estimates were not reported here. We chose to evaluate the risk of bias of each study indicating only the study design and number of participants. After data extraction, authors of this review determined that the studies were too heterogeneous to be quantitatively synthesised. We decided to show only the direction of potential association between the outcome and R/S variable instead of any specific summary measures.

3. Results

A total of 66 eligible abstracts were identified during PubMed search (see flowchart; Figure 1).

During the first stage of screening, abstracts were grouped according to the following outcomes of interest: (1) religiosity or spirituality as an intervention or co-variate, and (2) treatment adherence or medication compliance. This enabled us to exclude 31 articles that did not satisfy the inclusion criteria of this review.

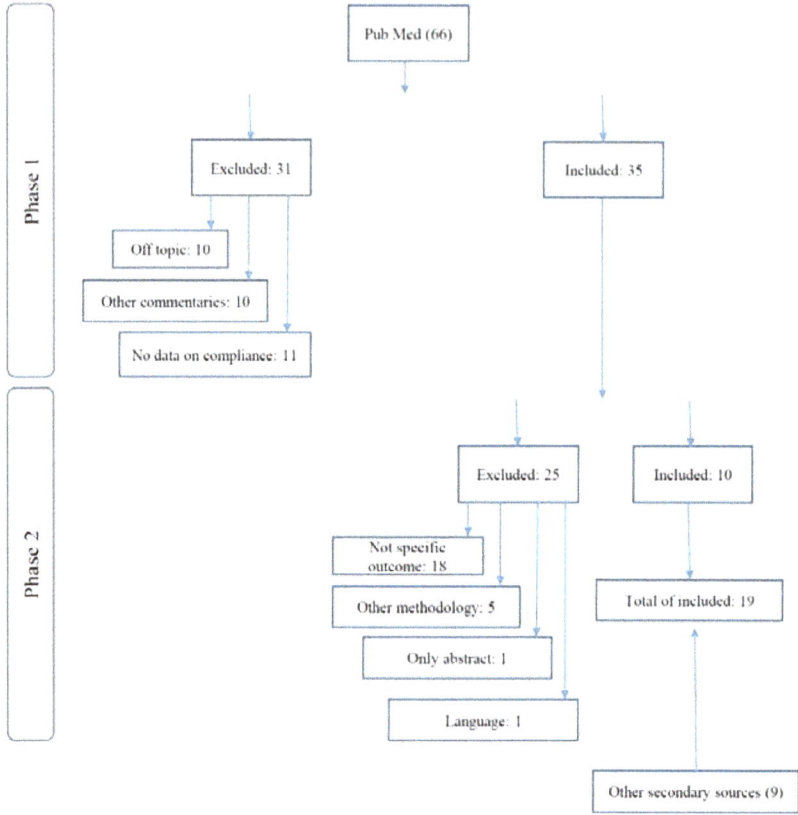

Figure 1. Flowchart of the selected studies.

The second, outcome-specific stage of screening included 35 potentially relevant papers that addressed medication compliance and R/S. A total of 10 full-text original papers and one review article were eventually identified as eligible for the review. Other 25 articles were excluded since they did not refer to the diseases of interest or medication compliance, presented psychiatric conditions that were not included in our search strategies (e.g., eating disorders), described research methodology, lacked abstract, or were not published in English.

Additional eight eligible studies were identified based on cross-reference check of review papers and books on spirituality. Therefore, a total of 18 original articles were eventually analyzed, along with one review paper referring to previous studies of treatment adherence and attendance (38).

3.1. Characteristics of Studies

General characteristics of identified studies, stratified according to the underlying mental illness, are summarized in Table 1. The studies included a total of 3449 patients with one of the diseases of interest, among them 132 individuals with depression, 125 with subclinical anxiety, 945 with schizophrenia, and 2777 with addictions.

Table 1. Characteristics of studies included in the review.

Mental Illness	Study	N of pts	Study Design	Tx / Exposure	Outcome	Effect
Depression	Koenig 2015	132	RCT*	religiously integrated cognitive behavioral therapy	adherence	no association
Anxiety	Rosmarin 2010	125	randomized controlled evaluation	spiritually integrated treatment	perceptions of treatment, treatment completion	positive
	Huguelet 2011	78	RCT	traditional treatment and a religious and spiritual assessment	treatment compliance	no association, better attendance
	Huguelet 2006	100	survey	religious beliefs	Synergy with psychiatric care	no association
	Caqueo-Urízar A 2015	253	survey	religious beliefs about causes of schizophrenia	medication attitudes	negative
Schizophrenia	Mohr 2012	276	survey	religious coping	compatibility with psychiatric treatment	positive
	McCann 2008	81	survey	religious beliefs/activities	neuroleptic taking	no association
	Kirov 1998	52	survey	religious faith after psychosis	compliance	positive
	Borras 2007	103	survey	religious and spiritual activities	blood level of the drug	negative
	D'Souza 2004	2	case series	SACBT (spirituality augmented)	treatment collaboration/relapse rate	positive
	Krentzman 2013	364	cohort	spirituality dimensions	AA participation	positive
	Kelly 2011	1726	cohort	spirituality religiousness	AA attendance	positive
	Arnold 2002	68	survey	spirituality	expectations/perceptions	positive
Addiction	Brown 2001	71	cohort	measures of religiosity	attendance	no association
	Stahler 2007	18	RCT	Church communities	treatment retention	positive
	Chi 2009	357	cohort	12-step/religiosity co-variate	abstinence	positive
	Margolin 2006	72	controlled study	3-S (Spiritual Self Schema therapy)	motivation for HIV prevention	positive
	Christo 1995	101	cohort	spiritual beliefs	NA (narcotics anonymous) attendance	no association
Mental Illness	Foulks 1986	60	cohort	patients' beliefs	compliance	no association

* RCT- Randomised Clinical Trial.

When stratified according to study design, the list eligible publications included 4 randomized studies, 1 controlled study, 4 cohort studies, 7 surveys, and 1 case series.

3.2. Interventions and/or Outcome Measures

Few studies were R/S intervention studies, and majority of papers address R/S as an influencing variable. The subset of experimental studies included a clinical trial in depression, randomized controlled evaluation in anxiety, randomized clinical trial in schizophrenia, community trial in cocaine addiction, and controlled study in drug users, one each.

The list of evaluated interventions included religiously integrated cognitive behavioral therapy that used patient's religious beliefs to identify and replace unhelpful thoughts and behaviors, in order to reduce depressive symptoms. Other spiritual approaches to intervention were spiritually integrated treatment including reading inspiring stories and excerpts from Jewish religious literature (study of anxiety in a Jewish community) and spiritual assessment by a psychiatrist followed by guidance and advice from a psychologist of religion (in schizophrenia patients). One study used spirituality-focused intervention based on a Buddhist framework. In another study, Bridges intervention consisting of interactions between church community and local activists or mentors was evaluated in a group of cocaine-dependent black women.

Non-experimental studies dealt with various measures or dimensions of spirituality/religiosity. Some studies involved specific validated questionnaires ("Multidimensional Measurement of Religiousness or Spirituality for Use in Health Research", "Religious Coping Index", "Spiritual Beliefs Questionnaire") or ad hoc semi-structured interviews developed by the authors. In a study of alcohol dependence, spirituality/religiousness were assessed with Religious Background and Behavior instrument. Other studies used some simple measures of spirituality/religiousness, such as the involvement in religious/spiritual activities or spiritual beliefs regarding the causes of mental illness ("magical-religious causes").

3.3. Outcomes and Associations

The list of eligible studies included only one randomized trial analyzing treatment adherence in depression. In this study, more religious patients presented with better adherence and had better treatment outcomes. Religiosity was shown to interact with treatment type: religiously-integrated CBT (RBCT) turned out to be slightly more effective in religious participants; also adherence to RCBT in this group was somehow better than in other study subjects (85.7% vs. 65.9%, $p = 0.10$) (20). Importantly, better adherence was not related to the intervention, but resulted from baseline intergroup differences in religiosity levels.

In a single randomized study of patients with anxiety, individuals subjected to spirituality-integrated treatment (SIT) reported higher levels of belief in treatment credibility, had greater expectations from treatment, and were more likely to complete the therapy than the controls offered progressive muscle relaxation (PMR) (35).

Only few eligible studies analyzed the effects of religion on medication compliance in schizophrenia. Noticeably, religious beliefs either exerted no effect or even negatively affected treatment adherence in patients with this condition.

In one clinical trial, schizophrenia patients were subjected to a spiritual assessment conducted by a psychiatrist, followed by a guidance and advice from a psychologist of religion. Although three months later, medication compliance and satisfaction with care in this group were similar as in the controls, the intervention contributed to significantly better appointment attendance during the follow-up period (15).

The authors of six surveys analyzed religious determinants of medication compliance in schizophrenia patients. Only few among one hundred individuals with this condition considered religious practice to be incompatible with treatment (16). However, this study did not provide sufficient evidence to support the role or religious beliefs as a determinant of better adherence. It showed only the neutral attitude among religious patients towards medication use. In only one study, medication compliance was determined not only based on the interview, but also through a systematic monitoring of drug levels in patients' blood. The study showed that religious representations of illness were more prominent in non-adherent subjects (2). Also a survey of 276 outpatients with a DSM-IV diagnosis of schizophrenia or schizoaffective disorder demonstrated that religion may sometimes interfere with psychiatric treatment (29).

Another study analyzed opinions on the causes of schizophrenia in 253 patients with this condition and in their caregivers. Stronger magical-religious beliefs turned out to be associated with higher incidence of positive symptoms and less favorable attitudes to pharmacotherapy. Patients' belief system turned out to be a significant predictor of medication attitude. Furthermore, a significant correlation was found between the medication attitudes and PANSS scores, which points to a likely link between treatment compliance and symptom severity (4). However, a small study of 81 patients with schizophrenia did not demonstrate an association between the level of involvement in religious or spiritual practices and medication compliance (28). In another study, 61% out of 52 patients used religion to cope with their psychotic illness. Importantly, these patients had a better insight into their disease, and were more compliant with antipsychotic therapy (19).

Finally, according to one published case report, a 56-year-old woman with psychotic depression re-involved in her life and showed complete treatment adherence after participation in a spiritually augmented cognitive behavioral therapy (SACBT) (8).

A better quality evidence originates from the research on addictions, as these studies included substantially larger number of participants, and typically (in 7 out of 8 studies) had a longitudinal design. In a controlled study analyzing the effects of spirituality-focused intervention in drug users, better treatment compliance was associated with greater involvement in spiritual practices and stronger motivation to prevent HIV infection. Moreover, participation in Spiritual Self Schema (3-S) therapy and stronger motivation to prevent HIV infection turned out to be associated with lower prevalence of HIV-risk behaviors (26).

In the largest of analyzed studies, involving a total of 1726 subjects with alcohol use disorders, participation in Alcoholic Anonymous (AA) meetings exerted a significant effect on future drinking outcomes, which was partially explained by an association between the involvement in AA movement and higher levels of spirituality/religiousness. This study has controlled confounding variables and found that "attending AA was associated with increases in spiritual practices" and that alcohol outcomes were "partially mediated by increases in spirituality". This implies that spirituality/religiousness may serve as a mechanism of AA-related change and contribute to better attendance in AA meetings (18). In another 18-month longitudinal study of 364 alcohol addicts, spiritual orientation was identified as an important aspect of recovery and a determinant of better treatment adherence (22). Further, a small preliminary study of 18 cocaine-dependent black women assigned randomly to Bridges treatment or standard residential therapy alone, demonstrated that the former approach was associated with significantly better treatment retention at six months (75% vs. 20%, as assessed by urinalysis) (36).

The results of a study conducted among 357 adolescents with chemical dependence imply that religious service attendance might exert a mediating effect on the relationship between post-treatment 12-Step affiliation (TSA) and 3-year outcomes (5). However, frequent religious service attendance was shown to mediate solely the relationship between TSA and drug abstinence, and exerted no effect on the association between TSA and alcohol abstinence.

In a small study of 71 patients participating in Narcotics Anonymous and/or AA meetings, frequent attenders did not differ from infrequent attenders and non-attenders in terms of their religiosity measures (3). However, a study of 101 drug users identified spiritual beliefs as a predictor of regular participation in Narcotics Anonymous (NA) meetings (6). In another, smaller study, the vast majority of 47 HIV-positive drug users declared their interest in receiving spirituality-focused treatment, and believed that combined with medical recommendations, this form of intervention may help them to reduce craving and HIV-risk behaviors, as well as to promote hopefulness (1).

The review paper included in the analysis referred to a study analyzing the role of patients' beliefs as a determinant of partial adherence to antipsychotic medications (27). Unfortunately, authors of this study did not specify the exact psychiatric diagnosis established in their participants, other than mentioning that they examined the subjects "treated in the outpatient psychiatric clinic". Nevertheless, the study did not show an association between patients' beliefs and medication compliance (9).

4. Discussion

This review showed that published evidence documenting the effects of religiosity on medication compliance in mental illness is quite limited.

The effects of religious interventions or religious exposure on treatment adherence vary depending on an underlying mental illness. While religious beliefs were associated with poor compliance in schizophrenia patients, spiritual orientation turned out to be an important aspect of recovery from addiction and a determinant of better treatment adherence in individuals with substance dependence. Better medication compliance was also observed in more religious patients with depression or anxiety, but available evidence is too limited for any ultimate conclusions in this matter.

Published evidence suggests that religious and spiritual interventions (RSI) may alleviate stress, alcoholism and depression. RCTs documented additional beneficial effects of RSI, among them attenuation of clinical symptoms (11). More religious persons seem to be more likely to involve in disease-screening practices and comply better with prescribed medical treatments (21). However, our review suggests that the same does not apply to individuals with mental illness.

4.1. Treatment Adherence in Schizophrenia

The lack of association or even an inverse relationship between religiosity and medication compliance seem to be particularly evident in schizophrenia patients. This points to an important role of insight in the context of mental illness. Relative lack of the insight may contribute to worse adherence (30). The term "insight" refers to patient's ability to recognize that his/her symptoms are associated with a mental illness and as such require an appropriate treatment. Lack of the insight is known to be associated with impaired cognitive function, and to predict poor medication compliance. This may be particularly challenging in psychotic patients in whom lack of the insight may interfere with both treatment and religious attitudes. Patients' opinion about the etiology of their mental disease usually reflects their general worldview, and not infrequently is also influenced by religious beliefs. Some more religious patients may accept a personalistic explanation of their illness, and believe that either its etiology or treatment extend beyond a natural world and involve some supernatural forces. Lack of the insight may dramatically alter medication compliance in patients with psychotic symptoms. Religion is often entangled in neurotic and psychotic disorders, and the content of delusions may be related to one's religious beliefs. Delusions may help to cope with some negative life events; however, they are often referred to as false beliefs, and probably do not produce a favorable effect in a longer perspective. Some proportion of people may experience psychotic symptoms, including auditory hallucinations. Such persons, especially more religious subjects, will probably try to make sense of these experiences; however, such religious delusions may negatively influence medication compliance.

4.2. Treatment Adherence in Addiction

The vast majority of identified studies of addictions demonstrated beneficial effects of religion and spirituality on treatment adherence. Most treatment protocols were based on 12-step programs and participation in AA meetings, i.e., therapeutic modalities in which spiritual elements constitute an integral component. Application of religious and spiritual issues to the therapy of addictions is relatively easy, owing moral aspects of substance abuse and important role of patient's will power as a determinant of persistent abstinence. Religion provides arguments against substance abuse, and gives motivation to involve in other activities than the addiction. Participants of the studies included in this review did not suffer from other mental comorbidities, and their cognitive skills and insight enabled them to rationally self-evaluate their situation and to continue the therapy. Therefore, inclusion of religious issues in therapeutic programs produced a beneficial effect in form of treatment retention.

4.3. Treatment Adherence in Depression and Anxiety

Only a limited number of studies dealing with depression and anxiety-related disorders satisfied criteria of this review. Although many previous studies analyzed the effects of spirituality and religiousness on treatment outcomes in depression, only one centered around a clearly defined level of treatment adherence (20). This randomized study demonstrated that beneficial effect of patient's religiosity is independent of a religious intervention; more religious patients benefited more form the therapy, showed higher levels of treatment adherence and better treatment retention. However, unless adjusted for patient's religiosity, treatment adherence levels in individuals subjected to religious (RCBT) and conventional therapy (CCBT) were essentially the same. Similar to depression, we have identified only one randomized study analyzing the effect of Internet-based therapy in individuals with subclinical anxiety. The study showed that the proportion of patients who completed a religious therapy was significantly higher than the percentage of subjects who fully adhered to a conventional treatment (35).

4.4. Quality of Evidence

Published evidence documenting beneficial effects of religiosity on treatment adherence is quite limited. Heterogeneity of patient populations and limitations in the study types made this review particularly challenging. Among all 19 eligible studies, there were only four in which the subjects were randomized to intervention. Experimental studies had a pilot character, included a small number of subjects (between 18 and 132), and were aimed at preliminary assessment of intervention outcomes. Randomized studies in schizophrenia and depression demonstrated that religiosity/spirituality had no effect on treatment adherence. We may conclude, then, if treatment compliance in schizophrenia and depression is related to religiosity and spirituality, it can't be influenced through intervention. While a few studies analyzed medication compliance, only one monitored blood level of the drug (15; 29; 28; 2). All these studies included patients with schizophrenia, i.e., condition in which medication compliance is of vital importance. In the study which analyzed blood level of the drug, an inverse relationship was found between religiosity and medication compliance (2). Studies of patients with addictions, including between 357 and 1,726 subjects, were the largest sources of evidence for this review (18; 22; 25). These studies were based on a 12-step program for recovery from addiction, including spiritual elements; participation in this form of intervention apparently stimulated involvement of patients in religious activities. This with no doubt hindered the analysis of a temporal relationship between religiosity and treatment outcomes. It is unclear if participation in AA therapy promoted religiousness, or it was religiousness which facilitated achieving desired therapeutic effects. Probably, both these mechanisms may be involved (10).

4.5. Limitations

Another important limitation of this study is heterogeneity of S/R measures. Whilst religiosity is relatively straight-forward to measure, spirituality is more difficult. The question of whether spirituality can be subjected to scientific research methodologies should be raised here. We did not differentiate spirituality from religion in this review. There are differences between attitudes and convictions on the one hand (belief in God, centrality, etc.) and engagement in S/R practices (church attendance, praying, meditation, etc.) on the other. Spiritual interventions can utilize the power of prayer and meditation, coping and transcendence, while religious approaches include specific traditions of Christians and Jews, conducted in pastoral services and therapeutic models. There are some aspects in philosophy and values of AA meetings that are not necessarily "spiritual". Looking for the strength to remain abstinent leads to healthier way of life that shares some common values with R/S but it is not spirituality itself.

5. Conclusions

This systematic review demonstrated that religiosity may influence treatment adherence in mental illness. With no doubt, inclusion of religious and spiritual components produces the most beneficial effects in the treatment of addictions. However, involvement of religiosity does not necessarily stimulate treatment adherence in patients with psychotic disorders and schizophrenia, and may even affect it negatively in the case of individuals with delusional interpretation of their illness etiology. There is no good quality evidence that religion may influence better compliance through intervention. Inclusion of religiosity and spirituality may be however necessary in the case of some patients with depression and anxiety, as it stimulates adherence, which eventually contributes to better treatment outcomes. These findings should motivate therapists and psychiatrists to routinely consider religiosity in treatment plans for their patients.

Acknowledgments: This work was supported by the Medical University of Gdansk (grant no.ST-20).

Author Contributions: Pawel Zagozdzon was responsible for the conception and design of the work, data analysis, interpretation and writing. Both authors Pawel Zagozdzon and Magdalena Wrotkowska contributed equally to literature search and data collection. Magdalena Wrotkowska was responsible for figures and bibliography for the article.

Conflicts of Interest: Pawel Zagozdzon and Magdalena Wrotkowska declared that there were no conflicts of interest in relation to the subject of this study.

References

1. Arnold, Ruth M., S. Kelly Avants, Arthur Margolin, and David Marcotte. 2002. Patient Attitudes Concerning the Inclusion of Spirituality into Addiction Treatment. *Journal of Substance Abuse Treatment* 23: 319–26. [CrossRef]
2. Borras, Laurence, S. Mohr, P.-Y. Brandt, C. Gilliéron, A. Eytan, and P. Huguelet. 2007. Religious Beliefs in Schizophrenia: Their Relevance for Adherence to Treatment. *Schizophrenia Bulletin* 33: 1238–46. [CrossRef] [PubMed]
3. Brown, Barry S., Kevin E. O'Grady, Eugene V. Farrell, Ilene S. Flechner, and David N. Nurco. 2001. Factors Associated with Frequency of 12-Step Attendance by Drug Abuse Clients. *The American Journal of Drug and Alcohol Abuse* 27: 147–60. [CrossRef] [PubMed]
4. Caqueo-Urízar, Alejandra, Laurent Boyer, Karine Baumstarck, and Stephen E. Gilman. 2015. The Relationships between Patients' and Caregivers' Beliefs about the Causes of Schizophrenia and Clinical Outcomes in Latin American Countries. *Psychiatry Research* 229: 440–46. [CrossRef] [PubMed]
5. Chi, Felicia W., Lee A. Kaskutas, Stacy Sterling, Cynthia I. Campbell, and Constance Weisner. 2009. Twelve-Step Affiliation and 3-Year Substance Use Outcomes among Adolescents: Social Support and Religious Service Attendance as Potential Mediators. *Addiction (Abingdon, England)* 104: 927–39. [CrossRef] [PubMed]
6. Christo, George, and Christine Franey. 1995. Drug Users' Spiritual Beliefs, Locus of Control and the Disease Concept in Relation to Narcotics Anonymous Attendance and Six-Month Outcomes. *Drug and Alcohol Dependence* 38: 51–56. [CrossRef]
7. Cramer, Joyce A., and Robert Rosenheck. 1998. Compliance with Medication Regimens for Mental and Physical Disorders. *Psychiatric Services (Washington, D.C.)* 49: 196–201. [CrossRef] [PubMed]
8. D'Souza, Russell F., and Angelo Rodrigo. 2004. Spiritually Augmented Cognitive Behavioural Therapy. *Australasian Psychiatry: Bulletin of Royal Australian and New Zealand College of Psychiatrists* 12: 148–52. [CrossRef] [PubMed]
9. Foulks, Edward F., J. B. Persons, and R. L. Merkel. 1986. The Effect of Patients' Beliefs about Their Illnesses on Compliance in Psychotherapy. *The American Journal of Psychiatry* 143: 340–44. [CrossRef] [PubMed]
10. Galanter, Marc, Helen Dermatis, Gregory Bunt, Caroline Williams, Manuel Trujillo, and Paul Steinke. 2007. Assessment of Spirituality and Its Relevance to Addiction Treatment. *Journal of Substance Abuse Treatment* 33: 257–64. [CrossRef] [PubMed]

11. Gonçalves, Juliane P. B., G. Lucchetti, P. R. Menezes, and H. Vallada. 2015. Religious and Spiritual Interventions in Mental Health Care: A Systematic Review and Meta-Analysis of Randomized Controlled Clinical Trials. *Psychological Medicine* 45: 2937–49. [CrossRef] [PubMed]

12. Haynes, R. Brian, David L. Sackett, D. Wayne Taylor, R. S. Roberts, and A. L. Johnson. 1977. Manipulation of the Therapeutic Regimen to Improve Compliance: Conceptions and Misconceptions. *Clinical Pharmacology and Therapeutics* 22: 125–30. [CrossRef] [PubMed]

13. Holzinger, Anita, Watter Loffler, Peter Muller, Stefan Priebe, and Matthias C. Angermeyer. 2002. Subjective Illness Theory and Antipsychotic Medication Compliance by Patients with Schizophrenia. *The Journal of Nervous and Mental Disease* 190: 597–603. [CrossRef] [PubMed]

14. Huguelet, Philippe, and Koenig Harold. 2009. Introduction: Key Concepts. In *Religion and Spirituality in Psychiatry*, 1st ed. Cambridge: Cambridge University Press, pp. 1–4.

15. Huguelet, Philippe, Sylvia Mohr, Carine Betrisey, Laurence Borras, Christiane Gillieron, Adham Mancini Marie, Isabelle Rieben, Nader Perroud, and Pierre-Yves Brandt. 2011. A Randomized Trial of Spiritual Assessment of Outpatients with Schizophrenia: Patients' and Clinicians' Experience. *Psychiatric Services (Washington, D.C.)* 62: 79–86. [CrossRef] [PubMed]

16. Huguelet, Philippe, Sylvia Mohr, Laurence Borras, Christiane Gillieron, and Pierre-Yves Brandt. 2006. Spirituality and Religious Practices among Outpatients with Schizophrenia and Their Clinicians. *Psychiatric Services (Washington, D.C.)* 57: 366–72. [CrossRef] [PubMed]

17. Van Rensburg, ABR Janse, C. P. H. Myburgh, C. P. Szabo, and M. Poggenpoel. 2013. The Role of Spirituality in Specialist Psychiatry: A Review of the Medical Literature. *African Journal of Psychiatry* 16: 247–55. [CrossRef]

18. Kelly, John F., Robert L. Stout, Molly Magill, J. Scott Tonigan, and Maria E. Pagano. 2011. Spirituality in Recovery: A Lagged Mediational Analysis of Alcoholics Anonymous' Principal Theoretical Mechanism of Behavior Change. *Alcoholism, Clinical and Experimental Research* 35: 454–63. [CrossRef] [PubMed]

19. Kirov, George, R. Kemp, K. Kirov, and A. S. David. 1998. Religious Faith after Psychotic Illness. *Psychopathology* 31: 234–45. [CrossRef] [PubMed]

20. Koenig, Harold G., Michelle J. Pearce, Bruce Nelson, Sally F. Shaw, Clive J. Robins, Noha S. Daher, Harvey Jay Cohen, L. S. Berk, D. L. Bellinger, K. I. Pargament, and et al. 2015. Religious vs. Conventional Cognitive Behavioral Therapy for Major Depression in Persons with Chronic Medical Illness: A Pilot Randomized Trial. *The Journal of Nervous and Mental Disease* 203: 243–51. [CrossRef] [PubMed]

21. Koenig, Harold, Dana King, and Verna B. Carson. 2012. Psychological, Social, and Behavioral Pathways. In *Handbook of Religion and Health*, 2nd ed. Oxford and New York: Oxford University Press, pp. 579–99.

22. Krentzman, Amy R., James A. Cranford, and Elizabeth A. R. Robinson. 2013. Multiple Dimensions of Spirituality in Recovery: A Lagged Mediational Analysis of Alcoholics Anonymous' Principal Theoretical Mechanism of Behavior Change. *Substance Abuse* 34: 20–32. [CrossRef] [PubMed]

23. Lacro, Jonathan P., Laura B. Dunn, Christian R. Dolder, Susan G. Leckband, and Dilip V. Jeste. 2002. Prevalence of and Risk Factors for Medication Nonadherence in Patients with Schizophrenia: A Comprehensive Review of Recent Literature. *The Journal of Clinical Psychiatry* 63: 892–909. [CrossRef] [PubMed]

24. Lieberman, Jeffrey A., Brian Sheitman, Miranda Chakos, Delbert Robinson, Nina Schooler, and Sam Keith. 1998. The Development of Treatment Resistance in Patients with Schizophrenia: A Clinical and Pathophysiologic Perspective. *Journal of Clinical Psychopharmacology* 18: 20S–4S. [CrossRef]

25. Lin, Shuai-Ting, Cheng-Chung Chen, Hin-Yeung Tsang, Chee-Siong Lee, Pinchen Yang, Kai-Da Cheng, Dian-Jeng Li, Chin-Jen Wang, Yung-Chi Hsieh, and Wei-Cheng Yang. 2014. Association between Antipsychotic Use and Risk of Acute Myocardial Infarction: A Nationwide Case-Crossover Study. *Circulation* 130: 235–43. [CrossRef] [PubMed]

26. Margolin, Arthur, Mark Beitel, Zev Schuman-Olivier, and S. Kelly Avants. 2006. A Controlled Study of a Spirituality-Focused Intervention for Increasing Motivation for HIV Prevention among Drug Users. *AIDS Education and Prevention: Official Publication of the International Society for AIDS Education* 18: 311–22. [CrossRef] [PubMed]

27. Masand, Prakash S., Miquel Roca, Martin S. Turner, and John M. Kane. 2009. Partial Adherence to Antipsychotic Medication Impacts the Course of Illness in Patients with Schizophrenia: A Review. *Primary Care Companion to the Journal of Clinical Psychiatry* 11: 147–54. [CrossRef] [PubMed]

28. McCann, Terence V., Cecil Deans, Eileen Clark, and Sai Lu. 2008. A Comparative Study of Antipsychotic Medication Taking in People with Schizophrenia. *International Journal of Mental Health Nursing* 17: 428–38. [CrossRef] [PubMed]

29. Mohr, Sylvia, Laurence Borras, Jennifer Nolan, Christiane Gillieron, Pierre-Yves Brandt, Ariel Eytan, Claude Leclerc, Nader Perroud, Kathryn Whetten, and Carl Pieper. 2012. Spirituality and Religion in Outpatients with Schizophrenia: A Multi-Site Comparative Study of Switzerland, Canada, and the United States. *International Journal of Psychiatry in Medicine* 44: 29–52. [CrossRef] [PubMed]

30. Mutsatsa, Stan H., E. M. Joyce, S. B. Hutton, E. Webb, H. Gibbins, S. Paul, and T. R. E. Barnes. 2003. Clinical Correlates of Early Medication Adherence: West London First Episode Schizophrenia Study. *Acta Psychiatrica Scandinavica* 108: 439–46. [CrossRef] [PubMed]

31. Olfson, Mark, David Mechanic, Stephen Hansell, Carol A. Boyer, James Walkup, and Peter J. Weiden. 2000. Predicting Medication Noncompliance After Hospital Discharge Among Patients With Schizophrenia. *Psychiatric Services* 51: 216–22. [CrossRef] [PubMed]

32. O Sarri, Katerina, Siobhan Higgins, and Anthony G. Kafatos. 2005. Are Religions "Healthy"? A Review on Religious Recommendations on Diet and Lifestyle. *Human Ecology Special Issue* 14: 7–20.

33. Pargament, Kenneth I., and James W. Lomax. 2013. Understanding and Addressing Religion among People with Mental Illness. *World Psychiatry: Official Journal of the World Psychiatric Association (WPA)* 12: 26–32. [CrossRef] [PubMed]

34. Perkins, D. O. 2002. Predictors of noncompliance in patients with schizophrenia. *Journal of Clinical Psychiatry* 63: 1121–28.

35. Rosmarin, David H., Kenneth I. Pargament, Steven Pirutinsky, and Annette Mahoney. 2010. A Randomized Controlled Evaluation of a Spiritually Integrated Treatment for Subclinical Anxiety in the Jewish Community, Delivered via the Internet. *Journal of Anxiety Disorders* 24: 799–808. [CrossRef] [PubMed]

36. Stahler, Gerald J., Kimberly C. Kirby, and MaryLouise E. Kerwin. 2007. A Faith-Based Intervention for Cocaine-Dependent Black Women. *Journal of Psychoactive Drugs* 39: 183–90. [CrossRef] [PubMed]

37. Wyatt, Richard Jed. 1991. Neuroleptics and the Natural Course of Schizophrenia. *Schizophrenia Bulletin* 17: 325–51. [CrossRef] [PubMed]

38. Zivin, Kara, and Helen C. Kales. 2008. Adherence to Depression Treatment in Older Adults: A Narrative Review. *Drugs & Aging* 25: 559–71.

39. Zolnierek, Kelly B. Haskard, and M. Robin Dimatteo. 2009. Physician Communication and Patient Adherence to Treatment: A Meta-Analysis. *Medical Care* 47: 826–34. [CrossRef] [PubMed]

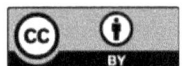

Chapter 3
Health Care Professionals and Spirituality

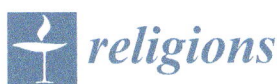

Conference Report

Spiritual Care Education of Health Care Professionals

Donia Baldacchino [1,2,3]

[1] Faculty of Health Sciences, University of Malta, Msida MSD 2090, Malta; donia.baldacchino@um.edu.mt;
Tel.: +356-2340-1847

[2] Department of Nursing, University of South Wales, Pontypridd Rhondda Cynon Taff CF37 4BE, Wales, UK

[3] Department of Nursing, Johns Hopkins University, Baltimore, MD 21218, USA

Academic Editors: Arndt Büssing and Hefti René
Received: 2 February 2015; Accepted: 16 April 2015; Published: 8 May 2015

Abstract: Nurses and health care professionals should have an active role in meeting the spiritual needs of patients in collaboration with the family and the chaplain. Literature criticizes the impaired holistic care because the spiritual dimension is often overlooked by health care professionals. This could be due to feelings of incompetence due to lack of education on spiritual care; lack of inter-professional education (IPE); work overload; lack of time; different cultures; lack of attention to personal spirituality; ethical issues and unwillingness to deliver spiritual care. Literature defines spiritual care as recognizing, respecting, and meeting patients' spiritual needs; facilitating participation in religious rituals; communicating through listening and talking with clients; *being with* the patient by caring, supporting, and showing empathy; promoting a sense of well-being by helping them to find meaning and purpose in their illness and overall life; and referring them to other professionals, including the chaplain/pastor. This paper outlines the systematic mode of intra-professional theoretical education on spiritual care and its integration into their clinical practice; supported by role modeling. Examples will be given from the author's creative and innovative ways of teaching spiritual care to undergraduate and post-graduate students. The essence of spiritual care is *being* in *doing* whereby personal spirituality and therapeutic use of self contribute towards effective holistic care. While taking into consideration the factors that may inhibit and enhance the delivery of spiritual care, recommendations are proposed to the education, clinical, and management sectors for further research and personal spirituality to ameliorate patient holistic care.

Keywords: spiritual care; holistic care; education; Benner's Theory; Kolb's Theory; ASSET model; role modeling; students; health care professionals; intra/inter-professional education

---

1. Introduction

The International Council of Nurses (ICN) Code of Ethics ([1], p. 5) specifies the nurse's role of promoting "an environment in which the human rights, values, customs and spiritual beliefs of the individual, family and community are respected". The Malta Code of Ethics supports this for nurses and midwives [2], stating that the nurse is to "recognize and respect the uniqueness of every patient/client's biological, psychological, social and spiritual status and needs". Since patients are attended by different members of the multi-disciplinary team, these codes of ethics also address the holistic care of health care professionals that contribute towards patients' safety. Examples of some heroes in nursing are given, whereby, their *being* in care generated signs of spirituality in their attempts to address patients' needs, while their caring attitude instilled hope and healing.

Nightingale [3] proposed that the environment should do no harm to patients. In this paper, the environment is provided by the presence of nurses and health care professionals, including the ward management personnel who attempt to deliver care holistically. Patients' safety may be achieved by individualized spiritual care, whereby care is given according to the patients' biological, psychological, social, cultural, and spiritual needs [4]. Mary Seacole (1805–1881) nursed sick soldiers in the Crimean War so kindly that she was known as "Mother Seacole". Mary was exposed to prejudice and racism, as her mother was from the Caribbean island of Jamaica and her father was Scottish. However, courageously, Mary made her own way in the world, as a single woman and as a person of mixed race. Mary mixed medicine with kindness and thus she is an admired role model to nurses and health caregivers [5]. Elisabeth Cadwa-ladyr from Wales volunteered to nurse sick soldiers in the Crimean War with Florence Nightingale in 1854. Betsy was devoutly religious and the small Welsh Bible, given to her when she was young, remained her "constant companion" and appeared to help her overcome the disappointments of her distorted plans in life and accept her situation in life [6].

During the last twenty-five years, care of patients has been criticized for neglecting the spiritual dimension in patient care [7]. This may be due to various reasons such as, secularization of contemporary society, unwillingness to deliver spiritual care, lack of time, work overload, feelings of incompetence to deliver spiritual care, lack of education in undergraduate and post-graduate curricula, and lack of inter-professional education, which generate omission of spiritual care [8–10]. Additionally, the medical model addresses primarily the illness of the patient and its progress to cure, while overlooking the religious and spiritual needs, and, consequently, threatens holistic care.

2. Definition of Spirituality in Illness

Spirituality is derived from the Latin word *spiritus*; *spirit* is the important part of the person that controls the mind, and the mind controls the body [11]. Religion may shed light on the interpretation of this spirit. For example, as a Roman Catholic person, I relate this spirit to the spirit of God within me, which gives me life day by day. Spirituality is also the power within a person that motivates that person to find meaning, purpose, and fulfillment in life; suffering and death; and fosters hope for one's will to live [12]. It infers that spirituality is the vital life force that unifies all aspects of the human being, including the religious component [13].

However, spirituality goes beyond religious affiliation, as it strives for inspirations, meaning and purpose in life, even in those who do not believe in any god/higher power [14,15]. Consequently, spirituality applies to both believers and non-believers, including the presence of different cultural and religious beliefs. Thus, when a person is more in tune with the vital, unifying, life force of the spiritual dimension, a will gain a more balanced state of physical, mental and social well-being, as a result [16].

3. Definition of Spiritual Care

Spiritual care is part of the art of nursing and professional care [17]. Spiritual care is defined by the literature as recognizing, respecting, and meeting patients' spiritual needs; facilitating participation in religious rituals; communicating through listening and talking with clients; *being with* the patient by caring, supporting, and showing empathy; promoting a sense of well-being by helping them to find meaning and purpose in their illness and overall life; and referring them to other professionals, including chaplains/pastors [18]. The outcome of spiritual care was found to enable patients to count their blessings in life, achieve inner peace and explore coping strategies to overcome obstacles during illness and crisis situations [19–21]. Spiritual care may also help patients to find a new equilibrium in faith by re-conceptualizing the self as one who is known and loved by God in the context of their specific illness [22,23].

The essence of spiritual care is *being* rather than simply *doing* [24]. Thus, therapeutic use of self is of utmost importance [25]. The role of the multidisciplinary team is to help patients find meaning in illness and purpose in life with a positive outlook to life and/or afterlife. Thus, in spiritual care it is not merely the delivery of care that matters, but it also includes the *heart and the spirit* by which holistic care is given [26].

In order to address spiritual needs both in health and in illness, competences are needed to guide the education of the health care professionals.

Religions **2015**, *6*, 594–613

4. Aim

The aim of this paper is to present the theories and methods of clinical education on spiritual care of health care professionals and students, and outline the dimensions of spiritual leadership to sustain the learning process.

5. Competences in Spiritual Care

The Nursing and Midwifery Council (NMC) in the UK [27] in line with the European Qualifications Framework (EQF) [28] defines competence as "the proven ability to use knowledge, skills and personal, social and/or methodological abilities in the work or study situations and in professional and personal development" ([28], p. 11) referred to as "responsibility and autonomy" ([28], p. 11).

Benner's Theory "From Novice to Expert" [29] defined nursing competency as the ability to perform a task with desirable outcomes under the varied circumstances of the real world. Benner placed competence in the middle of the continuum ranging from: novice to advanced beginner, to competent, to proficient, to expert. Competent practitioners are consciously able to plan their actions, but lack flexibility and speed [30]. The practitioner is described as "tolerably good but less than expert" because when practitioners are considered competent, they would still have something more to achieve for them to reach the level of proficiency and expertise [31]. This is highly applicable to the education of health care professionals. While considering the characteristics of the students who are undertaking the nursing, medical and paramedical education programs, who are young, with a lack of personal life experiences and with minimum attention to spiritual issues in life, it is very important not only to equip students with loads of *information*, but also attention needs to be given to their personal *formation* as spiritual individuals, who find meaning and purpose in their profession, and to help them develop the necessary skills and attitudes across their education programs in class and in the clinical practice. This process will contribute towards *transformation* into a professional health care *being* who becomes *responsible* and *accountable* for holistic patient care *including* the spiritual dimension of care.

Students and health care professionals need to achieve competence, *i.e.*, acquiring knowledge, skills and attitudes. Spiritual care competence is defined as an *active* ongoing process characterized by three interrelated elements which involve a growing awareness of one's value, developing an empathic understanding of the client's world view and the ability to implement individualized interventions appropriate to each client [32].

Research on competences in spiritual care is growing. An exploratory study in Malta that collected qualitative data from nurses, hospital and community chaplains as well as patients with heart attack revealed the following seven *generic* competences: integrating the individual person within the role of the nurse as a professional; assisting the search for meaning of illness and acceptance of illness; maintaining trustful relationship with patients and family; communicating with patients, inter-disciplinary team and clinical/educational Organizations; delivering spiritual care by the four stages of the nursing process that is, assessment, planning, implementation and evaluation; controlling ethical issues in care such as, confidentiality, data protection issues; and delivering holistic care [33].

These findings supported the three core themes derived from an extensive literature review which revealed *three core* domains of competences for spiritual care namely, awareness and use of self; spiritual dimensions of the nursing process (assessment, planning, implementation and evaluation of care); and assurance and quality expertise [34].

Research has shown that the strongest predictor for effective spiritual care is *personal* spirituality. *No one can give from what he/she does not possess.* This indicates the importance of maintaining the integrity between the individual person and the role of health care professionals to address and meet patients' needs holistically [35]. Therefore, health care professionals can both provide spiritual care and can also provide care spiritually [36]. Since, competence in professional practice incorporates knowledge, skills and attitudes with achievable outcomes [37], additional to knowledge, the *active* presence of the health care professional, that is *being* in *doing*, not simply *doing*, is needed to meet patients' spiritual needs and to generate the holistic doing of spiritual care. Therefore, the therapeutic use of self could be very helpful as it may enhance a trustful helping relationship.

Research recommends that health care professionals should take an *active* role in meeting patients' spiritual needs and not simply refer them to a chaplain [38]. However, it is argued that when patients need help in their *theological* beliefs and conflicts, then the chaplain, an expert with Clinical Pastoral Education should deliver this kind of specialized spiritual care [39]. Hence, the importance of considering the hospital chaplain/pastor as an important collaborator in the inter-disciplinary team [40], especially when prepared educationally for a chaplain's role [41].

While considering the importance of the responsibility of the health care professionals, research shows the concern of the nurses and health care professionals who consider themselves as incompetent to deliver spiritual care [42].

6. Education on Spiritual Care/Modes of Clinical Education on Spiritual Care

An overview of the theoretical and practical education on spiritual care is included based on a literature review following a literature search using the keywords: "spiritual care", "holistic care", "education", "Benner's Theory", "Kolb's Theory", "ASSET model", "role modelling", "students", "nurses", "health care professionals", and "intra/inter-professional education". Additionally, the author's teaching experience in Malta and in various foreign universities presented some examples of innovative teaching methods adopted to teach spirituality and spiritual care to undergraduate and post-graduate students. Spiritual care contributes towards holistic care, which demands a multi-disciplinary team approach to care, including the chaplain. This may be enhanced by intra- and inter-professional education on spiritual care as it may foster teamwork and team learning.

6.1. Intra-Professional and/or Inter-Professional Education on Spiritual Care

Intra-professional education is when students from different levels of education in the same profession are taught together. For example, currently, at the Faculty of Health Sciences in Malta, final year nursing students work in their clinical placements with first year students under the same mentor in preparation for the formative and summative clinical assessment. Feedback from both the first and final year students is generally very satisfactory and the intra-professional clinical experience is considered a rich learning opportunity. This experience supports project results in clinical simulation, which support intra-professional nursing student education [43].

Inter-professional education (IPE) is also known as multi-professional education, common learning, shared learning, and interdisciplinary learning [44]. Therefore, inter-professional education refers to students from different professions learning *from* each other, *with* each other, and *about* each other. The WHO-Study Group, consisting of 30 education, practice and policy experts, issued the WHO Framework for Action on Inter-professional Education and collaborative Practice [45]. The framework highlights:

- The current status of inter-professional collaboration around the world; identifies the mechanisms that shape successful collaborative teamwork; outlines a series of action items that policy makers can apply within their local health system; and
- Provides strategies and ideas that can help health policymakers implement the elements of inter-professional education and collaborative practice that will be most beneficial in their own jurisdiction.

The effectiveness of inter-professional education in enabling collaborative practice is still debatable. Some evidence was found by research studies on, for example 'death and dying learning' [46], and systematic reviews [47], and on the effectiveness in changing attitudes [48]. However, more longitudinal research is needed to identify the possible effects on service quality and patients' and service users' experiences.

Religions **2015**, *6*, 594–613

Inter-professional education (IPE) was also implemented to teach different professions, such as social workers and chaplains; also IPE was adopted on students from different professions such as medicine, nursing, chaplaincy and social work [49]. *Online* learning and interactive simulation modes of teaching were adopted. Educational programs on spiritual and cultural aspects of palliative care and spiritual assessment demonstrated that concepts of spirituality and basics of spiritual assessment may be taught and learned while students were found to develop an understanding and respect for the role of chaplains, social workers and physicians. Evaluation of these programs suggests that this innovative, inter-professional educational course may be transferable for use in other educational settings [50]. In addition to the physical presence of students together in class, *online forums* enable learners to discuss and outline the contribution of each discipline to spiritual care and holistic care of a patient case study. Thus, *online forums* may enhance understanding and appreciation of the precious contribution of each member of the interdisciplinary team to holistic care.

6.2. Areas Essential for Learning Spiritual Care

A literature review identified four main areas as essential for learning spiritual care:

a. importance of learning in *real-life* situations with repeated exposure to patients in the clinical placements supported by role modeling and mentorship;

b. use of pedagogical methods that assist students to understand, work with and reflect on patient's spirituality such as, reflective journals, written reflective accounts; writing care plans, which include spiritual interventions; role plays to practice spiritual assessment, including values, beliefs, and spiritual needs; group discussions on the relationship between religion, spirituality and health; analysis of case studies; reading literature and analyzing research on spirituality in illness and care;

c. awareness of and overcoming conditions inhibiting spiritual care learning, such as, lack of knowledge about spirituality; uncertainty about the health care professional's role in spiritual care; unawareness about one's own spirituality; having a different faith from that of the patient; incompetence in addressing spiritual needs; lack of role models; lack of time; and work overload; and

d. evaluation of students' spiritual care learning related to how students are prepared and how they are followed up after clinical studies by, for example, post clinical-reflection sessions; sharing of stories with fellow students, teachers and chaplains; supporting their learning by literature and research on spiritual care; reflective exercises and debriefing sessions to enhance safety of students and safe patient care' [51].

These are reflected in the ASSET Model for (Actioning Spirituality and Spiritual Care Education and Training) for teaching spiritual care [52].

The ASSET model incorporates a tripod of structure content, process of learning and outcome of education. First, the *structure content* encompasses self-awareness, spirituality and spiritual dimensions of care. Second, the *process* of teaching and learning incorporates experiential learning related to value clarification, holism, a broad perspective of spirituality, the four stages of the nursing process, and evaluation of teaching and learning. Third, the *outcome* of education, which is measured by value clarification, knowledge and competence in the delivery of spiritual care.

The foundation of this model lies on the importance of nurses' self-awareness about their *personal* spiritual beliefs, communication skills, and assessment procedures. Spirituality in this model has a Judeo-Christian perspective. However, it is argued that the present era of displaced individuals and refugees with different religions demands inclusion of other religions. Culture and interdisciplinary teamwork including the chaplain play an important role in this model.

Culture may challenge both the students and the educator. In summer 2013 and 2014, I was invited to teach various groups of students undertaking undergraduate courses such as nursing, psychology and tourism; and post-graduate students undertaking counseling, pastoral care, theology, and psychology programs at two Pontifical Catholic Universities in Parana' Brazil. Following analysis of the definition of the concept of spirituality to a group of forty five students undertaking BA Psychology, a student asked me, *"What has motivated you to tackle spirituality and spiritual care?"* Having a class of young students in a quite secularized class environment, I explained my personal spirituality regarding what gives me meaning and purpose in my life. This was oriented towards my Catholic religious background, my affiliation with the Society of Christian Education, and my clinical experience in Intensive Care Unit (ITU), and also my clinical care of an Arabic patient in a British hospital whose prayers calmed him down post-operatively [53]. At the end of the session, several young students shared with me *privately* their religious and/or their spiritual experiences in life. These sessions appeared to stimulate ten students, (six were aged 19–22 years; four were mature, over 23 years), to attend also the research group session because they wished to investigate spirituality in their research project.

Culture was again prominent in my teaching visit at the University of Pardubice, Czech Republic in 2014. It was interesting to note that a paramedic male student, aged 20 years asked me the same question! *"What motivated you to tackle spirituality and spiritual care?"* Having referred to my research findings on Maltese patients' spiritual coping strategies, of which some were religious coping, students with an atheistic background asked me *"Who is God?* What is the relationship between God's plans in life and 'destiny' and 'coincidence' in life?" These profound questions generated discussions across the whole week of my stay at the university.

Therefore, education of health care professionals should prepare students to recognize and act on spiritual cues; and build a trusting relationship and communicate respectfully and sensitively to patients to discover what is important to patients. Education should focus on holistic patient care with attention to spiritual and existential themes throughout the nursing program to help students integrate learning into the clinical practice [54].

Research could also be a medium of learning to explore the real experiences of patients and a resource of learning on spirituality in illness and care. Thus, the author tried to give the opportunity to patients with acute and chronic illness and healthcare professionals, consisting of hospital/community chaplains and qualified nurses working in medical and surgical wards, to participate in various research studies. While giving voice to patients and health care professionals, they contributed additional knowledge on the importance of spirituality and culture in care [55,56].

6.3. Integrating Theoretical Learning on Spiritual Care into the Clinical Practice

Literature review on how to develop a clinical learning culture emphasizes the importance of role model attitudes and behaviors of the health care professionals [57]. Role modeling in spiritual care is a concept that is still theoretical in nature because of various reasons, such as feelings of incompetence to deliver spiritual care and secularization of the contemporary society. It is argued that spiritual care may be "caught rather than taught" [58]. However, research shows that both theoretical teaching and clinical practice are needed in the education on spiritual care [59,60]. The clinical environment fosters integration of knowledge, clinical reasoning and formation of students [61]. Practice facilitates students' discovery of professional beliefs, values and attitudes and it assists them in integrating relevant knowledge and theories [62].

Experiential learning and *voluntary work* could also be a resource of learning for health care professionals [63]. As presented earlier on the inter-professional educational programs, core study units and organization of short- or long-term voluntary activities facilitate students from various disciplines to learn together and share their learning experiences. Optional study units at the University of Malta are open to all university students. However, timetables may clash with other study units rendering a limited mix of students.

Voluntary work may play an important role in students' learning in the form of community outreach. Voluntary work is acknowledged by the University of Malta Degree*Plus*. Thus, a study unit of 2 European Credits Transfer System (ECTS) on Spiritual Care for Health Caregivers (NUR3903) offers the students to do a minimum of five hours voluntary care in the community or accompany patients on a pilgrimage, such as to Lourdes in France. The experience of a group of seven students consisting of four nursing and three midwifery students was impressive! It was a means of self-reflection with enhancement of altruism. They confirmed the principle of *giving and receiving* as they were impressed by the patients' religious faith to travel so far to a sacred place, with an outcome of empowerment to cope with their illness [64].

Voluntary work also took the format of a health promotion activity to groups of adults, mostly older persons in the community by a small group of three to five undergraduate nursing students. The program consisted of students' delivery of a 20-minute Power Point presentation on preventive measures and care of diabetes or hypertension; and they answered the queries of the audience under the author's supervision or a parish nurse. The audience themselves were then asked to teach the group of students, by stating and interpreting proverbs or life principles of which spirituality was prominent. Finally, the blood pressure was measured by students on voluntary basis. Following the community outreach session, all students (average of 20 students) sit around and share their experiences using Gibb's Theory of Reflection [65]. Finally, a written reflective account formed part of the study unit assessment strategy where students reflected on such an inter-generational teaching and learning experience, which was usually a very positive experience.

This learning experience may take the format of a small group of three to four nursing students paying a visit to a family taking care of a person with terminal illness at home; or visiting an older person living alone at home while being supported by a relative/neighbor as an informal caregiver and/or community service. Such a learning experience on how the patient and family coped in their past and current life by the use of various religious and/or spiritual coping methods was usually interpreted by students as *"an experience which I will treasure for life"*.

These health promotion activities in the community were further extended to students' participation on a one-hour weekly radio program: *Il-Kuragg nofs il-Fejqan* (*Courage doubles the healing process*) on Radio Maria in Malta. A small group of three to four nursing students delivered a teaching session on health promotion in my presence and the author responded *live* to the public queries on telephone and text messages. This experience helped them to confirm the nurse's educational role in the community.

6.4. The Use of Arts in Identifying the Spiritual Dimension of the Role of the Nurse in Holistic Care

Towards the end of the introductory study units (NUR0118/NUR1116) for first year nursing students on foundations in nursing, they were invited to identify the spiritual dimension of the role of the nurse in providing holistic care by drawing their thoughts on a piece of white paper. A brief explanation was written by students on the back of the picture. This arts exercise helped them to explain and analyze the complexity of the spiritual dimension in holistic care. After three years that is, at the end of their nursing course program, a focus group of 12 nursing students discussed the differences they noticed between the perceived version and the observed real-life holistic care. This exercise enabled students to identify the preciousness and inaccuracies in the observed delivery of holistic care and the importance of addressing patients' spiritual needs to facilitate holistic care.

An experiential learning was conducted on first year students in their clinical placement with institutionalized older persons. Only few clients from each ward attend the activity center, leaving the majority of older persons passive, sitting all day, waiting for their meals to be served and perhaps waiting for someone to visit and communicate with them. On paying a visit to these students under the author's link-mentorship, students were found at the nurses' station discussing together the patients' documented care, which was also a learning resource for them. However, students could not understand the possible feelings of boredom and isolation experienced by older persons every day, day in day out, until they could pass through this experience.

Permission was granted by the respective hospital and ward administration and following individual's written consent, a group of fifteen first year nursing students were invited to experience an hour of *aloneness, segregated in a room alone for an hour* on the same day without having the wall clock. Using Kolb's Theory of experiential learning [66], each student stayed alone in a deserted room on their respective ward, coordinated by their respective mentor and the author. Each student was asked to enter the room without the uniform clock and without her/his mobile phone. During that hour, students were asked to reflect on their experience and write notes on a piece of paper. The majority of students experienced boredom due to lack of time orientation and communication system. They became frustrated as that hour was eternity for them. The common exclamation of students on coming out of that room was: *"how boring! Poor them!"* During the follow-up focus group discussion, this experience was applied to the older persons' aloneness on the ward and confirmed the importance of communication and activity exercises to help them live with dignity. Thus, transfer of knowledge appeared to be facilitated by this experiential learning session. A written reflective account of their critical experience was submitted as part of their clinical portfolio and followed up by counseling as deemed necessary.

The ability *to be present* is crucial in spiritual care. Availability, concentration at work and reflection allow students to bear witness to patients' suffering and do something meaningfully about it *without getting immune* to patient's suffering. Ability to listen to unspoken words accompanied by compassion and sensitivity is part of professional presence and spiritual care. Thus, the nurses' and health care professionals' connection and rapport with patients are fundamental for spiritual care [67]. Assignment of a mentor in the clinical environment fosters individual follow up system on a one-to-one basis to help students to identify spirituality as part of the fabric of everyday patient care. This also demands good collaboration between students, lecturers, health care professionals, and clinical mentors for optimal learning outcomes. Furthermore, leadership in the clinical environment plays a key role in maintaining holistic and creating a good learning environment [68].

6.5. Creating a Clinical Environment Conducive to Learning Spiritual Care

The *Personal* spirituality of the caregiver was found by research as the strongest predictor for perceiving ability to provide spiritual care as no one can give from what he/she does not possess [69,70]. Personal spirituality enables caregivers to be sensitive to patients' cultural and spiritual needs in their holistic care [71–73]. Hence, the importance for students to be helped to reflect and explore their own spirituality as it allows students to be more sensitive to the spirituality of others [74–76]. Research shows that students reported discomfort with self-reflection, but it provided them with access to their own growth [77].

Since health care professionals form the major part of the clinical environment of patients, attention needs to be given to the spiritual dimension and the holistic perspective of the health care professionals at the workplace [78,79]. Personal spirituality refers to an attitude and/or a lifestyle of an individual, which recognizes his/her own spiritual dimension of one's life. When personal spirituality is acknowledged, teamwork will generate a peaceful environment with enhanced patient care, incorporating also the individual patients' spirituality in their care. Implementation of spirituality in the clinical and the academic environments may motivate health care professionals to search meaning and purpose in their work, understand the value of work and become aware of their personal belief system [80]. The education system both in the clinical and the faculty sectors need highly motivated educators who radiate happiness and peacefulness to others, including students, colleagues and patients [81]. To sustain such an environment conducive to learning and self-development, the managers need to link their personal life values and educators' values to the respective university values, which may eventually pass on these values to students resulting in spiritual growth of both students and educators [82,83].

Literature suggests that a successful learning environment is created through inspirational leadership, reflective management and creation of a positive partnership between the clinical setting and the educational organization [84–87].

The spiritual leadership theory was adopted as a guide for such an inspirational leadership in the education of spiritual care. This is based on an intrinsic motivation model and on characteristics such as, faith, hope and altruism, which may generate homogeneous vision and values at the individual, team, and organizational levels [88]. These values may eventually generate higher levels of commitment to holistic care supported by spiritual leadership [89].

Fry identifies seven dimensions of spiritual leadership that may be applied to an environment conducive to learning, which are *vision, altruistic love, hope/faith, membership, meaning/calling, organizational commitment and productivity.*

Vision: As a result of the advancement of technology, patient care may be enhanced but at the same time health care professionals may be distracted from the actual holistic care of the person under their care [90]. The vision looks to the future goal to be reached, which gives meaning to the organization's aspirations, and fosters hope and faith [91]. Ideally, undergraduates and post-graduate learners need to be grouped together and learn together in classrooms and clinical seminar rooms about holistic care of specific patients. Methods of education are consistently changing such as, the introduction of *online* course programs that may facilitate interdisciplinary education.

Altruism: is a set of values, of going beyond one's needs to deliver care to others, and ways of thinking that are morally right, and are shared by group members and taught to new members. These values may be taught theoretically, but also by role models, during patient care and communication with colleagues.

Hope/Faith: During this pathway of looking to the future, hope and faith in the ability of the educators and the students themselves may help actualization of the set vision and goals to be achieved successfully in the proposed mission. The individuals' spiritual belief system may generate empowerment along this pathway.

Membership: The diversity of religious affiliations, spiritual beliefs, culture and social structures, demands efforts to try to understand each other and appreciate each other's strengths and tolerate each other's limitations with the intention to generate self-development and team work. This collegial process stems from the interactions and communication between the members of the multidisciplinary team and also the development of therapeutic relationship with the patient [92,93].

Meaning/Calling: Educators in the faculty and clinical placements identify the "calling"/vocational aspect as the sacred part of the profession, which may yield a transcendent experience, while becoming aware of the related empowerment to dedicate oneself to the care of others professionally. Eventually, educators may realize the worth of serving others, the wealth of making a difference in students' and patients' lives. Hopefully, through reflection, educators may realize that while they are *giving to others*, they *are also receiving*. Consequently, meaning and purpose in life is created along the pathway of learning from each other. Thus, the actual work environment is transformed into a workplace with a social meaning and value and not simply a job of people, or just seeking competence and knowledge [94].

Organizational Commitment: The practice of altruism, safe belongingness, and a sense of meaning at work will contribute towards a healthy environment, enhanced collegiality and collaboration, with less stress-induced sick leave, higher motivation and faithfulness to their individual "calling"/vocation in their respective profession. Thus an environment with a culture based on values and altruism may generate role-models to teach spiritual care and feelings of peace and security at work [95].

Productivity: Productivity is interpreted as an intelligent process of implementing interventions based on research evidence, creativity and innovations to achieve the set goals. Consistent reflection *in* and *on* action may lessen mistakes in care, one of which is the neglect of the spiritual dimension in care [96].

These characteristics may foster learning by role models generated from an environment of cooperation, trust, commitment and effectiveness of collegial work [97]. This environment may be inhibited by various factors, such as work overload, lack of time, incomplete staff complement, lack of job security [98], impaired personal spirituality, and career motivation system [99]. Motivation supported by personal spirituality was found positively related with better performance due to achievement of goals at work and collegial relationship in the education and delivery of holistic care [100].

7. Conclusions

Research identifies the active role of the nurses and health care professionals in meeting the spiritual needs of patients in collaboration with the family and the chaplain. However, it is well documented that nurses and health care professionals have overlooked the spiritual dimension in care with the consequence of threatening holistic care. While considering the complexity of spirituality and spiritual care, and the barriers to the delivery of spiritual care documented in the literature, the author presented various innovative teaching methods, which were introduced in various undergraduate and post-graduate course programs of nurses and health care professionals in Malta and foreign universities. The teaching methods integrated within the theoretical and clinical dimensions were guided by conceptual models to enhance learning such as, Benner's theory: *From Novice to Expert: Excellence and Power in Clinical Nursing Practice*; Kolb's experiential learning theory; Gibbs theory of reflective learning; and the ASSET model for Actioning Spirituality and Spiritual care Education and Training in nursing. Experiential learning, visits in the community, reflective exercises and reflective written accounts, use of arts for expression of the complex concepts of spiritual care, discussions on observed delivery of holistic care, participation in research, tutorials, and role modeling were identified as beneficial resources of learning. Various factors were identified which may influence students' education on spiritual care, such as characteristics of students, the extent to which the academic and clinical environments in hospital and in community are conducive to learning, and culture. This paper identifies the essence of spiritual care, which is *being in doing*, whereby personal spirituality and therapeutic use of self may contribute towards the education and delivery of spiritual care and holistic care.

8. Recommendations

The following *recommendations* are set for the education, clinical, and management sectors; personal spirituality; and further research to enhance education on spiritual care.

8.1. Education

Students tend to be *examination-oriented* so they tend to prefer to study for their examinations. Thus, examining clinical skills in spiritual care would identify the degree of acquisition of competence in spiritual care. Therefore, a framework on competences in spiritual care needs to be developed as a guide for the education and clinical sectors.

Literature confirmed that theoretical study units on spiritual care may be effective to the nurses' and midwives' perceived competence in spiritual care. Continuous professional development (CPD) is mandatory by reading literature and research, attending seminars, conferences, CPD courses on spiritual care in order to achieve competence and maintain high quality holistic care [101–103].

8.2. Clinical Practice

Literature discusses spiritual care learning as part of a total curriculum program emphasizing the clinical studies and ways of facilitating reflection in practice together with clinical tutorials as important in the students' learning process. Thus, students need to be provided with "teachable moments" by reflecting with students on patient care so that they can learn and approach new encounters with greater awareness and appropriate action [104].

Clinical practice presents students with diverse and rich opportunities to learn about the reality and nature of patients' spiritual needs and spiritual well-being in real-life situations. Students need to practice before they can fully understand the theoretical component. Thus *role-modeling* by health care professionals and mentors in the clinical placements is of utmost importance to help students to understand and to implement spiritual care. Furthermore, an effective dialogue between the clinical settings and the educational organizations is needed to maximize learning opportunities for students.

Spirituality and spiritual care are complex concepts, especially when faced with the diverse religions held by patients in hospital and the community. Learning about the relationship between religion and health care is of utmost importance especially in this era of immigrants with different religious affiliations who are admitted to hospital. Additionally, addressing spiritual distress and spiritual needs may involve various ethical issues, such as confidentiality in documenting certain aspects of spiritual assessment. Thus, support groups are needed for debriefing sessions to express feelings, biases and address ethical issues involved in spiritual care.

8.3. Management

Spiritual leadership is needed to develop a clinical environment conducive to learning spiritual care by facilitating holistic care and teamwork, which foster spirituality at the workplace.

Awareness of the sacredness of the caring profession and clinical environment is essential.

"When comparing the hospital to a sanctuary, the patient is the tabernacle", whereby the patient is the center of holistic care [105].

8.4. Further Research

Further transcultural longitudinal research is needed to identify the most appropriate and effective pedagogical approaches to teach spiritual care to students [106], such as by *online* and interactive simulation by intra-professional and inter-professional educational programs.

8.5. Personal Spirituality

The frequency of attending religious services and spiritual experiences were found to contribute towards the students' positive attitude towards spiritual care [107]. Thus, further research is suggested to identify the possible impact of personal characteristics, such as age, gender, personality traits, religious practices and life experiences on holistic care.

Personal religiosity and spirituality of students, their mentors and health care professionals may foster a healthy spiritual clinical environment. Thus, *organization of spiritual retreats, prayer meetings for students and health care professionals* may be beneficial to both the caregiver and the recipient of their care. Finally, the richness of both the theoretical presentations and socio-religious events during the European Conference on Religion Spirituality and Health in Malta in 2014, may enhance motivation to become *change agents* with the possible ultimate ripple beneficial effects of spiritual care:

If you reform your *spiritual-self*, you will reform your *professional care*;
If you reform your *professional care*, you will reform your *holistic care*;
If you reform your *holistic care*, you will reform the care *spiritually*.

Acknowledgments: The author appreciates the cooperation of Roberta Sammut, Head of the Nursing Department, Faculty of Health Sciences; the hospitals'/residences' managers; the Catholic church authorities of the day centers in the community; the Caritas and related Agencies; the Scientific Committee of the ECRSH 2014 Conference; the nursing students who undertook the study units related to spiritual care; Lilian Bonello for proof reading; Family Attard for providing a quiet reflective seaside environment to write this manuscript; and the three anonymous reviewers.

Conflicts of Interest: The author declares no conflict of interest.

References

1. International Council for Nurses (ICN). *Code of Ethics for Nurses*. Geneva: ICN, 2000.
2. Nursing and Midwifery Board. *Maltese Code of Ethics for Nurses and Midwives*. Valletta: Nursing and Midwifery Board, 2001.

3. Florence Nightingale. *Notes on Nursing: What Is Nursing and What Is Not.* New York: Dover Publications Inc., 1860.

4. Donia Baldacchino. *Spirituality in Illness and Care.* Blata l-Bajda: Preca Library, 2003.

5. BBC. "Why Is Mary Seacole Famous? The History of Mary Seacole." 2015. Available online: http://www.bbc.co.uk/schools/primaryhistory/famouspeople/mary_seacole/ (accessed on 30 March 2014).

6. Jane Williams. *Betsy Cadwaladyr: A Balaclave Nurse. An Autobiography of Elisabeth Davis.* Dinas Powys: Dinefwr Press, 2007.

7. Wilfred McSherry, and Linda Ross. *Spiritual Assessment in Healthcare Practice.* Cumbria: M & K Update Ltd., 2010.

8. Wendy Cadge, Elaine Howard Ecklund, and Nicholas Short. "Religion and Spirituality: A barrier and a bridge in everyday professional work of Paediatric Physicians." *Journal of Social Problems* 56 (2009): 702–21.

9. Susan Ronaldson, Lilian Hayes, Christina Aggar, Jennifer Green, and Michele Carey. "Spirituality and Spiritual Caring: Nurses' Perspectives and Practice in Palliative and Acute Care Environments." *Journal of Clinical Nursing* 21 (2012): 2126–35.

10. Michael J. Balboni, Adam Sullivan, Andrea C. Enzinger, Zachary D. Epstein-Peterson, Yolanda D. Tseng, Christine Mitchell, Joshua Niska, Angelika Zollfrank, Tyler J. Vanderweele, and Tracy A. Balboni. "Nurse and physician barriers to spiritual care provision at end of life." *Journal of Pain Symptom Management* 48 (2014): 400–10.

11. Betty Neuman. *The Neuman Systems Model.* Norwalk: Appleton and Lange, 2010.

12. Larry F. Renetzky. "The fourth dimension: Applications to the social services." In *Spiritual Well-Being. Sociological Perspectives.* Edited by David O. Moberg. New York: University Press of America, 1979.

13. Donia Baldacchino, and Peter Draper. "Spiritual coping strategies: A review of the nursing research literature." *Journal of Advanced Nursing* 34 (2001): 833–41.

14. Ruth Murray, and Judith Proctor Zentner. *Nursing Concepts for Health Promotion.* London: Prentice Hall, 1989.

15. Kristina Torskenes, Donia Baldacchino, Tracey Baldacchino, Josette Borg, Marica Falzon, and Mary Kalfoss. "Nurses' and informal caregivers' definition of spirituality from the Christian perspective: A comparative study between Malta and Norway." *Journal of Advanced Nursing* 23 (2013): 39–53.

16. Carolyn Young, and Cyndie Koopsen. *Spirituality, Health, and Healing: An Integrative Approach*, 2nd ed. Sudbury: Jones & Bartlett Learning, 2011.

17. Donia Baldacchino. "Spiritual Care: Is it the nurse's role? " *Spirituality & Health International* 9 (2009): 270–84.

18. Linda Ross. *Nurses' Perceptions of Spiritual Care.* Avebury: Aldershot, 1997.

19. Mohsen Saffari, Harold Koenig, Ghader Ghanizadeh, Amir H. Pakpour, and Donia R. Baldacchino. "Psychometric Properties of the Persian Spiritual Coping Strategies Scale in Haemodialysis Patients." *Journal of Religion & Health* 53 (2013): 1025–35.

20. Mohsen Saffari, Amir H. Pakpour, Maryam K. Naderi, Harold Koenig, Donia R. Baldacchino, and Chrystal N. Piper. "Spiritual coping, religiosity and quality of life: A study on Muslim clients on haemodialyis." *Nephrology* 18 (2013): 269–75.

21. Cynthia Kociszewski. "A Phenomenological pilot study of the nurses' experience providing spiritual care." *Journal of Holistic Nursing* 21 (2003): 131–48.

22. Leslie van Dover, and Jane Pfeiffe. "Patients of parish nurses experience renewed spiritual identity: A grounded theory study." *Journal of Advanced Nursing* 68 (2011): 1824–33.

23. Terry L. Koenig. "Caregivers use of spirituality in ethical decision-making." *Journal of Gerontological Social Work* 45 (2014): 155–72.

24. Tracy A. Balboni, Mary E. Paulk, Michael J. Balboni, Andrea C. Phelps, Elisabeth T. Loggers, Alexi A. Wright, Susan D. Block, Eldrin F. Lewis, John R. Peteet, and Holly G. Prigerson. "Provision of spiritual care to patients with advanced cancer: Associations with medical care and quality of life near death." *Journal of Clinical Oncology* 28 (2010): 445–52.

25. Dawn Freshwater. "The Therapeutic Use of Self in Nursing." 2002. Available online: http://www.uk.sagepub.com/upm-data/9470_011394Ch1.pdf (accessed on 5 April 2015).

26. Ann Bradshaw. *Lighting the Lamp. The Spiritual Dimension of Nursing Care.* Middlesex: Scutari Press, 1994.

27. The Nursing and Midwifery Council. *The Nursing and Midwifery Council (NMC) in the UK Requirements for Pre-Registration Nursing Programme.* London: NMC, 2002.

28. "The European Qualifications Framework for Lifelong Learning." In *The European Qualifications Framework for Lifelong Learning*. Belgium: European Commission Press, 2008.
29. Patricia Benner. "Issues in competency-based training." *Nursing Outlook* 30 (1982): 303–09.
30. Patricia Benner. *From Novice to Expert: Excellence and Power in Clinical Nursing Practice*. Menlo Park: Addison-Wesley, 1984.
31. Michael Eraut. *Developing Professional Knowledge and Competence*. London: Falmer Press, 1994.
32. David R. Hodge. "Developing cultural competence with Evangelical Christians." *Families in Societies* 85 (2004): 251–60.
33. Donia Baldacchino. "Nursing competencies for spiritual care." *Journal of Clinical Nursing* 15 (2006): 885–96.
34. Rene van Leeuwen, and Barth Cusveller. "Nursing competencies for spiritual care." *Journal of Advanced Nursing* 48 (2004): 234–46.
35. Mikael Lundmark. "Attitudes to spiritual care among nursing staff in a Swedish oncology clinic." *Journal of Clinical Nursing* 15 (2006): 863–74.
36. Denise Miner-Williams. "Putting a puzzle together: Making spirituality meaningful for nursing using an evolving theoretical framework." *Journal of Clinical Nursing* 15 (2006): 811–21.
37. William M. Sullivan. "Medicine under threat: Professionalism and professional identity." *Canadian Medical Association Journal* 162 (2000): 1–7.
38. Josephine Attard, and Donia Baldacchino. "The demand for competencies in Spiritual care in nursing and midwifery education: A literature review." *Revista Pistis Praxis, Teologia Pastorale* 6 (2014): 671–91.
39. Gowri Anandarajah, and Ellen Hight. "Spirituality and medical practice: Using the HOPE Questions as a practical tool for spiritual assessment." *American Family Physician* 63 (2001): 81–89.
40. Donia Baldacchino. "The nurse's role in spiritual care: A comparative study between perceptions of patients with first myocardial infarction and health carers in Malta." In *Nursing Today*. Edited by L. Beldean, U. Zeitler and L. Rogozea. Editura: Alma Mater, 2005, pp. 137–46.
41. Emily M. Cramer, and Kelly E. Tenzek. "The Chaplain profession from the employer perspective: An analysis of hospice chaplain Job Advertisements." *Journal of Health Care Chaplaincy* 18 (2012): 133–50.
42. Linda Ross, Rene van Leeuwen, Donia Baldacchino, Tove Giske, Wilfred McSherry, Aru Narayanasamy, Carmel Downes, Paul Jarvis, and Annemiek Schep-Akkerman. "Student nurses perceptions of spirituality and competence in delivering spiritual care: A European pilot study." *Nurse Education Today* 34 (2014): 697–702.
43. Brenda Leonard, Elaine L. H. Shuhaibar, and Ruth Chen. "Nursing student perceptions of intra-professional team education using high-fidelity simulation." *Journal of Health Care Chaplaincy* 49 (2010): 628–31.
44. Centre for the Advancement of Inter-professional Education (CAIPE). *Inter-Professional Education—A Definition*. London: CAIPE Bulletin, 1997, vol. 13, p. 19.
45. Health Professions Networks, Nursing and Midwifery, and Human Resources for Health. *Framework for Action on Inter-Professional Education and Collaborative Practice*; Geneva: W.H.O. Press, 2010. Available online: http://whqlibdoc.who.int/hq/2010/WHO_HRH_HPN_10.3_eng.pdf (accessed on 10 May 2014).
46. Louisa McIlwaine, Valentine Scarlett, Alan Venters, and Jean Ker. "The different levels of learning about dying and death: An evaluation of a personal, professional and inter-professional learning journey." *Medical Teaching* 29 (2007): 151–59.
47. Marilyn Hammick, Della Freeth, Ivan Koppel, Scott Reeves, and Hugh Barr. "A best evidence systematic review of inter-professional education: BEME Guide No 9." *Medical Teaching* 29 (2007): 735–51.
48. Katherine Pollard, and Margaret E. Miers. "From students to professionals: Results of a longitudinal study of attitudes to pre-qualifying collaborative learning and working in health and social care in the United Kingdom." *Journal of Interprofessional Care* 22 (2008): 399–416.
49. Robin Lennon-Dearing, Joseph A. Florence, Helen Halvorsin, and James T. Pollard. "An interprofessional educational approach to teaching spiritual assessment." *Journal of Healthcare Chaplain* 18 (2012): 121–32.
50. Matthew S. Ellman, Dena Schulman-Green, Leslie Blatt, Susan Asher, Diane Viveiros, Joshua Clark, and Margaret Bia. "Using online learning and interactive simulation to teach spiritual and cultural aspects of palliative care to inter-professional students." *Journal of Palliative Medicine* 15 (2012): 1240–47.
51. Tove Giske. "How undergraduate nursing students learn to care for patients spiritually in clinical studies—A review of literature." *Journal of Nursing Management* 20 (2012): 1–9.

52. Aru Narayanasamy. "ASSET: A model for actioning spirituality and spiritual care education and training in nursing." *Nurse Education Today* 19 (1999): 274–85.
53. Donia Baldacchino. *Spiritual Care: Being in Doing*. Blata l-Bajda: Preca Library, 2010.
54. Pamela P. Cone, and Tove Giske. "Teaching spiritual care—A grounded theory study among undergraduate nursing educators." *Journal of Clinical Nursing* 22 (2012): 1951–60.
55. Donia Baldacchino. "Spiritual Care Education of Health Care Professionals." Available online: www.ecrsh. eu/mm/Baldacchino_-_Keynote_ECRSH14 (accessed on 22 May 2014).
56. Donia Baldacchino, Kristina B. Torskenes, Josette Borg, Mary Kalfoss, Aaron Tonna, Clifford Debattista, Neville Decelis, and Rodianne Mifsud. "Spiritual coping of clients on rehabilitation: A comparative study between Malta and Norway (Part I)." *British Journal of Nursing* 22 (2013): 16–20.
57. Amanda J. Henderson, Joanna Briggs, Sue Schoonbeek, and Karen Paterson. "A framework to develop a clinical learning culture in health facilities: Ideas from the literature." *International Nursing Review* 58 (2011): 196–202.
58. Ann Bradshaw. "Teaching spiritual care to nurses: An alternative approach." *International Journal of Palliative Nursing* 3 (1997): 51–57.
59. Josephine Attard, Donia R. Baldacchino, and Liberato Camilleri. "Nurses' and midwives' acquisition of competency in spiritual care: A focus on education." *Nurse Education Today* 26 (2014): 1460–66.
60. Donia R. Baldacchino. "Teaching on 'The Spiritual Dimension in Care': The perceived impact on undergraduate nursing students." *Nurse Education Today* 28 (2008): 501–12.
61. Patricia Benner, and Molly Sutphen. "Learning across the professions: The clergy, a case in point." *Journal of Nursing Education* 46 (2007): 103–08.
62. Tove Giske, and Pamela Cone. "Opening up to learning spiritual care of patients: A grounded theory study of nursing students." *Journal of Clinical Nursing* 21 (2012): 2006–15.
63. Ann Purdie, Louisa Sheward, and Elaine Gifford. "Student nurse placements take a new direction." *Nurse Education in Practice* 8 (2008): 315–20.
64. Donia Baldacchino. "Caring in Lourdes: An innovation in students' clinical placement." *British Journal of Nursing* 19 (2010): 352–66.
65. Graham Gibbs. *Learning by Doing: A Guide to Teaching and Learning Methods*. Oxford: Oxford Polytechnic, 1988.
66. David Kolb. *Experiential Learning: Experience as the Source of Learning and Development*. Englewood Cliffs: Prentice-Hall, Inc., 1984.
67. Dee Marie Zyblock. "Nursing presence in contemporary nursing practice." *Nursing Forum* 45 (2010): 120–24.
68. Cleda Meyer. "Mentoring for spiritual caregiving: What factors enable nursing students or new graduated to provide spiritual care? " *Journal of Christian Nursing* 22 (2005): 38–40.
69. Barbara Pesut. "The development of nursing students' spirituality and spiritual care-giving." *Nurse Education Today* 22 (2002): 128–35.
70. Denise L. Mitchell, Marsha J. Bennett, and Linda Manfrin-Leder. "Spiritual development of nursing students: Developing competence to provide spiritual care to patients at the end of life." *Journal of Nursing Education* 45 (2006): 365–70.
71. Aru Narayanasamy. "The impact of empirical studies of spirituality and culture on nurse education." *Journal of Clinical Nursing* 15 (2006): 840–51.
72. Joseph D. Cortis. "Meeting the needs of minority ethnic patients." *Journal of Advanced Nursing* 48 (2004): 51–58.
73. Bruce D. Feldstein, Marita Grudzen, Art Johnson, and Samuel LeBaron. "Integrating Spirituality and Culture with End-of-Life Care in Medical Education." *Clinical Gerontologist* 31 (2008): 71–82.
74. Corinne Lemmer. "Teaching the spiritual dimension of nursing care: A survey of US baccalaureate nursing programs." *Journal of Nursing Education* 41 (2002): 482–90.
75. Lynn Clark Callister, Elaine A. Bond, Gerry Matsumura, and Sandra Mangum. "Threading spirituality throughout nursing education." *Holistic Nursing Practicen* 18 (2004): 160–66.
76. Elisabeth A. Rankin, and Mary B. DeLashmutt. "Finding spirituality and nursing presence: The student's challenge." *Journal of Holistic Nursing* 24 (2006): 282–88.
77. Ana Maria Catanzaro, and Kathleen A. McMullen. "Increasing nursing students' spiritual sensitivity." *Nurse Educator* 26 (2001): 221–26.

78. John Milliman, Andrew J. Czaplewski, and Jeffery Ferguson. "Workplace spirituality and employee work attitudes. An exploratory empirical assessment." *Journal of Organisation Change Management* 16 (2003): 426–47.
79. Don Grant, Kathleen O'Neil, and Laura Stephens. "Spirituality in the Workplace: New Empirical Directions in the Study of the Sacred." *Sociology of Religion* 65 (2004): 265–83.
80. Jamil Sadeghifar, Mohammed Bahadori, Donia Baldacchino, Mehdi Radaabadi, and Mehdi Jafari. "Relationship between Career Motivation and Perceived Spiritual Leadership in Health Professional Educators: A Correlational Study in Iran." *Global Journal of Health Science* 6 (2013): 145–54.
81. John Fisher, and David Brumley. "Nurses' and carers' spiritual wellbeing in the workplace." *Australian Journal of Advanced Nursing* 25 (2007): 49–57.
82. Joanna Crossman. "Conceptualising spiritual leadership in secular organizational contexts and its relation to transformational, servant and environmental leadership." *Leadership & Organization Development Journal* 31 (2010): 596–608.
83. Judi Neal. *Handbook of Faith and Spirituality in the Workplace—Emerging Research and Practice.* London: Springer, 2013, pp. 3–18.
84. Stephen G. Post, Christina M. Puchalaiski, and David Larson. "Physicians and patient spirituality: Professional Boundaries, competency and Ethics." *American College of Psysicians, American Society of Internal Medicine* 132 (2000): 578–83.
85. Christina M. Puchalski. "Spirituality and health: the art of compassionate medicine." *Hospital Physician* 37 (2001): 30–36.
86. Dee W. Ford, Lois Downey, Ruth Engelberg, Anthony L. Back, and Curtis J. Randall. "Discussing religion and spirituality is an advanced communication skill: An exploratory structural equation model of physician trainee self-ratings." *Journal of Palliative Medicine* 15 (2012): 63–70.
87. Michael Balboni, Adam Sullivan, Adaugo Amobi, Andrea C. Phelps, Daniel P. Gorman, Angelika Zollfrank, John Peteet, Holly P. Briggerson, Tyler J. Vanderweele, and Tracy A. Balboni. "Why is spiritual care infrequent at the end of life? Spiritual care perceptions among patients, nurses, and physicians and the role of training." *Journal of Clinical Oncology* 31 (2013): 461–67.
88. Lesley W. Fry. "Towards a theory of spiritual leadership." *The Leadership Quarterly* 14 (2003): 693–727.
89. Gary Geroy, Mario Fernando, and Frederick Beale. "The spiritual dimension in leadership at Dilmah Tea." *Leadership & Organization Development Journal* 30 (2009): 522–39.
90. Mary Carolyn Cooper. "The intersection of technology and care in the ICU." *Advances in Nursing Science* 15 (1993): 23–32.
91. Louis W. Fry, Sean T. Hannah, Michael Noel, and Fred O. Walumbwa. "Impact of spiritual leadership on unit performance." *The Leadership Quarterly* 22 (2011): 259–70.
92. Jeanne Siddiqui. "The Therapeutic relationship in midwifery." *British Journal of Midwifery* 7 (1999): 111–14.
93. Agneta Schreurs. *Psychotherapy and Spirituality: Integrating the Spiritual Dimension into Therapeutic Practice.* London: Jessica Kingsley Publishers, 2002.
94. Jeffery Pfeffer. *Business and the Spirit. Handbook of Workplace Spirituality and Organizational Performance.* New York: ME Sharpe, 2003, pp. 29–45.
95. John Arnold, Ray Randall, Joanne Silvester, Fiona Patterson, Ivan Robertson, Cary Cooper, Bernard Burnes, Don Harris, Carolyn Axtell, and Deanne Den Hartog. *Work Psychology. Understanding Human Behaviour in the Workplace*, 4th ed. Madrid: Pearson Education Limited, 2005.
96. William McEwan. "Spirituality in nursing." *Orthopaedic Nursing* 23 (2004): 321–36.
97. Afsaneh Mohammadi, Zohreh Vanaki, and Ashraf Mohammadi. "Effect of Implementation of Motivational Program Based on 'Expectancy Theory' by Head Nurses on Patients' Satisfaction." *Hayat* 18 (2012): 47–60.
98. Ali Khan Khuwaja, Riaz Qureshi, Marie Andrades, Zafar Fatmi, and Nadia Kha Khuwaja. "Comparison of job satisfaction and stress among male and female doctors in teaching hospitals of Karachi." *Journal of Ayub Medical College, Abbottabad* 16 (2003): 23–27.
99. Gilbert W. Fairholm. "Spiritual leadership: Fulfilling whole-self needs at work." *Leadership & Organization Development Journal* 17 (1996): 11–17.
100. Ahmed Al-Rfou, and Khalaf Trawneh. "Achieve Competitive Advantage through Job Motivation." *Journal of Social Sciences* 20 (2007): 105–07.
101. George Handzo, and Harold G. Koenig. "Spiritual Care: Whose job is it anyway?" *Southern Medical Journal* 97 (2004): 1242–44.

102. Christopher Levison. "Partners in care." *Nursing Management* 12 (2005): 18–21.

103. Rene van Leeuwen, Lucas Tiesinga, Doeke Post, and Henke Jochemsen. "Spiritual care: Implications for nurses' professional responsibility." *Journal of Clinical Nursing* 15 (2006): 875–84.

104. Cynthia Johnston, and Ann E. Mohide. "Addressing diversity in clinical nursing education: Support for preceptors." *Nurse Education in Practice* 9 (2009): 340–47.

105. Jason Azzopardi. "The sacredness of patient care." *Il-Mument* 3 (2010): 13–15.

106. Linda Ross. "Spiritual care in nursing: An overview of the research to date." *Journal of Clinical Nursing* 15 (2006): 852–62.

107. Neil Cockell, and Wilfred McSherry. "Spiritual care in nursing: An overview of published international research." *Journal of Nursing Management* 20 (2012): 958–69.

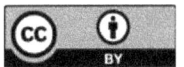

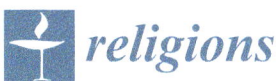

Article

The Spiritual Care Team: Enabling the Practice of Whole Person Medicine

Harold G. Koenig [1,2,3]

[1]   Department of Psychiatry & Behavioral Sciences; Department of Medicine, Duke University Medical Center, Durham, NC 27710, USA; Harold.Koenig@duke.edu; Tel.: +1-919-681-6633
[2]   Department of Medicine, King Abdulaziz University, Jeddah 21531, Saudi Arabia
[3]   School of Public Health, Ningxia Medical University, Yinchuan 750004, China

External Editor: Arndt Büssing
Received: 13 October 2014; in revised form: 9 November 2014; Accepted: 25 November 2014; Published: 9 December 2014

Abstract: We will soon be piloting a project titled "Integrating Spirituality into Patient Care" that will form "spiritual care teams" to assess and address patients' spiritual needs in physician outpatient practices within Adventist Health System, the largest Protestant healthcare system in the United States. This paper describes the goals, the rationale, and the structure of the spiritual care teams that will soon be implemented, and discusses the barriers to providing spiritual care that health professionals are likely to encounter. Spiritual care teams may operate in an outpatient or an inpatient setting, and their purpose is to provide health professionals with resources necessary to practice whole person healthcare that includes spiritual care. We believe that this project will serve as a model for faith-based health systems seeking to visibly demonstrate their mission in a way that makes them unique and expresses their values. Not only does this model have the potential to be cost-effective, but also the capacity to increase the quality of patient care and the satisfaction that health professionals derive from providing care. If successful, this model could spread beyond faith-based systems to secular systems as well both in the U.S. and worldwide.

Keywords: spirituality; religion; spiritual history; spiritual care; spiritual care team

1. Introduction

Research is rapidly accumulating that demonstrates a link between religious involvement and health [1]. As a result, clinicians are searching for ways to apply the findings from these studies to patient care. Perhaps just in time. Healthcare systems and healthcare professionals are struggling. As public health measures improve and healthcare becomes more widely available, people are living longer. Consequently, healthcare systems around the world are beginning to feel the strain involved in caring for more and more patients with chronic health problems as people advance in years. This is especially true in countries such as China, India, the Middle East, and some of the African and South American countries as well [2–5]. The problem is becoming particularly acute in developed countries, such as the United States, where rising healthcare costs are threatening to bankrupt the nation [6], leaving little room for other government-sponsored programs (social security, Medicaid, *etc.*) and encroaching on budgets to preserve the environment, invest in education, infrastructure and research, public safety and security, and defense [7].

Healthcare systems have sought to adapt to increasing numbers of patients by increasing the volume of patients that providers see, creating stress on providers and resulting in an estimated 30%–40% of physicians in the U.S. experiencing burnout (figures which are now about five years old, and the situation has worsened since then) [8]. The stressful healthcare environment limits clinicians' ability to provide whole person care that considers the physical, psychological, social, and spiritual needs of those with chronic disabling illness. These needs are closely interconnected, as research in the field of psychoneuroimmunology is demonstrating [9]. The mind, the body, the social environment, and people's spiritual beliefs and practices all influence each other in complex ways that make focusing on the physical body alone—especially when illness is chronic—incomplete and less effective than might otherwise be. In the days when diseases were primarily acute and occurred in the young or middle-aged, treating the physical body was often enough. That is not the case today, however, with chronic illnesses that may last many years and not only increase medical costs, but cause functional disability, adversely affect quality of life (of both the afflicted person and their family), and often raise questions about the meaning and purpose of life [10].

2. The Spiritual Care Team and Its Goals

The "spiritual care team" (SCT), a phrase coined by Emmer and Brown [11], is made up of a group of health professionals and staff who seek to integrate spirituality into patient care in a way that enhances their ability to provide "whole-person" healthcare that includes "spiritual care". The model described here is being developed at Duke University's Center for Spirituality, Theology and Health for implementation in the Adventist Health System, the largest Protestant healthcare system in the United States [12]. The goals of the SCT are to: (1) identify the spiritual needs of patients related to medical illness; (2) competently address those spiritual needs; (3) create an atmosphere where patients feel comfortable talking about their spiritual needs with the physician and other team members; (4) address the whole-person needs of healthcare team members related to patient care; and (5) provide whole-person health care to all patients they serve. Spiritual needs are those related to the Transcendent (however that is understood by the patient). For example, a patient may feel that their medical condition is a punishment from God or that God has deserted them or that their faith community has abandoned them. Alternatively, a patient may be struggling with where he or she is going after death, fearful perhaps of going to hell or concerned that there actually is a hereafter. A patient may have a need for prayer or a desire to be visited by members of their faith community. These are examples of spiritual needs.

3. The Rationale

Why should health professionals take the time to form SCTs to assess and address the spiritual needs of patients? The rationale is both theoretical and concrete, and relates to the interconnectedness of mind, body, and spirit. First, many patients have spiritual needs related to illness, and addressing those needs affects satisfaction with care, quality of life, and interestingly, healthcare costs [13–15]. Furthermore, clinical trials have reported that when physicians conduct a spiritual assessment, patient outcomes improve, including compliance with clinic visits, reduction of depressive symptoms, increased functional well-being, and improved the doctor-patient relationship (sense of personal caring from the physician) [16,17]. Second, religious beliefs influence coping with illness and may affect the patient's emotional state and motivation towards recovery, affecting their ability to provide self-care [18]. Third, religious beliefs affect important health-related behaviors and likely influence medical outcomes, as is increasingly being documented [19]. Fourth, religious beliefs influence medical decisions made by *both* patients [20,21] *and* physicians [22]; these decisions often involve the use of expensive, high tech treatments, especially towards the end of life [23].

Fifth, the "standard of care" put forth by the Joint Commission for the Accreditation of Hospital Organizations (JCAHO) in the U.S. requires that providers respect patients' cultural and spiritual beliefs [24]. Specifically, the regulations for hospitals (for all patients) say: "The hospital respects the patient's cultural and personal values, beliefs and preferences" (RI.01.01.01 EP 6) and "The hospital accommodates the patient's right to religious and other spiritual services" (RI.01.01.01 EP 9). The regulations are even more specific about respecting the spiritual beliefs of patients in end-of-life care, those being treated for alcohol and substance use, and those receiving treatment for emotional or behavioral disorders (PC.01.02.01 EP 4, PC.01.02.11 EP 5, and PC 01.02.13 EP3, respectively). Assessment is the only way to know the nature of these beliefs.

Sixth, support from a religious community may increase patient monitoring and improve compliance with treatment, resulting in more timely healthcare that is always less expensive than acute emergency care. Finally, addressing spiritual issues may benefit the health professional as well by providing intrinsic rewards associated with delivering whole-person healthcare.

There is also scientific rationale for assessing and addressing patients' spiritual needs. I will briefly review some of that research here. However, for a more detailed examination of these studies, readers are referred to the *Handbook of Religion and Health*, which contains a systematic review of quantitative studies published in academic peer-reviewed journals through 2010 [1]. I begin with mental health, and then move on to social health, health behaviors, and physical health.

First, in some areas of the U.S. and elsewhere in the world, up to 90% of medical patients rely on religion to cope [18]. High levels of stress, such as those experienced after the September 11 terrorist attacks, often cause people to turn to religion for comfort and control during such events [25]. In the overwhelming majority of over 400 studies that have now examined this (not including most qualitative studies), people say that religion helps them to cope better [1]. Religious beliefs are commonly used to endure the distress caused by health problems, giving meaning to illness, promoting hope for recovery, and providing rituals and behaviors that bring individuals together and settle anxiety (such as prayer). Similarly, beliefs of this kind have been repeatedly linked with better mental health in medical patients [26–28].

How is religious involvement related to mental health more generally and to social health? In brief, religiosity or spirituality is related to less depression in over 60% of 444 quantitative studies; greater well-being and happiness in nearly 80% of 326 studies; greater meaning and purpose in over 90% of 45 studies; greater hope and optimism in over 75% of 72 studies; and because they convey greater meaning, purpose and hope, religious beliefs and activities are related to less suicide, fewer suicide attempts, and more negative attitudes toward suicide in 75% of 141 studies. Religiosity was also found to be related to less alcohol or drug use/abuse in over 85% of nearly 300 studies, and greater social support, marital stability, and prosocial behavior in more than 80% of 257 studies.

What about health behaviors, such as exercise, diet, cigarette smoking, sexual activity, and weight control that are responsible for nearly 80% of all chronic medical illness? The research shows that religious persons were more likely to exercise or be physically active in nearly 70% of 37 studies; eat a better diet in over 60% of 21 studies; have lower cholesterol in over 50% of 23 studies; participate in less extra-marital sex in 86% of 95 studies, and were less likely to smoke cigarettes in 90% of 137 studies. Unfortunately, those who are more religious had lower weight in less than 20% of studies and were heavier than non-religious persons in nearly 40% of studies. Yes, those potluck suppers!

Despite this, however, religious persons have tended to have better physical health than non-religious persons in the majority of studies so far. This includes better immune function in over 50% of 25 studies; better endocrine function in nearly 75% of 31 studies; better cardiovascular functions in close to 70% of 16 studies; less coronary heart disease in nearly two-thirds of 19 studies; lower blood pressure in nearly 60% of 63 studies; less cancer or a better prognosis in more than half of 25 studies, and greater longevity overall in 68% of 121 studies, including over 75% of the most rigorously designed studies. Finally, research indicates that when spiritual needs have not been addressed by the medical team, this not only reduces the patient's quality of life and satisfaction with care, but may *double or triple healthcare costs*, at least towards the end of life [15].

In conclusion, based on this review of the available research, religion is often used to cope with stress in general and medical illness in particular; religious or spiritual involvement is associated with greater well-being, less emotional disorder, less substance abuse, greater social support, and better health behaviors; religiosity is related to less physical illness, better medical outcomes, and greater longevity; spiritual needs are widespread in medical settings, especially in those with serious, life-threatening disease; and assessing and addressing patients' spiritual needs is related to greater satisfaction with care, better QOL, less depression, fewer unnecessary health services, better functioning, and a better doctor-patient relationship. Much more research is needed to better understand relationships between religion and health; determine the underlying biological mechanisms involved; and develop new interventions that harness these effects. However, given the results of research already done, there is *every reason* for health professionals to assess and address the spiritual needs of patients.

4. Structure of the Spiritual Care Team

The members of the SCT and their roles will vary depending on whether the setting of care is outpatient or inpatient. For outpatient settings, the SCT will likely consist of a physician, a spiritual care coordinator (nurse or clinic manager), a chaplain or pastoral counselor, and a receptionist. In hospital settings, the SCT will include a social worker or case manager. The roles of each member of the team are distinct.

Physician. The physician's responsibility on the SCT is to conduct a brief "spiritual assessment" in order to identify spiritual needs. Once spiritual needs are identified, the physician will then arrange for someone to address those needs, follow up to ensure that spiritual needs are met, and be available to discuss this subject with patients as needed. The spiritual assessment done by the physician involves asking a few simple questions to identify spiritual needs related to medical illness. The purpose is to make the physician aware of the patient's religious background; determine if the patient has religious or spiritual support; identify beliefs that might influence medical decisions and affect compliance with the medical care plan; identify unmet spiritual needs related to medical illness; determine if engagement of the "spiritual care team" is necessary; and create an atmosphere where the patient feels comfortable talking with their physician about spiritual needs affecting medical care. The spiritual assessment consists of three questions:

1. Do you have a religious or spiritual support system to help you in times of need?
2. Do you have any religious beliefs that might influence your medical decisions?
3. Do you have any other spiritual concerns that you would like someone to address?

The physician will then document the patient's responses in the medical record, elaborating on any "yes" responses. If spiritual needs are identified, the physician will alert the Spiritual Care Coordinator (see below) so that arrangements can be made to address those needs. Finally, there should be follow-up down the road to determine if spiritual needs have been adequately addressed. The SCT will assist in this regard, although the physician is responsible for ensuring that such follow-up occurs. This is the minimum requirement that we are requesting of physicians. The spiritual assessment, however, is NOT a one-time event. Whenever there is a significant change in the patient's condition, the physician will want to check whether any new spiritual needs have arisen that the patient needs help with. Patients may not disclose a spiritual need or wish to discuss spiritual concerns, especially during a first visit. However, once the patient learns that the physician is receptive to discussing such issues, he or she may bring up the topic if needed during a future visit.

Do all patients need a spiritual assessment? No. There are five categories of patients where a spiritual assessment is indicated: patients with serious, life-threatening conditions; patients with chronic, disabling medical illness; patients with depression or significant anxiety; patients newly admitted to the hospital or to a nursing home; and patients being seen for a well-patient exam when time is available to address social issues. Those who do not need a spiritual assessment are patients seen for an acute problem without long-term implications, such as an upper respiratory infection, minor surgical procedure, routine pelvic exam, or some other specific, well-defined condition; patients seen for follow-up of a time-limited problem where there is no significant disability or challenges to coping; children, teenagers or young adults without chronic illness, life-threatening conditions, or disabling serious medical problem; and patients who are not religious or spiritual and so this area is not relevant to them.

Spiritual Care Coordinator (SCC). The SCC is often a nurse or a clinic manager. If the physician is the leader of the spiritual care team, then the SCC could be considered the "coach" of the team. The SCC has multiple duties. The first duty is to review the results of the physician's spiritual assessment, and identify and prioritize the spiritual needs that require addressing. The SCC does not conduct the assessment. The physician's assessment cannot be deferred to the SCC, since the physician needs to collect this information first hand. Next, the SCC manages each step to ensure that the patients' spiritual needs are addressed, providing resources as needed (for example, information on local faith communities, spiritual reading materials, information on pastoral care services, and so forth).

If a chaplain or pastoral care referral is necessary, the SCC prepares the patient to see the chaplain, *i.e.*, explains the reasons for the referral, describes the training that a chaplain has, and discusses what the chaplain will do. The SCC also prepares the chaplain (or pastoral counselor) for the referral, informing him or her about the spiritual needs identified and why the physician or SCC is referring the patient. After the chaplain referral is completed, the SCC follows up to obtain feedback from chaplain on the results of the evaluation and information about spiritual care plan, and then communicates this to the physician. The SCC then helps the chaplain follow-up with patient to ensure that spiritual needs identified during the physician's assessment were adequately addressed by the spiritual care plan. Finally, together with the chaplain, the SCC provides spiritual support to the physician and other members of the team, helping them to provide whole-person care to their patients. If, on the other hand, a patient prefers to address spiritual concerns with their own clergy, other member of their faith community, or other member of the healthcare team, the SCC will make the arrangements for such a meeting to occur.

The Chaplain. The chaplain likewise plays many roles, but there is one that is completely unique. The chaplain is the only person on the SCT *trained* to comprehensively assess and address the spiritual needs of patients. After receiving a referral, the chaplain will do a spiritual assessment that is quite different from physician's brief "screening" assessment. The chaplain will clarify spiritual needs that are present and will then develop a "spiritual care plan" to address those needs. The chaplain will work with the social worker (if available) to implement the spiritual care plan after discharge from the hospital or from the clinic. He or she will also follow up to ensure that spiritual needs are met and provide feedback to the team. Finally, the chaplain will work with the Spiritual Care Coordinator to address the spiritual needs of team members that are related to patient care. More specifically, what is involved in the chaplain's assessment and what types of interventions are then implemented?

The chaplain's assessment will differ depending on her or his individual style. Generally, though, the chaplain will make contact with the patient and spend time forming a relationship. During this time, the chaplain learns the "spiritual language" of the patient, which may or may not be religious. Much of the assessment will be spent listening to the patient talk about his or her struggles. No advice or spiritual counsel is usually offered during this time, which is often called the "ministry of presence". After that, the chaplain may ask questions about the patient's religious or spiritual background, and inquire about positive and negative experiences with religion. When the assessment has been completed, the chaplain will develop a spiritual care plan to address the spiritual needs identified.

The spiritual care plan will involve one or more specific interventions by the chaplain. Note that the "ministry of presence", which involves simply sitting with the patient and listening, is a powerful intervention by itself. The chaplain, however, may do other things besides simply listen. The chaplain may or may not pray with the patient, depending on the patient's preference. The chaplain may or may not read a Holy Scripture related to the patient's illness, again depending on the patient's preference. The chaplain may or may not provide spiritual advice, depending on patient's request and on the patient's readiness for such advice. The chaplain may provide religious resources to the patient, by request, such as spiritual reading materials, prayer beads, a prayer rug, *etc*. The chaplain may contact the patient's clergy or mobilize the patient's faith community for support, after obtaining explicit consent from the patient. All of this activity is highly patient-centered and focused on the patient's particular religious tradition or humanistic worldview. Finally, the chaplain will re-contact the patient at some future time to get follow-up on how effective the interventions were in addressing the patient's spiritual needs.

The chaplain may also engage in other activities, such as listening to, counseling, praying with, or providing spiritual and emotional support to family members. The chaplain may do the same for other members of the SCT. In hospital settings, the chaplain may hold chapel services and administer sacraments or perform other rituals at the bedside. The chaplain may also serve on the ethics committees or the institutional review board at the hospital. Finally, the chaplain works with community clergy, who may be trained to fill in for the chaplain during emergencies or during situations where the chaplain is absent.

Whether in an outpatient or inpatient setting, the chaplain should be fully integrated into the healthcare team. As noted above, the chaplain or pastoral counselor is at the core of the spiritual care team because he or she is the only person fully trained to address spiritual needs. Consequently, the chaplain should be actively involved in hospital rounds and in discussions involving patients in the clinic. Unfortunately, many hospital and outpatient settings do not have enough healthcare chaplains to meet the need. In a survey of 1591 patients at the Mayo Clinic [29], researchers found that 70% of hospitalized patients wanted to see a chaplain, but only 43% were visited by a chaplain, which is over double the national rate in the U.S. (*i.e.*, 20%) [30]. The proportion of outpatients seen by a chaplain or pastoral counselor is probably in the single digits. Note that over 80% of patients visited by a chaplain in the Mayo Clinic study said that the visit was important to them.

If a chaplain is not available, as may be the case in some outpatient settings, the Spiritual Care Coordinator would arrange a visit with a pastoral counselor or other person trained to address the spiritual needs of medical patients. If spiritual needs are urgent and trained clergy are not immediately available, then the SCC or other spiritual care team member might have to do their best to address the spiritual needs of the patient (primarily by listening and providing resources) and then make arrangements for follow-up by a religious professional at a later date. For this reason, all members of the spiritual care team, including the physician, should receive some training on providing "spiritual first aid" in the event that such care is needed.

Social Worker. In hospital settings, chaplains often have a close relationship with the team social worker, and some hospitals have actually combined pastoral care and social services into a single department. The reason is that spiritual needs are often closely linked with social issues. As a result, the social worker may provide important input to the spiritual care plan.

In this regard, the social worker may contact members of the patient's faith community for support after hospital discharge; identify a local faith community for the patient, if desired; identify a pastoral counselor after discharge and set up appointments; or help the chaplain follow-up to determine whether spiritual needs were effectively addressed.

There are many other contributions that the social worker can make to the spiritual care team. These include identifying spiritual needs during routine social assessment (however, this would not replace the physician's assessment); arranging referral to the chaplain or pastoral counselor if the Spiritual Care Coordinator is not available (or may work with the SCC to arrange the referral); and addressing simple spiritual needs if a chaplain is unavailable or is refused by the patient (this applies only to "simple" spiritual needs, since most social workers are not trained to address such needs). The social worker may also connect the patient with a mental health professional trained to integrate spiritual and emotional needs, as might be the case for trauma survivors and others with serious mental health problems.

The Receptionist. The receptionist in the physician's clinic or ward clerk in the hospital plays an important role on the spiritual care team. The duty of the receptionist is to record the patient's religious affiliation (specific denomination or religious group) in the medical record so that the physician can access it easily. This will save the physician time in conducting the spiritual assessment.

5. Spiritual Care

A major goal of the spiritual care team is to provide "spiritual care" to all patients as part of whole-person medicine. What is spiritual care? Although assessing and addressing the spiritual needs of patients is an important part of it, spiritual care goes far beyond that. The way that *ordinary health care* is provided by the physician and other members of the healthcare can be "spiritual". By that, I mean recognizing the sacred nature of the person being cared for and the holy obligation and privilege that health professionals have. More specifically, this means providing care with respect for the individual patient, a person with a unique life story; inquiring about how the patient wishes to be cared for, rather than providing the same care in the same way to everyone; providing care in a kind and gentle manner; providing care in a "competent" manner; and taking extra time with patients who really need it.

Spiritual care is the heart of what whole-person healthcare is really about, and has the potential to bring vitality back into the patient and into the practice of healthcare. However, it is not easy to do. Research indicates that only about 10% of physicians regularly conduct a spiritual assessment (and nearly 50% never do one) [31]. Why is this so? The following are 10 barriers that stand in the way of spiritual care. These barriers are based on research by the Harvard oncology group at the Dana Farber Institute [32]. They asked oncologists and oncology nurses why they did not routinely assess and address the spiritual needs of patients. Here is how they responded. After each barrier, I will suggest how to overcome it:

(1) *Lack of Time.* Spiritual care is just one more thing that health professionals are now being asked to do. They barely have enough time to perform required duties and document the results. Many are concerned about opening Pandora's box and not having adequate time to address the issues uncovered. There is temptation, then, to eliminate this "optional" activity (or defer it to others).

How to overcome: Doing a brief spiritual assessment must be a priority for the physician and addressing those needs a priority for the spiritual care team. This is not an optional activity, but central to providing "whole-person" medical care. The spiritual assessment can actually save time, improve the relationship with the patient, improve compliance, and make the physician's work more rewarding. The physician, as the director of the spiritual care team, cannot defer the spiritual assessment to anyone else. The spiritual care team, though, must be ready to fully address the patient's spiritual needs as their part of whole-person care.

(2) *Discomfort.* Many health professionals are not comfortable addressing this topic, particularly if they are not religious or particularly spiritual. Few health professionals have training on how to assess or address the spiritual needs of patients in a sensible and timely manner, or what to do if spiritual needs are identified.

How to overcome: Comfort comes with training and practice. Sometimes health professionals must do things that are not comfortable with to improve the quality of care that patients receive.

(3) *Making Patient Uncomfortable.* Health professionals may fear that asking such questions will make the patient feel uncomfortable, or may not know how to respond if the patient says: "Why are you asking these questions?"

How to overcome: Research shows that most patients, especially when seriously ill, are not offended or made uncomfortable when the physician performs a spiritual assessment, and in fact, the majority would like health professionals to do so [21,33]. If a patient asks why these questions are being asked, an appropriate response would be: "We are doing this routinely as a show of respect for the beliefs and values of patients, which may influence their medical care".

(4) *Spirituality Not Important.* Because spirituality is not important to the health professional, there is fear that the patient will ask about his or her own beliefs.

How to overcome: First, patients seldom ask health professionals about their personal beliefs. If they do ask, then a brief or general response usually satisfies the patient. The reason why most patients ask is that they are worried about how the clinician will treat their beliefs. Reassuring the patient that their beliefs will always be respected and honored usually allays this concern.

(5) *Topic Too Personal*. Health professionals feel that this topic is too personal to ask about, or they are concerned that they don't have a private space to discuss it.

How to overcome: Clinicians deal with other sensitive areas related to health much more personal than asking about religious beliefs. Sensitive areas include sexual behavior or personal health habits, such as smoking, drinking, diet, or weight control. Fear that these areas are too personal does not prevent health professionals from thoroughly assessing them.

(6) *Done Better by Others*. The physician believes that the spiritual assessment is done better by others.

How to overcome: Recognize that the physician is the leader of the healthcare team and needs to know about factors that could affect the patient's health and their compliance with the medical care plan.

(7) *Patients Don't Want Spiritual Care from Doctors/Nurses*. Health professionals believe that patients don't want them to address these issues.

How to overcome: As noted above, patient surveys indicate that only a minority of patients show resistance to inquiry about spiritual needs, or wish to keep medicine and religion separate [21,33]. Furthermore, doctors are usually only responsible for *assessment* in this model. Once spiritual needs are identified, the chaplain or pastoral counselor is the health professional who addresses them. One large study even found that when patients who did not want a visit from a chaplain and received one anyway, actually reported more satisfaction with their overall healthcare than did non-visited patients [34].

(8) *Power Inequality*. There is concern that the power inequality between patient and health professional might lead to coercion.

How to overcome: Realize that coercion in this area is unethical and a violation of civil rights. Thus, it is never appropriate to do so. I will discuss this boundary issue further in the next section.

(9) *Religious Beliefs Differ*. The religious beliefs of the healthcare provider differ from those of the patient.

How to overcome: Realize that in this era of patient-centered medicine, the focus should always be on respecting and supporting the spiritual beliefs of the patient, whether or not the health professional agrees with those beliefs.

(10) *Not Health Professional's Role*. Healthcare providers feel that assessing and addressing spiritual needs related to medical care is not part of their role.

How to overcome: Realize that providing whole-person care *is* part of the health professional's role and whole-person care includes addressing this area.

All of these barriers could be overcome through training and practice. Future research, however, will be needed to determine whether training, careful dividing up tasks among team members, and practice will make health professionals comfortable and fluent in spiritual care. In the Duke-Adventist Health collaborative study, we plan to systematically examine exactly this—whether the forming and training of spiritual care teams to assess and address patients' spiritual needs will affect health professionals' attitudes and behaviors (which will be measured at baseline and then 3 and 12 months afterwards).

6. Boundaries

There are, however, boundaries to providing spiritual care. Sometimes health professionals go beyond their expertise and perform actions that are neither sensible nor ethically justifiable. Here are five behaviors that healthcare providers should almost never do. First, don't prescribe religion to non-religious patients. Even though religious involvement may be good for health, non-believers should not be encouraged to become religious. Furthermore, the spiritual assessment should be conducted in such a way that patients who do not consider themselves spiritual do not feel devalued. As noted above, the spiritual assessment should be framed in such a way that the patient understands that such questions are being asked as a matter of routine in order to provide whole person care to those who do have spiritual needs. Second, and related to the latter, don't force a spiritual assessment if the patient is not religious. In that case, quickly switch to asking about what gives life meaning and purpose in the context of illness and how this can be supported. For these individuals, issues related to demoralization or death anxiety should be dealt with in a broad way using a holistic model grounded on humanistic beliefs and values. Third, don't pray with a patient before doing a spiritual assessment *and* unless the patient asks. While more than two-thirds to three-quarters of patients would like to pray with a health professional and deeply appreciate this [35,36], others might not. Fourth, in general, don't provide spiritual counsel to patients. Instead, always refer the patient to a trained professional chaplain or a pastoral counselor. As noted earlier, the only exceptions might be if the health professional has pastoral care training, or if addressing spiritual issues is urgent and the patient refuses pastoral care or pastoral care is not available. Finally, don't do any activity that is not patient-centered and patient-directed. Remember, it's about the patient—not the health professional. Addressing spiritual issues is like a ballroom dance. The patient leads and the health professional tries not to step on his or her toes.

Finally, in order for the physician and other team members to deliver whole-person spiritual care to patients, they need to be whole-persons themselves. The difficult task of caring for sick patients day-in and day-out challenges the physical, emotional and spiritual resources of most providers. For that reason, one major task of the spiritual care team is to support each other's spiritual needs that arise during the course of providing healthcare. Part of the role of the spiritual care coordinator and the chaplain is to ensure that the spiritual needs of team members are met. There are numerous spiritual resources that may help in this regard, depending on the provider's faith tradition [37–40].

Models, such as the one proposed here, and similar ones proposed by others [41], will need to be adapted to the unique settings and cultural environments that health professionals find themselves in—particularly as these models begin to be applied in non-Western countries (and in hospital settings that may not reflect the religious values of the Adventist Health System).

7. Conclusions

The following are the main points that this paper has been trying to convey. First, there is every reason to assess and address spiritual needs related to medical care—based on common sense, good clinical practice, and a firm scientific rationale. Second, the *physician* is responsible for a brief spiritual assessment that is designed to identify spiritual needs and create an atmosphere where spiritual needs related to medical care can be discussed. Third, the rest of the spiritual care team, led by the spiritual care coordinator, supports the physician by ensuring that the spiritual needs identified are effectively addressed. Fourth, the chaplain or pastoral counselor is at the core of the spiritual care team, and is responsible for conducting a comprehensive spiritual assessment to clarify spiritual needs and develop a spiritual care plan to address them. Finally, in hospital settings, the social worker helps the chaplain to develop and implement the spiritual care plan, and to arrange for follow-up to ensure that spiritual needs are met. For a more comprehensive resource on assessing and addressing the spiritual needs of patients, readers are referred elsewhere [42,43].

Conflicts of Interest: The author declares no conflicts of interest.

References

1. Harold G. Koenig, Dana E. King, and Verna B. Carson. *Handbook of Religion and Health*, 2nd ed. New York: Oxford University Press, 2012.
2. Michelle FlorCruz. "China's medical system strains both patients and doctors as hospital violence becomes increasingly common." *International Business Times*. 29 March 2014. Available online: http://www.ibtimes.com/chinas-medical-system-strains-both-patients-doctors-hospital-violence-becomes-increasingly-common (accessed on 15 September 2014).

3. David Lepeska. "Qatar's healthcare system under strain." *The National: World.* 9 July 2010. Available online: http://www.thenational.ae/news/world/middle-east/qatars-healthcare-system-under-strain (accessed on 15 September 2014).

4. Vanessa Furmans. "Germany strains to fund health care for all." *Wall Street Journal.* 18 November 2009. Available online: http://online.wsj.com/articles/SB125849684108252695 (accessed on 15 September 2014).

5. Jeb Blount. "Health care in Brazil on $300 a year." *World Policy.* 9 August 2010. Available online: http://www.worldpolicy.org/blog/health-care-brazil-300-year (accessed on 15 September 2014).

6. Wall Street Journal, and CNBC. "Report on Health Care Congress." *Clinical Psychiatry News*, 2005, 33, 86.

7. Avik Roy. "How health-care spending strains the U.S. military." *Forbes.* 12 March 2012. Available online: http://www.forbes.com/sites/aroy/2012/03/12/how-health-care-spending-strains-the-u-s-military/ (accessed on 15 September 2014).

8. Liselotte N. Dyrbye, and Tait D. Shanafelt. "Physician burnout: A potential threat to successful health care reform." *Journal of the American Medical Association* 305 (2011): 2009–10.

9. Harold G. Koenig, and Harvey Jay Cohen. *The Link between Religion and Health: Psychoneuroimmunology and the Faith Factor.* New York: Oxford University Press, 2002.

10. Wayne Katon, Elizabeth H.B. Lin, and Kurt Kroenke. "The association of depression and anxiety with medical symptom burden in patients with chronic medical illness." *General Hospital Psychiatry* 29 (2007): 147–55.

11. R. Emmer, and P. Browne. "Program helps nurses develop spiritual care skills." *Hospital Progress* 65 (1984): 64–66.

12. Harold G. Koenig, Ted Hamilton, and Kathy Perno. *Integrating Spirituality into Patient Care*; Durham: Duke University's Center for Spirituality, Theology and Health, Duke University Medical Center, 2014. Available online: http://www.spiritualityandhealth.duke.edu/ (accessed on 15 September 2014).

13. Tracy A. Balboni, Lauren C. Vanderwerker, Susan D. Block, M. Elizabeth Paulk, Christopher S. Lathan, John R. Peteet, and Holly G. Prigerson. "Religiousness and spiritual support among advanced cancer patients and associations with end-of-life treatment preferences and quality of life." *Journal of Clinical Oncology* 25 (2007): 555–60.

14. William D. Winkelman, Katharine Lauderdale, Michael J. Balboni, Andrea C. Phelps, John R. Peteet, Susan D. Block, Lisa A. Kachnic, Tyler J. VanderWeele, and Tracy A. Balboni. "The relationship of spiritual concerns to the quality of life of advanced cancer patients: Preliminary findings." *Journal of Palliative Medicine* 14 (2011): 1022–28.

15. Tracy A. Balboni, Michael J. Balboni, M. Elizabeth Paulk, Andrea C. Phelps, Alexi Wright, John R. Peteet, Susan D. Block, Christopher S. Lathan, Tyler J. Vanderweele, and Holly G. Prigerson. "Support of cancer patients' spiritual needs and associations with medical care costs at the end of life." *Cancer* 117 (2011): 5383–91.

16. Jean L. Kristeller, Mark Rhodes, Larry D. Cripe, and Virgil Sheets. "Oncologist Assisted Spiritual Intervention Study (OASIS): Patient acceptability and initial evidence of effects." *International Journal of Psychiatry in Medicine* 35 (2005): 329–47.

17. Philippe Huguelet, Sylvia Mohr, Carine Betrisey, Laurence Borras, Christiane Gillieron, Adham M. Marie, Isabelle Rieben, Nader Perroud, and Pierre-Yves Brandt. "A randomized trial of spiritual assessment of outpatients with schizophrenia: Patients' and clinicians' experience." *Psychiatric Services* 62 (2011): 79–86.

18. Harold G. Koenig. "Religious beliefs and practices of hospitalized medically ill older adults." *International Journal of Geriatric Psychiatry* 13 (1998): 213–24.

19. Harold G. Koenig. "Religion, spirituality and health: The research and clinical implications." *ISRN Psychiatry* 2012 Article 278730. (2012). [CrossRef]

20. John W. Ehman, Barbara B. Ott, Thomas H. Short, Ralph C. Ciampa, and John Hansen-Flaschen. "Do patients want physicians to inquire about their spiritual or religious beliefs if they become gravely ill? " *Archives of Internal Medicine* 159 (1999): 1803–06.

21. Gary McCord, Valerie J. Gilchrist, Steven D. Grossman, Bridget D. King, Kenelm F. McCormick, Allison M. Oprandi, Susan L. Schrop, Brian A. Selius, William D. Smucker, David L. Weldy, and *et al.* "Discussing spirituality with patients: A rational and ethical approach." *Annals of Family Medicine* 2 (2004): 356–61.

22. Farr A. Curlin, Ryan E. Lawrence, Marshal H. Chin, and John D. Lantos. "Religion, conscience, and controversial clinical practices." *New England Journal of Medicine* 356 (2007): 593–600.

23. Andrea C. Phelps, Paul K. Maciejewski, Mathew Nilsson, Tracy A. Balboni, Alexi A. Wright, M. Elizabeth Paulk, Elizabeth Trice, Deborah Schrag, John R. Peteet, Susan D. Block, and *et al.* "Religious coping and use of intensive life-prolonging care near death in patients with advanced cancer." *Journal of the American Medical Association* 301 (2009): 1140–47.

24. Information contained here on the standards are based on a series of communications between Dr. Harold G. Koenig and JCAHO staff, particularly Doreen Finn (DFinn@jointcommission.org), Senior Associate Director, JCAHO, Hospital Accreditation, e-mail communication, 6–12 January 2012, and the JCAHO Manual documenting the regulations.

25. Mark A. Schuster, Bradley D. Stein, Lisa H. Jaycox, Rebecca L. Collins, Grant N. Marshall, Marc N. Elliott, Annie J. Zhou, David E. Kanouse, Janina L. Morrison, and Sandra H. Berry. "A national survey of stress reactions after the September 11, 2001, terrorist attacks." *New England Journal of Medicine* 345 (2001): 1507–12.

26. Harold G. Koenig, Harvey Jay Cohen, Dan G. Blazer, Carl Pieper, Keith G. Meador, Frank Shelp, Veerainder Goli, and Robert DiPasquale. "Religious coping and depression in elderly hospitalized medically ill men." *American Journal of Psychiatry* 149 (1992): 1693–1700.

27. Harold G. Koenig, Linda K. George, and Bercedis L. Peterson. "Religiosity and remission from depression in medically ill older patients." *American Journal of Psychiatry* 155 (1998): 536–42.

28. Harold G. Koenig. "Religion and remission of depression in medical inpatients with heart failure/pulmonary disease." *Journal of Nervous and Mental Disease* 195 (2007): 389–95.

29. Katherine M. Piderman, Dean V. Marek, Sarah M. Jenkins, Mary E. Johnson, James F. Buryska, Tait D. Shanafelt, Floyd G. O'Bryan, Patrick D. Hansen, Priscilla H. Howick, Heidi L. Durland, and *et al.* "Predicting patients' expectations of hospital chaplains: A multi-site survey." *Mayo Clinic Proceedings* 85 (2010): 1002–10.

30. Kevin J. Flannelly, Katherine Galek, and George J. Handzo. "To what extent are the spiritual needs of hospital patients being met? " *International Journal of Psychiatry in Medicine* 35 (2005): 319–23.

31. Farr A. Curlin, Marshal H. Chin, Sarah A. Sellergren, Chad J. Roach, and John D. Lantos. "The association of physicians' religious characteristics with their attitudes and self-reported behaviors regarding religion and spirituality in the clinical encounter." *Medical Care* 44 (2006): 446–53.

32. Michael J. Balboni, Adam Sullivan, Andrea C. Enzinger, Zachary D. Epstein-Peterson, Yolanda D. Tseng, Christine Mitchell, Joshua Niska, Angelika Zollfrank, Tyler J. VanderWeele, and Tracy A. Balboni. "Nurse and physician barriers to spiritual care provision at the end of life." *Journal of Pain & Symptom Management* 48 (2014): 400–10.

33. Jennifer L. Hamilton, and Jeffrey P. Levine. "Neo-pagan patients' preferences regarding physician discussion of spirituality." *Family Medicine* 38 (2006): 83–84.

34. Joshua A. Williams, David Meltzer, Vineet Arora, Grace Chung, and Farr A. Curlin. "Attention to inpatients' religious and spiritual concerns: predictors and association with patient satisfaction." *Journal of General Internal Medicine* 26 (2011): 1265–71.

35. Oliver Oyama, and Harold G. Koenig. "Religious beliefs and practices in family medicine." *Archives of Family Medicine* 7 (1998): 431–35.

36. Harold G. Koenig, Mona Smiley, and Joann P. Gonzales. *Religion, Health, and Aging*. Westport: Greenwood Press, 1988, pp. 138–39.

37. Oswald Chambers. *My Utmost for His Highest*. Uhrichsville: Barbour Publishing, 1963.

38. David Winter. *Closer than a Brother*. Wheaton: Harold Shaw Publishers, 1971.

39. Aryeh Kaplan. *Jewish Meditation*. New York: Schocken, 2011.

40. Scott Kugle. *Sufi Meditation and Contemplation*. Lancaster: Omega Publications, 2013.

41. Michael J. Balboni, Christina M. Puchalski, and John R. Peteet. "The relationship between medicine, spirituality and religion: three models for integration." *Journal of Religion and Health* 53 (2014): 1586–98.

42. Harold G. Koenig. *Spirituality in Patient Care*, 3rd ed. Philadelphia: Templeton Press, 2013.

43. "Center for Spirituality, Theology and Health, Duke University Medical Center." Available online: http://www.spiritualityandhealth.duke.edu/ (accessed on 15 September 2014).

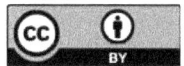

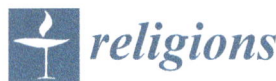

Article

How do Psychiatric Staffs Approach Religiosity/Spirituality in Clinical Practice? Differing Perceptions among Psychiatric Staff Members and Clinical Chaplains

Eunmi Lee [1,*], Anne Zahn [2] and Klaus Baumann [1]

[1] The Department of Caritas Science and Christian Social Welfare, Freiburg University,
Platz der Universitaet 3, D-79098 Freiburg, Germany; klaus.baumann@theol.uni-freiburg.de

[2] The Department of Psychiatry and Psychotherapy, Freiburg University Hospital, Hauptstrasse 5,
D-79104 Freiburg, Germany; anne.zahn@uniklinik-freiburg.de

* Author to whom correspondence should be addressed; eunmi.lee@theol.uni-freiburg.de;
Tel.: +49-761-203-2005; Fax: +49-761-203-2119.

Academic Editor: Arndt Büssing

Received: 20 May 2015; Accepted: 24 July 2015; Published: 3 August 2015

Abstract: The present study examined the perception of contemporary German psychiatric staff (*i.e.*, psychiatrists, psychotherapists and nurses) regarding their approach towards religious/spiritual issues in their clinical practice, and how clinical chaplains perceive attitudes and behaviors towards religiosity/spirituality of other psychiatric staff members. To answer these questions, two separate studies were conducted to include psychiatric staff and clinical chaplains. Curlin *et al.*'s questionnaire on *Religion and Spirituality in Medicine: Physicians' Perspectives* was the main instrument used for both studies. According to the self-assessment of psychiatric staff members, most contemporary German psychiatric staff members are prepared and open to dealing with religiosity/spirituality in therapeutic settings. To some extent, clinical chaplains agreed with this finding, but their overall perception significantly differs from the staff's own self-rating. Our results suggest that it may be helpful for psychiatric staff members and clinical chaplains to exchange their views on patients regarding religious/spiritual issues in therapeutic settings, and to reflect on how to apply such findings to clinical practice.

Keywords: religiosity/spirituality; psychiatric staff; chaplain; Germany; self-awareness

---

1. Introduction

When patients suffer from severe illnesses and mental crises, they frequently ask themselves why they have become a "victim" of such a difficult situation and why or whether they "deserve" it. It is not unusual for patients to ask existential questions and to reflect on and seek out the meaning of life [1,2]. Religious/spiritual people, in particular, try to find answers and deal with their hard times by turning to their belief systems and religious/spiritual practices, e.g., by reading the Bible or praying.

In the field of mental health, there are ambivalent attitudes regarding whether and how religion and/or spirituality should become a standard aspect of mental health care rather than being restricted to religious pastoral care. In continuity with a strong demarcation between psychiatry/psychology and religions/religious rituals in the 19th and most of 20th century [3–5], for instance, the Austrian Federal Ministry of Health on June 17th, 2014 edited guidelines for psychotherapists to (re-)establish boundaries against esoteric, spiritual and religious practices [6]. In addition to the stipulation to refrain from religious/spiritual methods and practices in psychiatric and psychotherapeutic practice, these guidelines also point to an increased yet perhaps unprofessional interest in esoteric and religious/spiritual issues in mental health practice. The mere avoidance of religious/spiritual practice in therapeutic settings does not yet resolve the question of how to perceive and deal with these issues in mental health care. Undoubtedly, religious/spiritual issues are part of the human mind and behavior in general—that is to say an object of behavioral sciences, psychiatry included—and they also play a role, for better or for worse, in the mental conditions of psychiatric patients.

In fact, there is a growing body of research and publications exploring the actual and potential role of religion and/or religiosity/spirituality in psychiatry and psychotherapy [7–11]. Research has shown that psychiatric patients sometimes indicate religious/spiritual needs during therapy [12–15]. There are patients receiving psychotherapeutic treatment who express a desire for their religious and spiritual needs to be taken into consideration by psychiatric staff members and to exercise their religious/spiritual activities without encountering prejudice. In addition, several empirical studies with psychiatric patients have found significant associations between religiosity/spirituality and mental health; e.g., depression [13,16–18], eating disorder [19], post-traumatic stress disorder [20–22] or schizophrenia [23], even though such studies have used different traits, tested various groups and accordingly shown inconsistent results. For instance, the American study of Miller *et al.* showed the protective relationship between maternal religiosity and having MDD (major depressive disorder) with $p < 0.005$ [17]. In a study with German patients, however, the depression measured by BDI (Beck's Depression Inventory) was not associated with RGH (Reliance of God's Help) [24].

Further studies have shown positive effects of religious and/or spiritual behaviors on mental health [22,25–27]. For example, the study with college-aged students in Wachholz and Pargament show that a spiritual meditation group shows significantly less anxiety in comparison to relaxation or secular group meditation (respectively, $p < 0.01$ and 0.05) [25]. Also, PPANS (positive mood; the Positive Affect Scale), but not NPANS (negative mood), showed a significant difference ($p < 0.01$). Plante (2008) was the first to distinguish between the intrinsic and extrinsic benefits of religious/spiritual behaviors: "Intrinsic benefits are benefits for the self helping to make someone a better and more well adjusted person [...] Extrinsic benefits involve advantages that are external to the self that benefit the person within community" [28]. In clinical settings, even in the era of secularized societies, various religious/spiritual tools based on religious/spiritual principles are frequently used, not necessarily in connection with any particular religion. Well-known therapeutic approaches are 12-step programs or diverse mindfulness-based meditations, such as the MBSR (The Mindfulness-Based Stress Reduction) or MBCT (Mindfulness-Based Cognitive Therapy).

Taking these elements into account, it is of increasing interest to assess how mental health care providers actually deal with religious/spiritual topics in their clinical practice. How do they approach their patients' religious/spiritual issues? According to empirical evidence, contemporary mental health specialists actually quite often encounter religious/spiritual aspects in clinical settings. Apart from pathological symptoms in the disguise of religious phenomena, they often observe positive effects from religiosity/spirituality in mental health care [29–32]. Generally, mental health specialists perceive themselves as being aware of their clients' religious/spiritual concerns. Yet, dealing with religious/spiritual matters in their clinical practice is not typically part of psychiatric staffs' "standard" repertoire, and they do not consider such issues to be their main responsibility [32–35]. For example, El-Nimr *et al.* surveyed psychiatric staffs in the UK [35] and found that (only) one quarter of psychiatrists and less than 20% of psychiatric nurses believed that psychiatrists should assess and provide spiritual care. Furthermore, over half of both groups thought that mental health professionals are not the appropriate professional group to deal with such issues. In a study by Huguelet *et al.*, only 36% of Swiss psychiatric staffs had ever discussed religious/spiritual topics with their patients [34].

While the presence of religious/spiritual factors in therapeutic settings requires further research and development, the international interest in religiosity/spirituality in mental health care, including its adequate integration into clinical practice, is increasing. In most German clinics, chaplains (or pastoral care providers) from different religious denominations are available to meet the explicit religious needs of patients (including rituals). The mutual perceptions, interactions and relationships between psychiatric staff and chaplains appear relevant, both for therapeutic processes (progress or regressions) as well as the spiritual "well-being" of patients. However, there are fewer studies dedicated to psychiatric staff, particularly in German-speaking countries, in comparison to the U.S. or other English-speaking countries. In addition, there are hardly any studies focusing on both of these mental health "specialists" [32,36], and, to our knowledge, no study that investigates the level of correspondence between the self-perception of psychiatric staff and the "outside" perception of clinical chaplains.

Therefore, within the scope of a larger research project, we aimed at surveying both psychiatric and psychotherapeutic staff members as well as clinical chaplains in the psychiatry department with regard to religiosity/spirituality in clinical practice. In particular, we addressed the following topics: How do contemporary German psychiatric staffs deal with religiosity/spirituality during therapy? How do clinical chaplains perceive the way other psychiatric staff members deal with religious/spiritual issues? Which similarities and differences exist in these perceptions?

2. Materials and Method

2.1. Respondents

To answer the aforementioned questions, we conducted two main studies. One study focused on psychiatric staff, and the other was directed towards clinical chaplains. All participants in these anonymously conducted studies were informed about the purpose of the study (to survey their various experiences with religious/spiritual issues in treatment processes in psychiatry and psychotherapy wards). They were also assured of confidentiality and their right to withdraw at any time.

2.1.1. Study with Psychiatric Staff

From October 2010 to February 2011, an anonymous survey was conducted in German university hospitals and faith-based clinics in 16 cities to explore the viewpoints of psychiatric staff in regard to religiosity/spirituality. In this study, we defined psychiatric staff as medical, (psycho-) therapeutic, nursing and also other team members (e.g., social worker, secretary) directly working with patients. A total of 32 German university hospitals and 21 faith-based clinics had been asked to take part in our study. Ultimately 21 clinics participated. The medical director of each psychiatric department distributed a paper-based questionnaire to relevant employees. A total of 404 questionnaires were returned (response rate = 24.43%; $n = 1654$): The response rate of 11 participating university hospitals was 29.54% ($n = 205$ of 694) and that of 10 participating faith-based clinics was 20.73% ($n = 199$ of 960). The detailed information as well as part of results have been published in several papers [29,30,37].

For the purpose of our analysis, we focused on three occupational groups: psychiatrists, psychotherapists and nurses. A total of 330 questionnaires were filled out by these groups. An isolated response rate could not be calculated for this group, as the total number of participants from each clinic could only be obtained at the beginning of the survey. There were 312 questionnaires used for the final analysis and 18 questionnaires were not included due to incomplete responses.

2.1.2. Study with Clinical Chaplains

For a comparative analysis, we conducted an anonymous survey among clinical chaplains working in psychiatry and psychotherapy departments. Among other goals, this study aimed to find out how chaplains perceive the attitudes as well as the behaviors of other psychiatric staff members towards religiosity/spirituality. First, we conducted a pilot study from November 2012 to February 2013. In the context of this pilot study, we began by locating all Catholic psychiatric chaplains in Baden-Württemberg (federal state in southern Germany). Subsequently, paper-based questionnaires were sent to these Catholic chaplains as well as their Protestant or other confessional colleagues working in the same clinics. The response rate was 59.38% (38 of 64 questionnaires).

From March 2014 to June 2014, a nationwide study was consequently conducted among all clinical chaplains who were at the time mainly working in the field of psychiatry and psychotherapy. Again, we began by first locating all Catholic psychiatric chaplains of German dioceses (beyond Baden-Württemberg): participation was requested of 23 German dioceses[1] and ultimately 15 dioceses participated in the survey. Each diocese provided a list of all enrolled Catholic chaplains via a dedicated contact person. Then, paper-based surveys were sent to them as well as the Protestant and other confessional chaplains working in the same hospitals. Contact information of Protestant and other confessional chaplains was either provided via reference of Catholic colleagues or researched on the relevant clinic's website. The response rate was 47.39% (100 of 211 questionnaires); the response rate of Catholic chaplains was 75.28% (67 of 89 questionnaires) and that of Protestant and other confessional chaplains was 27.05% (33 of 122 questionnaires).

Finally, the data collected from both studies were analyzed. Of the 275 distributed questionnaires, 138 were returned (response rate = 50.18%). Due to incomplete responses, the final sample included 124 questionnaires.

2.2. Measures

The main instrument used for the survey was the questionnaire from Curlin *et al.*, *Religion and Spirituality in Medicine: Physicians' Perspectives* [38]. F. Curlin and his colleagues primarily developed this instrument to measure the religious/spiritual characteristics of medical doctors, their observation/interpretation of the influence of religion and/or spirituality on patients' health, and also their attitudes/self-reported behaviors towards religion and/or spirituality in therapeutic settings. The questionnaire was developed using literature reviews and qualitative pilot studies, and tested through multiple iterations of expert panel reviews [39] More detailed information on how they developed and tested this questionnaire has been described in several papers [31,38,39].

To meet the requirements for a study in German-speaking territories, Curlin's questionnaire was translated into German (for the first time) and was slightly modified to suit the German language. This translation was then revised by a team of professionals. In 2009, a first pilot study was conducted in the department of psychiatry and psychotherapy of the University Medical Center Freiburg in Germany from December 2008 to January 2009 [40]. Based on respondents' comments, response options were modified to a 5-point ordinal scale and all questionnaire items were redesigned into statements. According to each category, all items were tested by principle component analysis as well as reliability (internal consistency) [29]. In addition, because the German term "religion" is generally limited to formal religious affiliation, we decided to use the expression "religiosity/spirituality" rather than the original terminology "religion/spirituality" in order to encompass all related subjective religious/spiritual issues. For the large part of the questionnaires, the format used in both studies was identical. In the study with the psychiatric staff, however, the meaning of the translated answer "unsure" was unclear for several respondents. According to these participants, the translated term conveyed an ambiguous meaning, such as "I have no idea" or "I am not sure", thereby leading to some confusion The number of respondents finding this term difficult was not negligible. After discussion with a team of professionals we decided that the translated answer "unsure" had to be removed from the mean analysis to ensure the accuracy of the ordinal scale. In the questionnaire of chaplains, this response option was presented separately. The remaining response options provided a 4-point ordinal scale.

In line with the aim of our analysis, we concentrated only on items concerning attitudes/self-reported behaviors towards religiosity/spirituality in therapeutic settings. Fully described items are listed in Tables accessed in the result part.

---

[1] There are 27 dioceses in Germany. Among them, two already participated in our pilot study. Another two dioceses do not have pastoral care especially dedicated psychiatry and psychotherapy.

2.3. Statistical Analysis

A total of 436 questionnaires were included in the final statistical analysis. All data were analyzed with SPSS 20.0 for Windows. To test the difference between groups and variables, cross-tabulation as well as Pearson's chi-squared-test, Levene's test, *t*-test, univariate analyses of variance (UNIANOVA), in addition to Scheffé's *post hoc* test and Spearman's rank correlation were used. Significance level was set at $p < 0.05$.

All questions were set on and analyzed as a 4-point ordinal scale (from 1-definitely not true to 4-definitely true of me). The response option "unsure" was tested separately to see if there were any significant differences according to demographic characteristics.

3. Results

3.1. Characteristics of Survey Respondents

On average, respondents were 43.15 years old (Table 1). Among the respondents, 54.4% were women. More than three-fourths of participants had a religious affiliation. Among chaplains, 65.3% were Catholic and 34.7% were Protestant (data not shown). Among psychiatric professionals, 67.6% indicated a religious affiliation[2]: 44.9% of them were Protestant and 41% were Catholic. In addition, among the psychiatric staff, 50.3% worked in university clinics and 49.7% in faith-based clinics (data not shown). The largest group of participants were nurses (33.9%) and clinical chaplains (28.4%). On average, respondents had 10.05 years of work experience in the fields of psychiatry and psychotherapy. The detailed results are described in Table 1.

Table 1. Characteristics of survey respondents.

Variable		Values (%)
Absolute Number		436
Age (years)		43.15 (±11.64 [a])
Sex	Female	237 (54.4)
	Male	199 (45.6)
Religious affiliation	Have a religious affiliation	335 (76.8)
	No religious affiliation [b]	101 (23.2)
Occupation	Doctor	118 (27.1)
	Psychotherapist	46 (10.6)
	Nurse	148 (33.9)
	Chaplain	124 (28.4)
Work experience in occupation (years)		15.94 (±10.95)
Work experience in psychiatry (years)		10.05 (±8.18)

[a] All numeric results were rounded up to the nearest hundredth; [b] Atheist, agnostic, and none.

In addition, we examined demographic differences between the respondents, particularly in terms of their occupation. A significant difference was found between different occupations (Table 2). Via Scheffé's *post hoc* test, we found that clinical chaplains differed significantly from other professions with regard to age and professional work experience. With regard to religious affiliation, as could be expected, there was also a significant difference between chaplains and psychiatric staff, while among

---

[2] This percentage is somewhat less than in the wider German population. According to "Religionsmonitor 2008", 26% of the German population has no religious affiliation [41]. The research of the EKD (*Protestant Church in Germany*) conducted in 2010 also showed that approximately 76% have a religious affiliation [42].

other psychiatric staff (*i.e.*, excepting chaplains) there was no significant difference. In psychiatric fields, nurses had the longest experience, significantly different from psychiatrists and psychotherapists (respectively $p < 0.01$).

Table 2. Demographic differences between professional groups.

		Psychiatrist (N = 118)	Psychotherapist (N = 46)	Nurse (N = 148)	Chaplain (N = 124)	P
Age (years)		38.78 ($\pm$ 7.96)	35.50 ($\pm$ 8.90)	39.78 ($\pm$ 11.41)	54.16 ($\pm$ 7.61)	<0.001 [a]
Sex (%)	Women	45.8	73.9	70.9	35.5	<0.001 [b]
	Men	54.2	26.1	29.1	64.5	
Religious affiliation (%)	No...	28.8	34.8	34.5	0.0	<0.001 [b]
	Have...	71.2	65.2	65.5	100.0	
Work experience in occupation (years)		10.56 ($\pm$8.01)	9.12 ($\pm$8.62)	17.75 ($\pm$11.79)	21.42 ($\pm$9.52)	<0.001 [a]
Work experience in psychiatry (years)		8.24 ($\pm$7.55)	7.10 ($\pm$7.07)	12.39 ($\pm$8.79)	10.08 ($\pm$7.66)	<0.001 [a]

[a] Results of UNIANOVA; each eta squared size is $\eta^2 = 0.368$ (age); $\eta^2 = 0.187$ (work experience) and $\eta^2 = 0.055$ (work in psychiatry); [b] Results of Pearson; s square test.

3.2. Psychiatric Staff's Attitudes and Self-Reported Behaviors Regarding Religiosity/Spirituality in Clinical Settings

3.2.1. Attitudes towards Religiosity/Spirituality

Among the psychiatric staff, almost 80% of respondents found it appropriate to ask patients about religion and/or spirituality, and nearly 90% found the discussion of religious/spiritual issues appropriate when patients address such topics. At the same time, it was considered inappropriate by 72.8% that staff members share or talk about their own religious/spiritual backgrounds. Concerning prayer with patients, more than 55% of respondents considered it absolutely unsuitable. Detailed information is provided in Table 3.

Table 3. Psychiatric staff's attitudes and self-rated behaviors regarding religiosity/spirituality.

Questionnaire Items	Values (%) [a]				
	Definitely True of Me	Tends to Be True	Tends Not to Be True	Definitely Not True	Unsure
Attitudes					
In general, it is appropriate for *psychiatric staff* to inquire about a patient's religion and/or spirituality.	116 (37.2)	130 (41.7)	35 (11.2)	14 (4.5)	17 (5.4)
In general, it is appropriate for *psychiatric staff* to discuss religious/spiritual issues, when a patient brings them up.	159 (51.0)	121 (38.8)	17 (5.4)	4 (1.3)	11 (3.5)
In general, it is appropriate for *psychiatric staff* to talk about his or her own religious beliefs or experiences with a patient.	8 (2.6)	60 (19.2)	112 (35.9)	115 (36.9)	17 (5.4)
In general, it is appropriate for *psychiatric staff* to pray with a patient together.	9 (2.9)	27 (8.7)	74 (23.7)	175 (56.1)	27 (8.7)
Behaviors [b]					
I listen carefully and empathetically.	229 (73.4)	74 (23.7)	5 (1.6)	0 (0.0)	4 (1.3)
I try to change the subject in a tactful way.	11 (3.5)	44 (14.1)	143 (45.8)	93 (29.8)	21 (6.7)
I encourage patients in their own religious/spiritual beliefs and practices.	72 (23.1)	152 (48.7)	36 (11.5)	11 (3.5)	41 (13.1)
I respectfully share *my* own religious ideas and experiences.	13 (4.2)	42 (13.5)	106 (34.0)	139 (44.6)	12 (3.8)
I pray with the patient.	9 (2.9)	17 (5.4)	49 (15.7)	229 (73.4)	8 (2.6)
I refer patients to chaplains.	100 (32.1)	160 (51.3)	25 (8.0)	9 (2.9)	18 (5.8)
It's not *my* responsibility.	19 (6.1)	36 (11.5)	87 (27.9)	150 (48.1)	20 (6.4)

[a] N = 312 (psychiatrists, psychotherapists and nurses); [b] Preceded by "when religious/spiritual issues come up in discussions with patients."

In the comparative analysis according to profession, particularly the nursing and medical staff showed a significant difference regarding the question of whether it is appropriate for staff members to share their own religious beliefs or related experiences (via the *post hoc* test; the highest possible score with 4.00,[3] *m* of nurses = 2.03 ± 0.90 *vs. m* of psychiatrists = 1.71 ± 0.73; *p* = 0.009). With regard to prayer with patients, the *post hoc* test again showed a significant difference between nurses and psychiatrists (*p* < 0.001) as well as psychotherapists (*p* = 0.001). The mean of each item as well as each occupational group is reported in Table 4.

Table 4. Psychiatric staff's self-reported attitudes and behaviors regarding religiosity/spirituality.

Questionnaire Items [a]	Psychiatrist	Psychotherapist	Nurse
Attitudes			
In general, it is appropriate for *psychiatric staff* to inquire about a patient's religion and/or spirituality.	3.17 ± 0.80	3.38 ± 0.65	3.12 ± 0.88
In general, it is appropriate for *psychiatric staff* to discuss religious/spiritual issues, when a patient brings them up.	3.45 ± 0.61	3.69 ± 0.47	3.37 ± 0.74
In general, it is appropriate for *psychiatric staff* to talk about his or her own religious beliefs or experiences with a patient.	1.71 ± 0.73	1.77 ± 0.75	2.03 ± 0.90
In general, it is appropriate for *psychiatric staff* to pray with a patient together.	1.27 ± 0.49	1.32 ± 0.57	1.84 ± 0.94
Behaviors [b]			
I listen carefully and empathetically.	3.75 ± 0.45	3.83 ± 0.38	3.68 ± 0.53
I try to change the subject in a tactful way.	1.84 ± 0.78	1.64 ± 0.61	2.05 ± 0.81
I encourage patients in their own religious/spiritual beliefs and practices.	3.18 ± 0.65	3.19 ± 0.74	2.91 ± 0.80
I respectfully share *my* own religious ideas and experiences.	1.59 ± 0.72	1.53 ± 0.66	1.99 ± 0.95
I pray with the patient.	1.13 ± 0.36	1.09 ± 0.29	1.64 ± 0.92
I refer patients to chaplains.	2.94 ± 0.72	2.90 ± 0.77	3.47 ± 0.58
It's not *my* responsibility.	1.76 ± 0.83	1.53 ± 0.74	1.79 ± 1.01

[a] Response categories are: 1 = definitely not true, 2 = tends not to be true, 3 = tends to be true, 4 = definitely true of me; [b] Preceded by "when religious/spiritual issues come up in discussions with patients".

3.2.2. Self-Reported Behaviors Regarding Religiosity/Spirituality

Nearly all respondents (97.1%) indicated that they listen carefully and empathetically to patients' religious/spiritual concerns, when these issues come up in the conversation (Table 3). This response corresponds strongly with professionally desired behavior. About 75% reported to not shy away from such topics. Furthermore, nearly 72% indicated that they encourage their patients to practice their religious/spiritual activities. A percentage of 83.4% of psychiatric staff members recommend patients to clinical chaplains. Approximately 79% of respondents, however, preferred not to share their own religious/spiritual backgrounds. About 90% did not find it appropriate to engage in prayer with patients (73.4% found it absolutely inappropriate).

---

[3]   In the mean analysis, the answer "unsure" was removed to ensure the nature of an ordinal scale in our German version. We tested for significant differences in regard to demographic characteristics (age, sex, occupation, religious affiliation, work experience and work in psychiatry) and the response "unsure". Only one significant difference was found: Younger participants tended to reply with "unsure" when asked whether it is generally appropriate to discuss religious/spiritual issues with patients (*p* = 0.013).

Among the staff, nurses were most inclined to change the subject when patients addressed religious/spiritual topics (Table 4). Especially in comparison to psychotherapists, the nursing staff showed a significant difference (of the highest possible score 4.00^4, *m* of nurses = 2.05 ± 0.81 *vs. m* of psychotherapists = 1.64 ± 0.61; $p = 0.01$). Again, the nursing staff was the most reluctant to encourage religious/spiritual practical activities. Particularly compared to psychiatrists, their mean differed significantly (*m* of nurses: 2.91 ± 0.80 *vs. m* of psychiatrists: 3.18 ± 0.65; $p = 0.019$). However, nurses were the most willing to suggest patients visit chaplains and the least reluctant to share their own religious beliefs or pray with patients, when compared to other groups (at least $p < 0.01$).

As an additional question, we asked psychiatric staff members about their experience with chaplains in clinical settings (data not shown). Of 312 participants, 83.3% reported having encountered chaplains in clinics, and the remaining 16.7% did not have any experience with them. In addition, having an experience with chaplains was significantly dependent on the occupation. More than 90% of the nursing staff and about 85% of psychiatrists reported having experience with chaplains. In contrast, only 52.2% of psychotherapists had ever come across chaplains in their clinical experience ($p < 0.001$).

3.3. Clinical Chaplains' Assessment of Other Staff's Attitudes as Well as Their Behaviors Regarding Religiosity/Spirituality in Clinical Setting

3.3.1. Attitudes towards Religiosity/Spirituality

Clinical chaplains perceived that psychiatric staff members *occasionally* regard it as appropriate to inquire or discuss religion and/or related topics. Each reply of occupational groups was slightly in the middle between *tends to be true* and *tends not to be true*, as mean scores were shown around 2.5 of 4.00. In comparison to psychiatric staff's self-assessment regarding these two questions (*i.e.*, inquiry and discussion), the perception of chaplains was significantly less positive (respectively $p < 0.001$; *cf.* Table 4). Particularly psychiatrists and psychotherapists indicated a strong tendency to discuss religious/spiritual issues with patients when patients address such topics. In contrast, chaplains rated the attitudes of psychiatrists and psychotherapists rather moderately. Based on subgroups of chaplains (age, sex, work experience in occupational field, work in psychiatry), chaplains' assessments of psychiatric staff's attitudes were not significantly different.

Concerning issues about sharing one's own religious/spiritual backgrounds and praying with patients, clinical chaplains assessed the attitudes of nurses most positively. In general, clinical chaplains' observation was not significantly different from other psychiatric staff's self-rated assessment. Only one significant difference was found: Clinical chaplains perceived nursing staff to have a more positive attitude towards sharing religious/spiritual background than the nurses themselves indicated (2.26 *vs.* 2.03; $p = 0.023$).

3.3.2. Behaviors Regarding Religiosity/Spirituality

According to chaplains, psychiatric personnel tend to listen carefully and empathetically when religious/spiritual themes are brought up, but not to a strong extent (Table 5). Chaplains reported that psychiatric staff members *occasionally* encourage their patients to practice religious/spiritual activities and usually refer patients to visit chaplains. By and large, clinical chaplains found that the nursing staff of a clinic has the most positive behavior towards patients' religiosity/spirituality.

---

[4] Again, the answer "unsure" was not included in the analysis of the mean. According to sex, occupation, religious affiliation and work experience in psychiatry, no significant difference was found. According to age, some significant differences were found: younger participants tended to be unsure whether they listen carefully, change religious/spiritual themes, encourage their patients to practice patients' religiosity/spirituality or share staff's own religious/spiritual backgrounds (respectively $p < 0.05$). Furthermore, participants with less work experience in their occupational field seemed to be unsure whether they encourage their patients to practice religious/spiritual activities or share staff's own religiosity/spirituality (respectively $p < 0.05$).

Table 5. Chaplains' assessment of other psychiatric staff's attitudes and self-reported behaviors regarding religiosity/spirituality in clinical settings.

Questionnaire Items [a]	Psychiatrist [b]	Psychotherapist [b]	Nurse [b]
Attitudes			
In general, it is appropriate for *psychiatric staff* to inquire about a patient's religion and/or spirituality.	2.44 ± 0.66 ***	2.52 ± 0.69 ***	2.69 ± 0.70 ***
In general, it is appropriate for *psychiatric staff* to discuss religious/spiritual issues, when a patient brings them up.	2.59 ± 0.77 ***	2.67 ± 0.71 ***	2.84 ± 0.68 ***
In general, it is appropriate for *psychiatric staff* to talk about his or her own religious beliefs or experiences with a patient.	1.81 ± 0.73	1.80 ± 0.71	2.26 ± 0.71 *
In general, it is appropriate for *psychiatric staff* to pray with a patient together.	1.37 ± 0.70	1.28 ± 0.56	1.84 ± 0.81
Behaviors [c]			
I listen carefully and empathetically.	2.73 ± 0.62 ***	2.85 ± 0.49 ***	2.99 ± 0.47 ***
I try to change the subject in a tactful way.	2.47 ± 0.77 ***	2.45 ± 0.72 ***	2.26 ± 0.59 *
I encourage patients in their own religious/spiritual beliefs and practices.	2.58 ± 0.74 ***	2.57 ± 0.70 ***	2.82 ± 0.60
I respectfully share my own religious ideas and experiences.	1.77 ± 0.69	1.73 ± 0.66	2.34 ± 0.68 **
I pray with the patient.	1.29 ± 0.53 *	1.25 ± 0.46 *	1.86 ± 0.83 *
I refer patients to chaplains.	3.32 ± 0.61 ***	3.16 ± 0.64 *	3.48 ± 0.55
It's not my responsibility.	2.98 ± 0.94 ***	2.94 ± 0.89 ***	2.68 ± 0.83 ***

[a] Response categories are: 1 = definitely not true, 2 = tends not to be true, 3 = tends to be true, 4 = definitely true of me; [b] In comparison to psychiatric staff's self-assessment (described in Table 4): * $p < 0.05$, ** $p < 0.01$, *** $p < 0.001$; [c] Preceded by "when religious/spiritual issues come up in discussions with patients".

By comparison, in fact, chaplains assessed other psychiatric staff member's behavior significantly less positively than the staff itself. For example, the psychiatric staff strongly agreed that they listen carefully and empathetically when patients address religious/spiritual issues (around 3.80 of 4.00). In contrast, clinical chaplains are more skeptical in this regard (the lowest result for psychiatrists with $m = 2.73$; the highest scores for nurses with $m = 2.99$). In addition, chaplains perceived that all subgroups of the psychiatric staff do not generally consider their patients' religiosity/spirituality to be part of their professional responsibility. In strong contrast, however, psychiatric staff personnel do believe that they are responsible for these topics. Finally, chaplains perceive a significantly lower level of readiness on the part of psychiatrists and psychotherapists to refer patients to the chaplain. Chaplains also had a significantly more negative perception regarding the psychiatric staff's encouragement of patients in their religious/spiritual beliefs and practices. These latter differences were not present for nurses.

Regarding other psychiatric staff's behaviors, chaplains reported significantly different perceptions depending on different characteristics, e.g., how long they had worked in the field of psychiatry.[5] For instance, clinical chaplains who had more years of experience replied more frequently that psychiatrists and psychotherapists do not regard religiosity/spirituality as their responsibility ($r = 0.259$ and $r = 0.276$) and that nursing staff refers patients to them ($r = 0.200$).

4. Discussion

The present study examined how contemporary German psychiatric staffs (*i.e.*, psychiatrists, psychotherapists and nurses) perceive their approach to religious/spiritual issues when such topics

---

[5] According to subgroups (age, occupational work experience and work experience in psychiatry) there were several significant correlations ($p < 0.05$). Via Spearman's 2-sided rank correlation, the following associations were found; age with the question "psychiatrists listen carefully and empathetically ($r = 0.196$)," "psychiatrists/psychotherapists refer patients to chaplains ($r = 0.206/r = 0.236$)" and "psychotherapists pray with the patient ($r = -0.219$)"; or the question "nurses refer patients to chaplains" was associated with chaplains' age and work experience in psychiatry ($r = 0.234/r = 0.190$).

arise in therapeutic settings. Moreover, we also investigated how clinical chaplains perceive other psychiatric staff member's attitudes and behaviors regarding religiosity/spirituality. Both perceptions are confronted with each other in this study.

Overall, psychiatric staff in our survey reported that they are considerably open to religion and/or spirituality when brought up by their patients. The majority of psychiatric staff members are ready to listen and discuss such topics with their patients. This does not differ remarkably from other studies' results [38]: in Curlin *et al.*'s study, 97% of psychiatrists considered it appropriate to discuss religious/spiritual issues when patients want. Despite such positive attitudes towards religious/spiritual issues, the personnel's self-assessment showed that they do not work proactively on religious/spiritual issues, and they engage even less in religious/spiritual activities with their patients. Respondents showed a particularly negative attitude towards prayer with patients, finding it generally inappropriate. Psychiatric staffs in other countries share this viewpoint and in part were even more strongly against it. For example, according to Curlin *et al.*, 94% of American psychiatrists rarely or never prayed with patients [38].

Interestingly, chaplains' perceptions differed significantly from the psychiatric staff's self-reports. Clinical chaplains agreed that psychiatric staff members neither reject nor ignore religious/spiritual issues when their patients want to address such topics in therapeutic settings. However, chaplains had significantly different perceptions than the psychiatric personnel themselves, especially regarding questions like whether these issues are part of the psychiatric staff's professional responsibility and how they actually care by listening carefully and empathetically. Similar skepticism is also found in their rating of the psychiatrists' and psychotherapists' readiness to refer patients to the chaplains for religious/spiritual issues. These differences suggest that there may be a need to improve both communication and cooperation between psychiatric staff and clinical chaplains. This may become especially valuable when psychiatric staff members perceive their own limited competence in this regard, or a need and obligation to remain neutral towards religious/spiritual issues in order to avoid unprofessional behavior develops.

Appropriate ways to deal with religious/spiritual issues may vary from person to person. Previous findings show that there are different needs among different groups of patients and it is important to find ways to approach such topics sensitively. Although it is important that a psychiatric staff is open and willing to integrate religious/spiritual issues and practices into its clinical practice, psychiatric methods of patient care with religious/spiritual or even esoteric methods should not be replaced. According to the results of our study, psychiatric staffs do consider religious/spiritual issues or their patients' religious/spiritual needs as part of their responsibility. The question remains how they can adequately deal with these issues and needs of their patients. There are various ideas on how to adequately integrate religiosity/spirituality into therapeutic settings, such as implicit and explicit integration, or spiritual care [43–46]. A first step, as frequently emphasized, may be a religious/spiritual assessment or to take a religious/spiritual history, which usually takes 2–5 min [47]. Such an assessment can enable psychiatric staff to recognize patients' religious/spiritual resources and difficulties. However, this is not yet a common practice in psychiatric fields. Patients' religious affiliation or related information is usually entered into the file by nurses [14].

For this reason, training programs addressing religious/spiritual issues should be conducted (more) regularly and with more specific content. In Germany and Europe, only few such training programs are available [48–50]. Accordingly, many psychiatric staff members do not have the possibility of participating in such a training program [29,50]; in a national study with German psychotherapists, more than 80% of respondents had rarely or never participated in such a program. Nevertheless, 62.5% of the therapeutic practitioners indicated that they would find training programs with religious/spiritual topics to be beneficial. Furthermore, the differences in perception between psychiatric staff and clinical chaplains suggest that these professional groups should become more aware of the role of the other and find ways to learn more about the way of thinking and attitudes of the other, to discuss these issues as well as to cooperate more effectively. Training programs with both professional groups may be one possibility to promote such interdisciplinary communication and cooperation. This might facilitate innovative interdisciplinary teamwork for the benefit of the patients above all, but also for all staff in psychiatry and psychotherapy, clinical chaplains included. In our study, the majority of psychiatric staff members reported that they refer their patients to clinical chaplains when confronted with religious/spiritual matters of patients. In contrast, the majority of psychiatrists in the UK (72%) had not suggested visiting chaplains or religious/spiritual advisors [14]. Chaplains as professional specialists for religious/spiritual issues can be considered an important resource for "holistic" patient care. Interestingly, the results of our study indicated that nurses were the least reluctant group to share their own religious/spiritual belief or experiences, or even to pray with patients together. This difference could perhaps be a result of nurses' more frequent contact with patients. In addition, this difference could originate from the different roles of psychiatric staff for patients, *i.e.*, for nurses especially as caregivers. Or does this difference reveal a varying level of competence or professional training between these groups?

In professional training programs it is common practice to undergo a self-assessment as well as an assessment by fellow trainees under the supervision of experts on specific issues (e.g., sensitivity). Based on the feedback of supervisors and other trainees, clinical staff can identify how consciously they deal with certain topics and learn how to work in a professionally appropriate manner while also being aware of and monitoring for potential prejudices [30]. In this sense, self-observation as well as self-experience concerning religious/spiritual issues should be developed and encouraged within training programs to improve psychiatric staff member's understanding of their attitudes towards religiosity/spirituality. Such measures are preconditions for competent neutrality and abstinence with regard to patients' religious/spiritual issues, whether needs, resources or problems.

In spite of our findings, this study has a number of limitations that should be considered alongside the results. First of all, minor content differences due to the translation of English into German cannot be ignored. In our translation, we accounted for different cultural and religious backgrounds between the USA and Germany and agreed on them with the author (Curlin). In the German version, the translated term of "unsure" was removed from the mean analysis, as it conveyed an ambiguous meaning. This implies some loss of information and a limitation in the analysis of the data obtained. Although Curlin's questionnaire has been used frequently, there is still a need for further formal validation of the instrument.

Secondly, some caution is necessary when generalizing these results to other populations of psychiatric and psychotherapeutic staff, even within Germany. First of all, the sample for the study among the psychiatric staff was limited to psychiatry and psychotherapy departments of university hospitals and faith-based clinics in Germany. Furthermore, the response rate among the psychiatric staff is relatively low with 24.43% of the hospitals ready to participate. In fact, the response rate for both university and faith-based clinics equally shows that only one-fourth of our targeted groups showed enough interest in religious/spiritual issues to dedicate some time to filling out the questionnaire (without other incentives) This may have skewed the results, as respondents could be a biased sample group and not representative of all German psychiatric staffs.

Similarly, the sample for the study among clinical chaplains was limited to chaplains belonging to Catholic German dioceses as well as their colleagues in other denominations. Other confessional chaplains ultimately showed a very low participation rate in comparison to Catholic chaplains. One possible explanation is that most of the Catholic chaplains were informed via their dioceses even before the survey, whereas other confessional chaplains were not. This shows a structural deficit in the sampling, and perhaps also varying levels of preparedness of both groups, and could possibly further skew the findings.

Third, additional studies are required, such as exploring the psychiatric staff's observation of how clinical chaplains deal with religious/spiritual issues. Finally, the patients themselves need to be asked how they perceive the care provided by different professional groups in regard to religiosity/spirituality. Such studies are underway and will allow for an even better picture and

Religions **2015**, *6*, 930–947

understanding of the opinions of all groups involved. This will help to implement and improve more interdisciplinary work in this field for the benefit of the patients. Notwithstanding the already growing range of research, further studies are needed to explore whether, which and how religiosity/spirituality and its adequate integration into therapeutic processes affects therapeutic outcomes.

5. Conclusions

In conclusion, this study finds that most contemporary German psychiatric staffs are open and willing to deal with religiosity/spirituality in therapeutic settings. To some extent, clinical chaplains agreed with this finding, but their assessment differed significantly from the staff's own self-rating in some regards. In the light of these results, we suggest that psychiatric staff and clinical chaplains should be provided with more opportunities to participate in interdisciplinary teamwork on religious/spiritual issues in therapeutic settings. Moreover, both psychiatric staff and clinical chaplains must reflect on their own attitudes and on how to apply such findings in clinical practice in order to provide more personalized patient care.

Acknowledgments: We sincerely thank all survey participants; in particular, we thank Mathias Berger as well as Ulrich Voderholzer (Dept. Psychiatry and Psychotherapy, the Freiburg University Hospital) for their support and cooperation. In addition, we would like to thank Karin Jors for her revision of the manuscript as a native speaker.

Author Contributions: In the research group of Baumann, Lee and Baumann designed this research, in cooperation with the dept. of psychiatry and psychotherapy of Freiburg university hospital, incl. Zahn. Mainly Lee collected data. Supervised by Baumann, Lee analyzed the data, outlined and wrote the first version of this article. Baumann and Zahn discussed and commented. All authors read and approved the final version improved by Lee and Baumann.

Conflicts of Interest: The authors declare no conflict of interest.

References

1. Susann Strang, Ingela Henoch, Ella Danielson, Maria Browall, and Christina Melin-Johansson. "Communication about existential issues with patients close to death-nurses' reflections on content, process and meaning." *Psycho-Oncology* 23 (2014): 562–68.

2. Scott Murray, Marilyn Kendall, Kirsty Boyd, Allison Worth, and T. Fred Benton. "Exploring the spiritual needs of people dying of lung cancer or heart failure: A prospective qualitative interview study of patients and their carers." *Palliative Medicine* 18 (2004): 39–45.

3. Klaus Baumann. "The Birth of Human Sciences, especially Psychology." In *L'uomo Moderno e la Chiesa—Atti del Congresso (Analecta Gregoriana, 317).* Edited by Paul Gilbert. Rome: Gregorian & Biblical Press, 2012, pp. 391–408.

4. Klaus Baumann. "Remarks on Religions and Psychiatry/Psychotherapies." In *Spirituality and Health. Selected Contributions on Conflicting Priorities in Research and Practice.* Edited by Rene Hefti and Jacqueline Bee. Frankfurt: Peter Lang, 2012, pp. 99–118.

5. Klaus Baumann. "Zwangsstörung und Religion aus heutiger Sicht." *Fortschritte der Neurologie Psychiatrie* 75 (2007): 587–92.

6. Federal Ministry of Health (Austria). "Guidelines for Psychotherapists." 17 June 2014. Available online: http://www.bmg.gv.at/cms/home/attachments/7/0/5/CH1002/CMS1415709133783/ richtlinieabgrenzungesoterik.pdf (accessed on 27 July 2015).

7. Klaus Baumann, and Frank-Gerald B. Pajonk. "Religions and Psychotherapies—Special Issue." *Religions* 5 (2014): 871–75.

8. Raphael M. Bonelli, and Harold G. Koenig. "Mental Disorders, Religion and Spirituality 1990 to 2010: A Systematic Evidence-Based Review." *Journal of Religion and Health* 52 (2013): 657–73.

9. Michael Utsch. "Spiritualität in der psychiatrisch-psychotherapeutischen Praxis: Eine verloren gegangene oder eine wiedergefundene Dimension? " In *Spiritualität und Seelische Gesundheit.* Edited by Jürgen Armbruster, Johannes Peter Petersen and Katharina Ratzke. Köln: Psychiatrie Verlag, 2013, pp. 27–47.

10. Harold G. Koenig, Dana E. King, and Verna B. Carson. *Handbook of Religion and Health*, 2nd ed. New York: Oxford University Press, 2012.

11. Peter Kaiser. *Religion in der Psychiatrie: Eine (un)bewusste Verdrängung?* Göttingen: V&R Unipress, 2007.

12. Michael Utsch, Raphael M. Bonelli, and Samuel Pfeifer. *Psychotherapie und Spiritualität. Mit Existentiellen Konflikten und Transzendenzfragen Professionell Umgehen*. Heidelberg: Springer, 2014.

13. Joanne Cunningham, Jo Anne Sirey, and Martha L. Bruce. "Matching Services to Patients' Beliefs about Depression in Dublin, Ireland." *Psychiatric Servicesh* 58 (2007): 696–99.

14. Robert M. Lawrence, Julia Head, Georgina Christodoulou, Biljana Andonovska, Samina Karamat, Anita Duggal, Jonathan Hillam, and Sarah Eagger. "Clinicians' attitudes to spirituality in old age psychiatry." *International Psychogeriatrics* 19 (2007): 962–73.

15. Tiburtius Koslander, and Barbro Arvidsson. "Patients' conceptions of how the spiritual dimension is addressed in mental health care: A qualitative study." *Journal of Advanced Nursing* 57 (2007): 597–604.

16. Lisa Miller, Priya Wickramaratne, Marc J. Gameroff, Mia Sage, Craig E. Tenke, and Myrna M. Weissman. "Religiosity and Major Depression in Adults at High Risk: A Ten-Year Prospective Study." *The American Journal of Psychiatry* 169 (2012): 89–94.

17. Lisa Miller, Virginia Warner, Priya Wickramaratne, and Myrna Weissman. "Religiosity and Depression: Ten-Year Follow-up of Depressed Mothers and Offspring." *Journal of the American Academy of Child and Adolescent Psychiatry* 36 (1997): 1416–25.

18. Rachel E. Dew, Stephanie S. Daniel, David B. Goldston, and Harold G. Koenig. "Religion, Spirituality, and Depression in Adolescent Psychiatric Outpatients." *The Journal of Nervous and Mental Disease* 196 (2008): 247–51.

19. Jennifer A. Boisvert, and W. Andrew Harrell. "The impact of spirituality on eating disorder symptomatology in ethnically diverse Canadian women." *International Journal of Social Psychiatry* 59 (2013): 729–38.

20. Joseph M. Currier, Jason M. Holland, and Kent D. Drescher. "Spirituality Factors in the Prediction of Outcomes of PTSD Treatment for U.S. Military Veterans." *Journal of Traumatic Stress* 28 (2015): 57–64.

21. Daniel N. McIntosh, Michael J. Poulin, Roxane Cohen Silver, and E. Alison Holman. "The distinct roles of spirituality and religiosity in physical and mental health after collective trauma: A national longitudinal study of responses to the 9/11 attacks." *Journal of Behavioral Medicine* 34 (2011): 497–507.

22. Jill E. Bormann, Steven Thorp, Julie L. Wetherell, and Shahrokh Golshan. "A Spiritually Based Group Intervention for Combat Veterans with Posttraumatic Stress Disorder: Feasibility Study." *Journal of Holistic Nursing* 26 (2008): 109–16.

23. Frank Röhrichta, Raphaela Basdekis-Jozsab, Juggy Sidhuc, Amer Mukhtarc, Iris Suzukic, and Stefan Priebed. "The association of religiosity, spirituality, and ethnic background with ego-pathology in acute schizophrenia." *Mental Health, Religion & Culture* 12 (2009): 515–26.

24. Arndt Büssing, and Götz Mundle. "Reliance on God's Help in Patients with Depressive and Addictive Disorder is not associated with Their Depressive Symptoms." *Religions* 3 (2012): 455–66.

25. Amy B. Wachholtz, and Kenneth I. Pargament. "Is Spirituality a Critical Ingredient of Meditation? Comparing the Effects of Spiritual Meditation, Secular Meditation, and Relaxation on Spiritual, Psychological, Cardiac, and Pain Outcomes." *Journal of Behavioral Medicine* 28 (2005): 369–84.

26. James Carmodya, George Reedb, Jean Kristellerc, and Phillip Merriamd. "Mindfulness, spirituality, and health-related symptoms." *Journal of Psychosomatic Research* 64 (2008): 393–403.

27. Katherine M. Piderman, Terry D. Schneekloth, V. Shane Pankratz, Susanna R. Stevens, and Steven I. Altchuler. "Spirituality during Alcoholism Treatment and continuous Abstinence for one year." *The International Journal of Psychiatry in Medicine* 38 (2008): 391–406.

28. Thomas G. Plante. "What Do the Spiritual and Religious Traditions Offer the Practicing Psychologist? " *Pastoral Psychology* 56 (2008): 492–44.

29. Eunmi Lee. *Religiosität bzw. Spiritualität in Psychiatrie und Psychotherapie. Ihre Bedeutung für psychiatrisches Wirken aus der Sicht des psychiatrischen Personals anhand einer bundesweiten Personalbefragung*. Wôrzburg: Echter Verlag, 2014.

30. Eunmi Lee, and Klaus Baumann. "German Psychiatrists' Observation and Interpretation of Religiosity/Spirituality." *Evidence-Based Complementary and Alternative Medicine* 2013 (2013): 1–8.

31. Farr A. Curlin, Sarah A. Sellergren, John D. Lantos, and Marshall H. Chin. "Physicians' Observations and Interpretations of the Influence of Religion and Spirituality on Health." *Archives of Internal Medicine* 167 (2007): 649–54.

32. John Fosketta, James Marriotta, and Fay Wilson-Rudda. "Mental health, religion and spirituality: Attitudes, experience and expertise among mental health professionals and leaders in Somerset." *Mental Health, Religion & Culture* 7 (2004): 5–22.

33. Glòria Durà;-Vilàa, Matthew Haggerb, Simon Deinc, and Gerard Leaveyd. "Ethnicity, religion and clinical practice: A qualitative study of beliefs and attitudes of psychiatrists in the United Kingdom." *Mental Health, Religion & Culture* 14 (2011): 53–64.

34. Philippe Huguelet, Sylvia Mohr, Laurence Borras, Christiane Gillieron, and Pierre-Yves Brandt. "Spirituality and Religious Practices among Outpatients with Schizophrenia and Their Clinicians." *Psychiatric Services* 57 (2006): 366–72.

35. George El-Nimr, Laura L. Green, and Emad Salib. "Spiritual care in psychiatry: Professionals' views." *Mental Health, Religion & Culture* 7 (2004): 165–70.

36. Mark R. McMinn, Steven J. Runner, Jennifer A. Fairchild, Joshua D. Lefler, and Rachel P. Suntay. "Factors Affection Clergy-Psychologist Referral Patterns." *Journal of Psychology and Theology* 33 (2005): 299–309.

37. Eunmi Lee, Anne Zahn, and Klaus Baumann. "Religiosity/Spirituality and Mental Health: Psychiatric Staff's Attitudes and Behaviors." *Open Journal of Social Science* 2 (2014): 7–13.

38. Farr A. Curlin, Ryan E. Lawrence, Shaun Odell, Marshall H. Chin, John D. Lantos, Harold G. Koenig, and Keith G. Meador. "Religion, Spirituality, and Medicine: Psychiatrists' and Other Physicians' differing Observations, Interpretations, and Clinical Approaches." *American Journal of Psychiatry* 164 (2007): 1825–31.

39. Farr A. Curlin, Marshall H. Chin, Sarah A. Sellergren, Chad J. Roach, and John D. Lantos. "The Association of physicians' religious characteristics with their attitudes and self-reported behaviors regarding religion and spirituality in the clinical encounter." *Medical Care* 44 (2006): 446–53.

40. Eunmi Lee, Anne Zahn, and Klaus Baumann. "Religion in Psychiatry and Psychotherapy? A Pilot Study: The Meaning of Religiosity/Spirituality from Staff's Perspective in Psychiatry and Psychotherapy." *Religions* 2 (2011): 525–35.

41. BertelsmannStiftung. *Religionsmonitor 2008*. München: Gütersloher Verlagshaus, 2007.

42. Bundeszentrale Politische Bildung. "Religionszugehörigkeit." Available online: http://www.bpb.de/nachschlagen/zahlen-und-fakten/soziale-situation-in-deutschland/145148/religionszugehoerigkeit (accessed on 17 June 2015).

43. Eckhard Frick. "Spiritual Care in der Humanmedizin: Profilierung und Vernetzung." In *Die Bedeutung von Religion für die Gesundheit*. Edited by Friedrich Balck, Hendrik Berth and Constantin Klein. Weinheim: Juventa, 2011, pp. 407–20.

44. George Handzo. "Spiritual Care for Palliative Patients." *Journal of Pediatric Nursing* 26 (2011): 34–43.

45. Harold G. Koenig. "Integrating Spirituality into Medical Practice: A New Era in Medicine." In *Spiritualität, Krankheit und Heilung—Bedeutung und Ausdrucksformen der Spiritualität in der Medizin*. Edited by Arndt Büssing, Thomas Ostermann, Michaela Glöckler and Peter F. Matthiessen. Frankfurt: Vas-Verlag für Akademische Schriften, 2006, pp. 232–41.

46. Siang-Yang Tan. "Religion in clinical practice: Implicit and explicit integration." In *Religion and the Clinical Practice of Psychology*. Edited by Edward P. Shafranske. Washington: American Psychological Association, 1996, pp. 365–87.

47. Harold G. Koenig. *Spirituality in Patient Care. Why, How, When and What*, 2nd ed. Philadelphia: Templeton Press, 2007.

48. Stephen R. Russell, and Mark A. Yarhouse. "Training in religion/spirituality with APA-accredited psychology predoctoral internships." *Professional Psychology: Research and Practice* 37 (2006): 430–36.

49. Rachel M. Schafer, Paul J. Handal, Peter A. Brawer, and Megan Ubinger. "Training and Education in religion/spirituality within APA-Accredited Clinical Psychology Programs: 8 Years Later." *Journal of Religion and Health* 50 (2011): 232–39.

50. Liane Hofmanna, and Harald Walachb. "Spirituality and religiosity in psychotherapy—A representative survey among German psychotherapists." *Psychotherapy Research* 21 (2011): 179–92.

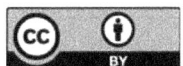

Chapter 4

Faith-Based Services and Programs in Health Care

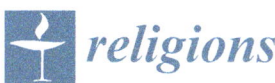

Article

Meaning-Making, Religiousness and Spirituality in Religiously Founded Substance Misuse Services—A Qualitative Study of Staff and Patients' Experiences

Torgeir Sørensen [1,2,*], **Lars Lien** [3,4], **Anne Landheim** [3] **and Lars J. Danbolt** [1,2]

1   MF Norwegian School of Theology, P.O. Box 5144 Majorstuen, Oslo 0302, Norway; post@mf.no
2   Centre for Psychology of Religion, Innlandet Hospital Trust, P.O. Box 68, Ottestad 2312, Norway; postmottak@sykehuset-innlandet.no
3   Norwegian National Advisory Unit on Concurrent Substance Abuse and Mental Health Disorders, Innlandet Hospital Trust, P.O. Box 104, Brumunddal 2381, Norway; post@rop.no
4   Faculty of Public Health, Hedmark University College, P.O. Box 400, Elverum 2418, Norway; postmottak@hihm.no
*   Author to whom correspondence should be addressed; torgeir.sorensen@mf.no; Tel.: +47-22-59-05-33; Fax: +47-22-59-05-05.

Academic Editor: René Hefti
Received: 5 November 2014; Accepted: 28 January 2015; Published: 2 February 2015

Abstract: The Norwegian health authorities buy one third of their addiction treatment from private institutions run by organizations and trusts. Several of these are founded on religious values. The aim of the study was to investigate such value-based treatment and the patients' experiences of spirituality and religiousness as factors of meaning-making in rehabilitation. The study was performed in an explorative qualitative design. Data were collected through focus-group interviews among therapists and in-patients at a religiously founded substance misuse service institution. The analysis was carried out by content analysis through systematic text-condensation. Through different activities and a basic attitude founded on religious values, the selected institution and the therapists facilitated a treatment framework which included a spiritual dimension and religious activity. The patients appreciated their free choice regarding treatment approaches, which helped them to make meaning of life in various collective and individual settings. Rituals and sacred spaces gave peace of mind and confidence in a situation that up to now had been chaotic and difficult. Sermons and wording in rituals contributed to themes of reflection and helped patients to revise attitudes and how other people were met. Private confessions functioned for several patients as turning point experiences influencing patients' relations to themselves and their surroundings. Spirituality and religious activity contributed to meaning-making among patients with substance use disorder and had significance for their rehabilitation.

Keywords: meaning-making; spirituality; religion; substance misuse services; Norway

---

1. Introduction

Several institutions facilitating substance misuse services are founded on religious value factors like meaning-making, spirituality and religion. In various forms and degrees these factors are integrated into these institutions' therapy approaches [1]. How institutions and their therapists arrange for such elements in therapy, their reasons for doing so, and patients experiences of these factors' importance in treatment are therefore of interest.

Substance misuse carries a large burden for the affected individual, and greatly impacts on several levels of society [2]. The prevalence of drug use disorders in EU and Norway ranges between 0.3% and 0.9% [3]. Lifetime prevalence of alcohol dependence/abuse is found to be 23% in a Norwegian sample [4]. In the treatment of these disorders, the concept of meaning-making may represent a fruitful approach to understanding substance misuse services [5]. For a person with addiction problems the intoxication can of itself represent meaning in life [6]. On the other hand, his or her life in general might be experienced as meaningless with low well-being scores [7]. The search for meaning in life is regarded as central in human experiences, and religion is assessed as a considerable provider of such a sense of significance by several contributors [8].

In Norway, the substance misuse services by the Pentecostal movement have assumed that Christian conversion, by changing object of significance from substance misuse to Christian faith [1], is a crucial starting point fundamental for successful treatment [9]. Other substance misuse services based on religious values do not necessarily view inclusion of religious and spiritual factors as intervention. Rather it is an offer in general, in terms of, for instance, church services and pastoral counselling at the institution. Religiousness and spirituality have a purpose of its own, and possibly for that reason it may have significance for patients' rehabilitation [10].

Orientations towards an immaterial, supernatural power are considered as "religion" when it occurs as organized with institutional components of faith traditions [11]. "Spirituality" addresses individuals' relationships with and search for the sacred. The sacred refers to God or higher powers, but also other aspects of life perceived as manifestations of the divine or features having divine-like qualities [12]. Spirituality may involve self-transcendence in a quite broad sense as long as it is a search for existential goals beyond one's immediate needs. Throughout this paper, both "religion" and "spirituality" as terms will be used. These are overlapping constructs, and both therapist and patients refer to elements related to traditional organized religion as well as individual's private search for the sacred independent of organized settings.

Meaning is considered central in human experience [13]. Humans face fundamental existential needs in life, like for instance self-regulation, control, comfort, identity, social acknowledgement, values and purpose. In meaning-making, people meet these needs adequately when they utilize the different sources of meaning [14]. If fundamental relations or conditions in life are broken, sources of meaning are used to restore the balance between the individual's expectations of life and the reality as it is experienced here and now. Such reappraisal and usage of sources of meaning are essential when it comes to handling demanding life situations, such as living with substance use disorder. According to Schnell [14], sources of meaning can be categorized in different groups. To target objects beyond one's immediate needs is designated as self-transcendence. "Vertical self-transcendence", consisting of religion and spirituality, is an orientation towards an immaterial supernatural power. "Horizontal self-transcendence" targets other people, knowledge of self, nature, health, *etc.* With use of "self-actualisation", one's own capacities are developed and challenged. "Order" is about relation to tested and durable values, traditions and practices. In "well-being and relatedness", individuals cultivate and enjoy what is good in life, both private and collectively.

Meaning-making can also be seen in the perspective of global meaning [13] where an overarching ideology or world-view can help individuals to see their lives in a larger context. Affiliation to, for instance, organized religion, with its overall understanding of existence, can serve as an important reference and may contribute to significant structures in life when experiencing demanding life situations.

Schnell's [14] concept of meaning-making takes a secular European context into account. To our knowledge, this perspective is not much used in investigations regarding meaning-making, religion and spirituality among patients with substance use disorder.

However, spirituality may be an important part of recovery from substance misuse [15]. For instance, among different relapse prevention strategies, it has been found that engaging in prayer or relying on a "higher power" were of importance for patients in their attempts to stay clean at a Chicago rehabilitation centre [16]. In a Canadian study, spirituality was one of the main themes when patients discussed what helped recovery, especially when spirituality was linked to nature, a supernatural power, the feeling of not being alone, and rituals [17].

Research regarding the significance of religion and spirituality as meaning-making in substance misuse services is needed for several reasons. Review of the international research literature shows limited knowledge [18], especially when studies of the 12-step program (Alcoholics Anonymous) and studies from America are excluded. Further, due to environmental, cultural, religious and health-related differences, findings from one context are not necessarily transferable to another [19]. Thus, knowledge from specific environments is needed. In the Norwegian case, the health authorities bought one third of their addiction treatment from private institutions run by organizations and trusts in 2012 [20]. Several of these are founded on religious values. Despite this considerable use of external services, little is known about the rationale behind such value-based treatment and patients' experiences in Norway.

Our aim was to investigate the significance and function of meaning-making, spirituality and religiousness in substance misuse services founded on religious values in a Norwegian context. Our research questions were: What is the treatment framework? What are the experiences of meaning-making, religiousness and spirituality in a treatment setting among the patients?

2. Methods

2.1. Design and Setting

The investigation was performed in an explorative qualitative design. The setting for the study was a private institution being part of and funded by the specialist healthcare service in South-East Norway. The institution provided a 12-month stay for all patients, independent of their individual progress of rehabilitation. An individual treatment approach were emphasized at the institution, where respect for the patient's participation and assessments were of importance. The institution employed professional therapists with various occupational backgrounds.

2.2. Sample

The sample consisted of both therapists and patients at the selected institution. The therapists were recruited through an enquiry from the investigators to the management of the institution who passed on an open invitation of participation to the employees. Among the 14 therapists willing to participate, specialist trained nurses, social workers, psychologists and a chaplain were present, allowing for maximum variation sampling [21]. Several of the therapists had previously led the social work of local parishes. Except for these last therapists and the chaplain, no special competence regarding religion and spirituality was present among the staff. On the other hand, most of the therapists had been employed at the institution for many years. Consequently, a positive basic attitude towards religion and spirituality had been handed over between colleagues and integrated among several staff members through internal seminars and clinical practice at the institution. Both genders were present in the sample, and their age was between 40 and 65.

The patients were recruited by the investigators through information and open invitation at a daily morning meeting at the institution. Of the 26 patients, one third was excluded because at least a four months' stay at the clinic was required, due to distance from intoxication and adaption to the treatment programme. Finally, eight patients were willing to participate, four women and four men aged between 20 and 50. Misuse of alcohol, different drugs, pills and mixed misuse were present in the group.

2.3. Data Collection

Data were collected through focus-group interviews, two sessions among therapists (seven plus seven informants) and one among patients (eight informants). Each session lasted for one hour and 30 minutes. The therapists' interviews were conducted in November 2013, the patients' interview in February 2014. Due to the focus-groups being a discussion-forum, only a handful of themes were selected. Based on an interview guide the therapists discussed treatment at the clinic in general, the function of meaning, meaning-making, spirituality and religiousness in treatment, their contribution as therapists, and the significance of the institution being founded on religious values. The patients discussed where they found meaning in life, what was important in treatment in general, the religious basis of the institution, in which way meaning-making, spirituality and religiousness could be significant in treatment, and the pastoral care at the institution.

2.4. Analysis

The availability of informants was higher among the therapists than among the patients. Therefore, two sessions were held among the therapists and analyzed as a whole. The patient session was analyzed separately. The analysis was carried out by qualitative content analysis through systematic text-condensation based on Giorgi's phenomenological analysis in a four-step model [22]. First, an overview of data was established, next meaning units were identified and sorted, further the content of these codes was condensed, and finally the condensate was synthesized into descriptions and concepts.

2.5. Ethics

Participation in this study was voluntary. Before participating, informants received information and signed an informed consent form. The study was approved by the Protection Officer at Oslo University Hospital in accordance with the Norwegian Personal Data Act.

3. Results

The intentions behind treatment, as well as experiences of treatment at the selected institution, were important as a whole when describing possible functions of meaning-making, spirituality and religion. From the content analysis, eight themes, two among the therapists and six among the patients, turned out to be central (see Table 1).

The presentation of the findings in the following is thus twofold. In Sections 3.1 and 3.2, the most prominent themes among the therapists are shown, with regard to values and arrangements at the institution. In Sections 3.3–3.8, we will present the patients' experiences of treatment, and the most prominent meaning-making, spirituality, and religious factors within it.

Table 1. Central themes arising from the content analysis among therapist and patients.

The therapists	The patients
The institution's values	Meaning in life
The institution's arrangements	To be met at the institution
	Violation of rules
	Choice of approaches in treatment
	Spiritual and religious activities
	The chaplain

3.1. The Therapists' vs. The Institution's Values

A long history of being an institution founded on religious values together with the staff members' professional considerations and practices set a treatment framework where emphasis on the spiritual dimension was essential. At the same time, the therapists stressed that patients' participation in explicit religious activity related to rituals and spiritual guidance by the chaplain was voluntary, due to demands from the funding authorities. The descriptions of the patients' perceptions and experiences presented later must be seen in this light. The common goal among the therapists was to help the patients to rediscover their own dignity. The basic attitude of the therapists was coloured by the fact that the majority of them had worked there for many years. The values of the institution had been handed over to new therapists and been incorporated among them. Such values were expressed through the therapists' fundamental attitude of openness towards the patients and included in their assessments of the patients' needs, for example in conjunction with rule violation.

> "If a patient has committed undesirable actions, the institution should actually react to it and in worst case discharge the patient. However, it is my assertion that the perspective of forgiveness and a new opportunity, anchored in the Christian view of values, is emphasized when assessing patients' violation of rules at this institution."

(Therapist # 6)

For the therapists, spirituality was first and foremost how they met and saw the patient in various ways and settings, based on a holistic view of human life. Spirituality as the fourth dimension in care was seen by the therapists as important for, and included in, the three other dimensions, the physical, the mental, and the social dimension. It was emphasized by a therapist that the practice and the awareness of spirituality in treatment was a reason for her to work at this very institution.

The therapists held a broad understanding of spirituality and defined it as for individuals (*i.e.*, the patients) to go beyond themselves and at the same time identify the core of themselves. Spirituality among the therapists was closely linked to values of different kinds, expressed in therapy as well as through everyday life situations at the institution. Care and benevolence were important factors in how they met patients.

> "Especially in the first weeks here, our patients bear quite a burden of shame, feelings of guilt, remorse, and such heavy stuff. At the same time it is important for them to receive hope, faith and forgiveness. And here at the institution it is an arena where they can get some help and support in that direction. Almost regardless of belief and faith I see that these factors makes them well."

(Therapist # 5)

The therapists aimed to be as unprejudiced as possible in meeting the patients on the patients' terms. Warmth and respect towards patients should as well be part of the institution's fundamental values manifested through the therapists. However, despite such ideals, the therapists could have relatively tough internal discussions concerning how to handle specific situations regarding patients' actions and how to confront them with, for instance, undesirable behaviour.

3.2. The Therapists' vs. The Institution's Arrangements

It was important for the therapists to facilitate spirituality and religiousness as part of different approaches of therapy; nevertheless, as with other therapeutic activities at the institution, it was the patients' choice what to make use of. For instance, it was up to the patients whether religious and/or spiritual questions should be part of the conversational therapy or not, following a mapping of their spiritual history on entering their stay.

At the institution, several artefacts, such as pictures with religious motives, proverbs, crosses and other Christian symbols were visible expressions of the institution's religious foundation. However, several of the therapists regarded the chapel and the rituals taking place there, like the morning prayers, the weekly service with Holy Communion and celebration of the church festivals as even more important. A therapist said she sometimes encouraged patients to take part saying that the morning prayers may be a good way of starting the day. Rituals and symbolism were assessed by the therapists as important to facilitate even though participation for patients was voluntary.

> "I will light a candle in that window (pointing at the chapel) every morning to convey to those in the square outside who maybe never participate in the chapel that there is something spiritual here, something about taking humans seriously, something about love. So, it is something we … I will show symbolism, then."

(Therapist # 3)

The chaplain functioned outside the therapist team when working with rituals and pastoral counselling. At the same time, he was an integrated part of the institution's total effort of treatment. The chaplain also arranged for conversation groups discussing existential questions, world view, and relevant themes at the institution such as "from shame to dignity", "from guilt to emancipation", and "in the landscape of grief".

3.3. The Patients' Experiences—Meaning in Life

When discussing meaning in life here and now, staying clean from drugs was the first and most conspicuous theme for the patients. They wanted to find solutions to their problems of misuse. As a basis for this project, several patients saw the need for long-term perspectives with something to reach out for in life, to have goals and dreams, and to have something meaningful to do in everyday life. "You can invest in your own future by doing good things", as a patient put it. Contact with nature helped clear thinking and making sensible choices. Support from and to relatives, friends and fellow patients gave meaning in life.

A superstructure in the effort of the patients' rehabilitation was to restore the different kinds of broken relationships that had arisen through many years as misusers. The patients found meaning in working with this complicated landscape of shame and guilt

> "What gives me meaning in life is to be clean, and if you get in contact especially with the family, and try to get in contact with former friends, maybe, (. . .)."
>
> (Patient # 1)

3.4. The Patients' Experiences—To Be Met at the Institution

Life as an addict had been demanding on several levels. The patients' identity in earlier life had been linked to what they did, connected to misuse, and not to who they were as individuals. They were lonely, isolated and frightened. Often they carried mental health problems like neuroses, anxiety and avoidant personality disorder. Such experiences stood in considerable contrast to how many of the patients experienced their arrival and stay at the institution.

> "I was really scared before I came. (. . .) When I arrived here, I met a therapist with a big heart expressing warmth and goodness. I felt confident together with her from the very beginning."
>
> (Patient # 7)

Those with positive experiences felt they were met and seen with an open mind. In these patients' view, the therapists and other workers at the institution expressed confidence through personal human qualities like care and love. Other patients did not have the same overall positive impression. These patients were quite selective regarding which therapist worked well for them or not regarding how they were met.

3.5. The Patients Experiences vs. Violation of Rules

Patients compared the institution's treatment with other institutions they had been to. A pronounced difference was, for instance, how this institution handled rule violation regarding remaining substance-free during the stay. At other institutions they would be exposed in front of others and had to tell in public what they had done. In contrast, here they would be protected and withdrawn from the other patients until the situation had been stabilized and the patients were ready to move on in the treatment.

> "If you crack you have to sit on a chair and everybody is sitting in a ring around you, and then you have to proclaim your sins. Here you will be protected and withdrawn."
>
> (Patient # 4)

The patients felt more confident with the last approach. They experienced that they were better taken care of with a withdrawal under such circumstances, and they thought it would have better effect on their rehabilitation in a long-term perspective compared to a confrontational mode.

3.6. The Patients' Experiences vs. Choice of Approaches in Treatment

Compared to detailed treatment programmes with rigid methodologies elsewhere, the patients found it more positive to have choices. Here, they could take responsibility for their own rehabilitation process. Quite different approaches and activities were available at the institution and the patients used those they experienced worked for them. Activities such as psychological treatment, conversation with other patients, pastoral counselling, group sessions, physical activity, hiking in the mountains, craft activities, creating things, going on trips, morning prayers and religious services helped them to face their challenges from different angles.

> "You could say about this institution that it is rehabilitation for advanced patients. In a way you have to take the case in your own hands. At the same time you have good helpers around."
>
> (Patient # 4)

3.7. The Patients' Experiences vs. Spiritual and Religious Activities

Even though patients participated in organized religious settings like morning prayers and services, faith seemed to appear at an individual level where patients needed to make their private decisions on what should be the content, and what faith meant to them personally. Still, the spiritual and religious activities facilitated by the institution had important functions for treatment experiences. According to some of the patients, the morning prayers and the weekly service led by the chaplain served as important places for processing different themes, helping several of the patients to relate to others and to reflect on demanding issues important for their state of rehabilitation. For one of the patients, this was especially exemplified through sermons, where she found help for how to ask for forgiveness. Other patients experienced the rituals and the chapel as invigorating, giving peace of mind and confidence in contrast to life with addiction problems.

> "We need some peace and tranquillity, right. There has been so much negativity, action and impulses and anxiety and things like that earlier. So, to get some peace of mind is cool, right."
>
> (Patient # 4)

However, it was important for the patients to stress that they had not come to the institution for religious salvation, but to become clean.

3.8. The Patients' Experiences vs. The Chaplain

The chaplain appeared as a kind of "holy person" with a certain role. He was described by the patients to be a symbol, a carrier and mediator of something bigger. This function was experienced in social settings and talks as well as in his formal role as chaplain administering services, morning prayers and pastoral counselling. His special, compassionate and respectful manner invited to conversations regarding existential questions in a wider sense.

> "He has an authority here at the institution, but actually he can . . . , he can go so deep that he places me as a patient . . . One time he asked me 'NN, in our next appointment, would you come here and teach me about forgiveness? How did you learn to forgive yourself?' And I just; wow (surprised and a bit frightened)! 'Are you asking me about that?' And it was so good. He is so non-judgemental. He is so . . . There is no harm in that man. And I

think that it is a big deal for us staying here and for us sitting here. The confidence he oozes out daily."

(Patient # 5)

The patients underlined that the chaplain's contribution was different to that of the therapists. He had a wider perspective. It was not his task to be restrictive. His independent role was important for the patients, with special emphasis on him administering a strict degree of professional secrecy. According to several of the patients, the chaplain would not share with others, e.g., therapists, what was said during pastoral counselling. Neither would the content of the conversation be analyzed, as it would be by the psychologist or another therapist. This facilitated open conversation where patients could raise subjects they possibly would not share in therapy. Consequently, in the patients' view, the chaplain contributed to treatment despite not being a therapist.

This was especially true when it came to confession. When introducing his work to newcomers, the chaplain gave information regarding the possibility for confession with respect to patients' possible needs of settlement and deliverance. Confession including absolution given by the chaplain represented a significant instrument in conversations and pastoral counselling. Even more important was its functioning as a symbol and ritual, and the power within it contributing to patients' processes of rehabilitation and leaving things behind.

"The chaplain is the spokesman of Jesus. If you struggle with such a heavy burden that you need a confession, this is a reassurance, if you have enough balls to dare it."

(Patient # 5)

Confession as a tool in rehabilitation was also desired by agnostics:

"So, the chaplain has a moral professional secrecy. That is important because I, for my part, have some things in my life that I have to come to terms with. And my plan is to use the chaplain for that purpose. But I am not ready yet. But I perceive that he is the only one, absolutely the only one I want to talk to about these things, then. And that is good to know."

(Patient # 3)

4. Discussion

In summary, we found that the therapists were influenced by the institution's set of values and their own faith histories. Despite differences, they shared a common commitment to integrate the spiritual dimension into treatment and everyday life at the institution in various ways. The patients stressed that they had not come to the selected institution seeking religious salvation, but to become clean. Still, several patients had positive experiences regarding the therapists' obligingness, care and love based on the spiritual foundation discussed. Activities related to spirituality and religiousness were among several patients regarded as important together with other factors contributing to treatment. Rituals and sacred spaces could give peace of mind and confidence in a situation that up to now had been chaotic and difficult. The importance of the chaplain's role was accentuated with regard to pastoral presence in social and conversational settings, and his administration of morning prayers, services, pastoral counselling and private confession. In total, it seems as if several factors contributed to meaning-making for the patients.

It was important for the patients to have the possibility of making their own choices regarding which of the activities offered at the institution they should utilize in their rehabilitation, concurrent with recent trends within addiction treatment [23]. On the other hand, confrontational methods are demanded by patients in other studies [17]. From a psycho-dynamic point of view, it could be questioned why the therapists at the institution want to present themselves to the patients as unprejudiced, or why they seek to protect and withdraw patients in cases of rule violation instead of confronting them with other patients present. However, several of the patients in the present study had negative experiences of confrontational therapies from other institutions. They found the current individual rehabilitation programme worked for them, with reference to emphasis on future expectations and social support in the therapy. In this respect, several of the patients had chosen the current institution, perceiving the fact that different therapies match with different patients. This is, however, not evidence of the quality or the effectiveness of the institution.

The patients related to religiousness and spirituality in a cognitive manner. Sermons with references to the Bible and the wording in the rituals contributed to themes of reflection regarding their own personal life histories helping them to revise attitudes and how they met other people. Equally important, however, were the non-verbal experiences. Religious spaces, artefacts, religious symbols and rituals such as morning prayers and service, perceived through the body and the senses, seemed to have importance as a resource, which also has been found in other studies [24]. Such non-cognitive experiences contributed to peace of mind and confidence in contrast to a chaotic life of substance misuse. As self-transcendence, patients in both cognitive and non-cognitive settings reached out for objects beyond their immediate needs. Despite different degrees of relating to a supernatural power, this connection to religion and spirituality had significance for patients and functioned as sources of meaning in general and more specifically in their rehabilitation processes. Situated in a vertical self-transcendence paradigm [14], this kind of meaning-making may enhance the probability of living a meaningful life compared to other sources of meaning [25]. Further, the factors discussed are seen by others as important for relapse prevention [16]. Consequently, religious and spiritual factors can be seen here as sources of meaning contributing to the patients' current desire to stay clean, which was most prominent when the patients discussed meaning in life in their present situations.

Morning prayers and services with Holy Communion were based on old texts and hymns and were expressions of long-standing traditions and ideology which may contribute to a global meaning system and set life into a frame of reference [13]. It contributes to meaning in life when adjustments in life can be made through rituals [14,25]. Consequently, moral issues are also part of individuals' appraisals in this matter, as emphasized by patients in this study. They saw the importance of doing good things which in turn generated good consequences for the patients and their surroundings. In the patient conversations, it came through that such moral considerations were based on ideologies like humanity, and to some extent also on religious values, with reference to global meaning systems [13].

A prominent finding in the material was the quite extensive use of private confession as an important way of putting negative life events and misdeeds behind them. Private confession within the frame of pastoral counselling by the chaplain and his strict vow to secrecy contributed to turning point experiences for the patients. The patients' articulation of their transgressions and the chaplain's proclamation of the forgiveness of sins could be important elements here. Also, the setting as a ritual and the actions associated with it, such as the chaplain's hand laid on the head of the patient, may have contributed to the patients' experience of this ritual being crucial and cleansing in their rehabilitation processes. An interesting parallel is First Nations women's positive experience of re-purification ceremonies for rehabilitation purposes [17]. The fact that agnostics also wanted to take part in private confession may show the importance of rituals in substance misuse services in general. As is the case for rites of passage in general, such *ad hoc* rituals in a therapeutic setting can mark a distinct transformation from one status to another, generating a sense of order, community and transition [26]. This may help patients to change object of significance in their lives [1]. Additionally, knowing that private confession is virtually absent in pastoral care in the setting of the majority church in Norway may be an expression of this ritual's pronounced significance and function within substance misuse services. People with addiction problems may to a larger degree than others find confession significant as a source of meaning due to their former lives bearing traces of guilt and shame, and the need to rebuild broken relationships.

To cultivate relationships is an important issue within meaning-making [14,25]. However, according to the patients, life as a substance misuser had in many cases led to broken relationships.

On the other hand, it was underlined that restoring these broken relationships gave meaning in life. Important issues within this process are forgiveness of others, to be forgiven and, not least, forgiveness of the self. In addition to making meaning, forgiveness of the self has been shown to be a predictor of favourable outcomes regarding future substance misuse [27]. As a source of meaning, such processes are closely connected with well-being where joy, love and comfort experienced in relation to family, friends and other relations are essential goals [14,25]. These factors were underlined as important by the patients when they described the long, demanding, but also positive process of restoring their relationships with their closest ones.

4.1. Limitations and Implications

A limitation of the present study may be that the interviews with the patients were performed in a therapeutic setting. How the informants will view these questions after their stay is difficult to predict. The sample of patients could be positively selected. On the other hand, after exclusion the patient sample consisted of about half of the potential participants at the institution. A focus-group interview approach may be criticized for a harmonizing presentation of the topic in question. However, the conversation climate among the participants gave room for disagreements. A focus-group interview approach was utilized because group dynamics were needed to generate knowledge on the present topic. It is also a limitation that this study collected data from one institution only. Consequently, it may be difficult to generalize the present findings to other Norwegian programs. Additionally, generalization of qualitative studies is difficult in general.

Despite obvious limitations concerning generalization, possible clinical implications and incentives for development of clinical practices can be seen on the grounds of the present study. Nevertheless, further research on the topic in comparable contexts is demanded. Religion and spirituality have value on their own. Additionally, this study may show that religious rituals, services, and symbolism through art and architecture *etc.* had significance for peace of mind and comfort and thus made meaning in life among those affiliated to these factors. Facilitation of such practices within institutions may be a first step towards an integration of religious and spiritual factors in clinical settings.

We have also seen in the material that religious wordings in sermons, rituals and hymns, and pastoral counselling together with private confession have led to reflections over former, present and future life and contributed to meaning-making in this respect. Meaning-making has generated new platforms for how patients can live their lives, how patients relate to broken relationships from the past and how they can relate to their family and friends in the future. To some extent, such aspects are taken care of today, but not all institutions have their own chaplains. An even more integrated strategy would be to include religious and spiritual factors in the therapeutic setting, if the patients find it relevant. However, therapists in general are in lack of competence regarding religion and spirituality. On the other hand, the most important part for the therapist is to have an open attitude towards the patients' possible religiousness and spirituality as resources in therapy. Patients with substance use disorder often suffer from broken relationships, guilt and shame. In this perspective, religious and spiritual factors in meaning-making may for this patient group, possibly more than for others, be a relevant perspective in the clinical setting.

5. Conclusions

Through different activities and a basic attitude founded on religious values, the selected institution and its therapists facilitated a treatment framework which included a spiritual dimension and religious activity. The patients appreciated their free choice regarding treatment approaches, which helped them to make meaning of life in various collective and individual settings. Rituals, especially private confession, could function as turning point experiences influencing their relation to themselves and their surroundings.

Religions **2015**, *6*, 92–106

Acknowledgments: The authors thank the therapists and patients at the selected institution for their participation in this study. We also thank Innlandet Hospital Trust for funding the study (grant # 150267).

Author Contributions: TS contributed to design of the study, acquisition of data, transcription, analyzing data, drafting and critical revision of the article and approval of the final version. LL, AL and LJD contributed to the design of the study, analyzing data, critical revision of the article and approval of the final version.

Conflicts of Interest: The authors declare no conflict of interest.

References

1. Berit Borgen. "Transformational turning points in the process of liberation." *Mental Health, Religion & Culture* 16 (2013): 463–88. [CrossRef]
2. Ann Kristin Knudsen, Samuel B. Harvey, Arnstein Mykletun, and Simon Øverland. "Common mental disorders and long-term sickness absence in a general working population. The Hordaland Health Study." *Acta Psychiatrica Scandinavica* 127 (2013): 287–97. [CrossRef]
3. Jürgen Rehm, Robin Room, Wim van den Brink, and Ludwig Kraus. "Problematic drug use and drug use disorders in EU countries and Norway: An overview of the epidemiology." *EuropeanNeuropsychopharmacology* 15 (2005): 389–97. [CrossRef]
4. Einar Kringlen, Svenn Torgersen, and Vicoria Cramer. "A Norwegian psychiatric epidemiological study." *American Journal of Psychiatry* 158 (2001): 1091–98.
5. Harold G. Koenig. "Concerns about measuring 'spirituality' in research." *The Journal of Nervous and Mental Disease* 196 (2008): 349–55. [CrossRef]
6. Valerie DeMarinis, Christina Scheffel-Birath, and Helen Hansagi. "Cultural analysis as a perspective for gender-informed alcohol treatment research in a Swedish context." *Alcohol and Alcoholism* 44 (2009): 615–19. [CrossRef]
7. Human-Friedrich Unterrainer, Andrew Lewis, Joanna Collicutt, and Andreas Fink. "Religious/Spiritual Well-Being, Coping Styles, and Personality Dimensions in People With Substance Use Disorders." *The International Journal for the Psychology of Religion* 23 (2013): 204–213.
8. Ralph W. Hood, Peter C. Hill, and Bernard Spilka. *The Psychology of Religion: An Empirical Approach*, 4th ed. New York: Guilford Press, 2009.
9. Olav H. Angell. *Ennå er det håp? Ei evaluering av Pinsevennenes evangeliesenter [There is Still Hope? An Evaluation of the Substance Misuse Services of the Pentacostal Movement]*. Oslo: Diakonhjemmet University College, 1996.
10. Tor Torbjørnsen. *'Gud hjelpe meg!' Religiøs mestring hos pasienter med hodgkins sykdom ['God Help Med!' Religious Coping among Patients with Hodgkin Diseas]*. Oslo: MF Norwegian School of Theology, 2011.
11. Carolyn Aldwin, Crystal L. Park, Yu-Jin Jeong, and Ritwik Nath. "Differing Pathways Between Religiousness, Spirituality, and Health: A Self-Regulation Perspective." *Psychology of Religion and Spirituality* 6 (2014): 9–21.
12. Kenneth I. Pargament, Annette Mahoney, Julie J. Exline, James Jones, and Edward Shafranske. "Envisioning an integrative paradigm for the psychology of religion and spirituality." In *APA Handbook Of Psychology, Religion, And Spirituality*. Edited by K.I. Pargament. Washington: American Psychology Association, 2013, pp. 3–19.
13. Crystal L. Park. "Religion and Meaning." In *Handbook for Psychology of Religion and Spirituality*, 2nd ed. Edited by Raymond F. Paloutzian and Crystal L. Park. New York: Guilford Press, 2013, pp. 357–79.
14. Tatjana Schnell. "The Sources of Meaning and Meaning in Life Questionnaire (SoMe): Relations to demographics and well-being." *The Journal of Positive Psychology* 4 (2009): 483–99.
15. Chris Cook. "Substance Misuse." In *Spirituality and Psychiatry*. Edited by Chris Cook, Andrew Powell and Andrew Sims. London: RCPsych, 2009, pp. 139–68.
16. Kristin E. Davis, and Sheila J. O'Neill. "A focus group analysis of relapse prevention strategies for persons with substance use and mental disorders." *Psychiatric Services* 56 (2005): 1288–91. [CrossRef]
17. Edward Kruk, and Kathryn Sandberg. "A home for body and soul: Substance using women in recovery." *Harm Reduction Journal* 10 (2013): 39. [CrossRef]
18. Harold G. Koenig, Dana E. King, and Verna B. Carson, eds. *Handbook of Religion and Health*, 2nd ed. Oxford and New York: Oxford University Press, 2012.

19. Torgeir Sørensen, Lars J. Danbolt, Jostein Holmen, Harold G. Koenig, and Lars Lien. "Does Death of a Family Member Moderate the Relationship between Religious Attendance and Depressive Symptoms? The HUNT Study, Norway." *Depression Research and Treatment* 2012 (2012): 396347. [CrossRef]

20. Ingrid M. Hatlebakk. "Spesialisthelsetjenester - Offentlig og privat rusbehandling [Special health care—Public and privat substance misuse treatment]." *Samfunnsspeilet*, 2014, 16–19.

21. Michael Quinn Patton. *Qualitative Research and Evaluation Methods*, 3rd ed. Thousand Oaks: Sage Publications, 2002.

22. Kirsti Malterud. "Systematic text condensation: A strategy for qualitative analysis." *Scandinavian Journal of Public Health* 40 (2012): 795–805. [CrossRef]

23. Katherine Van Wormer, and Diane R. Davis. *Addiction Treatment: A Strengths Perspective*. Pacific Grove: Brooks/Cole-Thomson, 2013.

24. Ronald L. Grimes. *Deeply into the Bone. Re-Inventing Rites of Passage*. Berkeley: California University Press, 2000, p. 391.

25. Tatjana Schnell. "Individual differences in meaning-making: Considering the variety of sources of meaning, their density and diversity." *Personal and Individual Differences* 51 (2011): 667–73.

26. Tom F. Driver. *Liberating Rites. Understanding the Transformative Power of Ritual*. Boulder: Westview Press, 1998, p. 270.

27. Elisabeth A.R. Robinson, Amy R. Krentzman, Jon R. Webb, and Kirk J. Brower. "Six-month changes in spirituality and religiousness in alcoholics predict drinking outcomes at nine months." *Journal of Studies on Alcohol and Drugs* 72 (2011): 660–668.

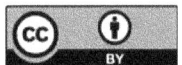

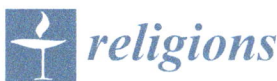

Article

Moving Forward in Their Journey: Participants' Experience of Taste & See, A Church-Based Programme to Develop a Healthy Relationship with Food

Riya Patel, Deborah Lycett *, Anne Coufopoulos and Andy Turner

Faculty of Health and Life Sciences, Coventry University, Priory Road, Coventry CV1 5FB, UK;
patelr34@uni.coventry.ac.uk (R.P.); Anne.Coufopoulos@coventry.ac.uk (A.C.); hsx116@coventry.ac.uk (A.T.)
* Correspondence: Deborah.lycett@coventry.ac.uk; Tel.: +44-247-765-5938

Academic Editors: Arndt Büssing and René Hefti
Received: 14 November 2016; Accepted: 12 January 2017; Published: 19 January 2017

Abstract: Quantitative evidence is beginning to document the successful outcomes achieved from holistic interventions that include a spiritual element as an approach to self-manage obesity in the community. However, qualitative research, which helps us understand the reasons behind their success, is scarce. Our aim was to explore participants' acceptance of and engagement with the Taste & See programme. Semi-structured interviews were carried out after participants had completed the Taste & See programme. Interviews were transcribed and analysed using deductive thematic analysis. Themes showing that 'God and food issues had been kept separate' at the start of the programme and that participants then 'Began to use faith as a resource' were identified. Also, while 'Eating freely was a challenge' initially, participants later found 'empowerment and enjoyment in freedom'. 'Addressing more than just a weight problem' was valued highly and there were benefits and difficulties that arose from 'Coping with other group members'. The rich level of evaluation provided through this study identifies that the participants found the programme a novel experience. The intervention was acceptable and participants engaged well with the programme content.

Keywords: obesity; weight; religion; spirituality; church-based; faith-based; Christian; intervention; feasibility trial; qualitative; acceptability; UK; engagement

---

1. Background

Obesity treatment is a high priority globally [1]. Evidence from cross-sectional studies indicates that religion and spirituality are positively associated with a better diet, which includes higher consumption of fruit and vegetables [2,3], higher fish intake [4] and lowered fat intake amongst specific Christian denominations (e.g., Seventh-Day Adventists) [3]. Systematic review evidence [5] is beginning to document the successful outcomes achieved from holistic interventions that include a spiritual element as an approach to self-manage obesity in the community. However, qualitative evidence that seeks to develop an understanding of why a spiritual element is important to participants in these programmes is limited [6]. According to the Medical Research Council (MRC) guidelines for the evaluation of complex interventions, an important part of an evaluation process is a qualitative exploration of the intervention. This can provide valuable insight into the successful and unsuccessful mechanisms of an intervention, as well as providing evidence of any unexpected outcomes that are not always easily disclosed using quantitative measures [7].

2. Aim

To explore participants' experience of participating in Taste & See, a Christian, church-based, healthy, intuitive eating, weight management programme in the United Kingdom.

Objectives

- To explore how participants engage with the programme, content and materials.
- To explore how acceptable participants find the programme.

3. Methods

This qualitative study was carried out as part of the Taste & See feasibility study, the protocol [8] and main results [9] of which are published elsewhere. Ethical approval was provided by Coventry University Research Ethics Committee. The paper is reported in accordance with the Consolidated Criteria for Reporting Qualitative Research [10].

3.1. Participants

Participants were recruited purposively, where all those who had taken part in the feasibility trial of the Taste & See programme were invited to participate in an interview. A total of 15 out of the 18 participants took part in semi-structured interviews post-intervention during July–August 2015. Three participants could not participate in interviews due to the time commitment involved. The interviews typically lasted between 30–40 min.

3.2. Data Collection

Before the trial began, an information session was held where participants were given the opportunity to ask what their participation would involve. They were given participant information sheets to take away and read. The following week participants were screened for eligibility to take part and invited to give consent to participate. During the final session of the programme, participants were reminded about the post-intervention interview. Interview schedules were given to participants ahead of the interview, so they could read and make notes around the schedule. The semi-structured interview schedule (Table 1) was designed and used as an aide-memoire during the interviews.

Table 1. Semi-structured interview schedule.

1. What did you think of this programme?
2. What were your initial expectations?
3. What did you find most helpful about this programme?
4. What did you find least helpful about this programme?
5. Could you please tell me how you found the religious and spiritual aspect of the programme?
6. Could you please tell me how you found the intuitive eating/non-dieting aspect of the programme?
7. Could you please tell me your thoughts about the programme being delivered at a church?
8. How helpful were the resources provided with the programme?
9. How does this programme compare with your previous attempts to diet?
10. What would you describe as the most successful part of this intervention?
11. Could you tell me about anything that you did not like about the programme?
12. How did you find the data collection for research purposes?
13. Overall, how would you describe your experience of the programme?
14 Before we finish, is there anything you would like to discuss about the programme that we haven't had a chance to discuss?

The majority of the interviews were conducted face-to-face; one participant did not want to participate in a face-to-face interview and chose to provide their feedback about the programme via e-mail. Riya Patel conducted the interviews under the supervision of Deborah Lycett; the interviews were carried out at the church where the intervention was delivered. Only the interviewers and participant were present during the interviews.

In line with realist research practice [11,12], during the interview the researcher summarised the key points covered to establish whether she had correctly interpreted the participant, this allowed participants to revise or clarify their views. Participants were also offered a chance to add to their answers at any point, and were provided an opportunity again at the end of their interviews. Transcripts were not returned to participants for checking and they were not asked to provide feedback on the results. This was because we wanted to explore how participants felt about the programme as soon after completing it as possible. With further time to reflect, these feelings may have changed; in particular, strong feelings important to the acceptance of the programme may have been diluted.

3.3. Data Analysis

All the interviews were audio-recorded and transcribed verbatim for analysis by Riya Patel. Transcripts were analysed using thematic analysis, as outlined by Braune and Clarke [13]. Each transcript was analysed separately and coded deductively at a semantic level. The researcher adopted a realist approach wherein the participant's experiences were taken at face value, as it was assumed that they were reporting the truth about their experiences of participating in the programme. Transcripts were read and re-read, and line-by-line coding was completed. Nvivo 10 (Qualitative Solutions and Research International, Doncaster, Victoria, Australia) data management software was used to organize and manage the data. The coding process progressed by moving back and forth across the dataset in an iterative process where comparisons were made between codes and phrases. Those with similar context or concepts were grouped together. Peer review was also performed by two of the co-authors (Deborah Lycett and Andy Turner), who agreed with the themes that were developed. Riya Patel also had frequent discussions with Deborah Lycett to ensure that the data interpretation was credible, valid and shared.

3.4. Reflexivity

Riya Patel is a Ph.D. student with a background in health psychology; this study was conducted as a part of her Ph.D. Riya Patel had established professional relationships with the participants through facilitating during the intervention and trial data collection.

Riya Patel identifies herself as an insider to the phenomena under focus, as she is a British Indian woman who belongs to the Christian faith and actively practices her faith by attending church weekly. She also has a personal, as well as academic, understanding of the weight-related issues (e.g., psychological issues like stigma, as well as eating for reasons like boredom) that participants discussed.

There are benefits to being an insider in qualitative research: an insider can share and identify with the experiences of participants, is equipped with insights into the phenomena, and possesses the ability to understand implied content [14]. With this in mind, issues with being an insider also arise, which include the risk of blurring boundaries due to the familiarised understanding that derives from the 'insider' researcher, imposing one's own beliefs through directing the interview and direction of participant's discussion, and over-disclosure of one's own experiences, which might shift the focus of the interview away from the participant [15].

To counter this, these issues were considered in the beginning prior to the research, and subsequent measures, such as journaling with engagement in deep reflexivity, plus continuously asking for clarification of participants' accounts, were taken to ensure the voice of the participant was not lost or misinterpreted. In particular, the researcher reflected on her role during the interviews and made changes in her approach, the questions asked and the manner they were phrased so that a clearer participant voice was heard in subsequent interviews.

Particular care was taken during the coding and analysis of data so that the deductive coding was completed in line with the clear aims of the study, rather than directed by researcher influence. The researcher refrained from insinuating meaning based on what the participants had said. A clear audit trail was created with annotations that highlighted the thought processes the researcher had when collating the codes into sub-themes and then themes.

4. Results

Of the 15 participants who took part in the interviews, the majority were females belonging to the Christian faith. The demographics of the participants are presented in Table 2.

Table 2. Participants' demographics.

Participant Characteristics		Interviewees		Those Not Interviewed	
		Mean	SD	Mean	SD
Age (Years)		48.1	13.8	43.3	21.8
		N (% Frequency)		N (% Frequency)	
Sex:	Male	2 (13)		1 (33)	
	Female	13 (87)		2 (67)	
Ethnicity:	White	13 (87)		3 (100)	
	Black	1 (6.5)		0 (0)	
	Asian	1(6.5)		0 (0)	
Religion:	Christian	13 (87)		3 (100)	
	Sikh	1 (6.5)		0 (0)	
	Spiritual, but not religious	1 (6.5)		0 (0)	
BMI category:	Healthy (with high TFEQ)	3 (20)		0 (0)	
	Overweight	3 (20)		1 (33)	
	Obese	6 (40)		2 (67)	
	Morbidly Obese	3 (20)		0 (0)	

Following close engagement with the data, seven super-ordinate themes were identified: 'God and food issues had been kept separate', 'Beginning to use faith as a resource', 'Eating freely was a challenge', 'There is empowerment and enjoyment in freedom', 'Addressing more than just a weight problem', 'Coping with other group members', and 'Journeying towards a healthier relationship with food'. All super-ordinate themes encapsulated sub-themes, all of which are illustrated with a series of extracts.

Theme 1: God and food issues had been kept separate

The spiritual component of this weight loss programme was a novel and salient experience for participants. The theme 'God and food issues were separate' illustrates the initial stages of participants' engagement with the spiritual component of the intervention. This theme captures participants' initial thoughts and feelings about where God and their spirituality fit within their eating behaviour. The data for this theme has been organised into three sub-themes, which are now explored in more detail.

Subtheme 1:   Food issues had never been taken to God before

Participants described how their faith was central to their lives; most of the participants actively engaged with their faith daily. At the start of the course, the idea of spirituality in relation to eating was a new concept that needed to be worked through as bringing God into their eating was not something they had previously considered.

"When it comes to . . . eating healthy and all of that, no, I'd never attached that [to] God"

[Extract 1, Participant 1]

Subtheme 2:   Food issues were considered too trivial for God

When participants started to consider the role that God played in their food-related struggles, many participants believed that the issues they experienced were too trivial for God to be interested in. Participants identified how they felt their eating behaviour was something they had to deal with by themselves, illustrating a reason why issues associated with food were not previously taken to God.

> "At the beginning I did find it difficult ... I felt it was trivial for God ... taking things about eating and dieting and weight to Him."
>
> [Extract 2, Participant 2]

> "Previously I would have thought [issues related to weight] are just too trivial for God to be bothered about, [and] actually it was my responsibility to sort them out."
>
> [Extract 3, Participant 3]

Subtheme 3:   Shame prevented participants from bringing God into their eating

For many participants, the issues they had with food and the problems they faced represented great failures in their lives, whereas their relationship with God was viewed positively. Accounts from the participants suggested that feelings of guilt and shame meant they deliberately kept God separate from their eating behaviour.

> "I never brought them together because as far as I'm concerned my eating is a big, well, a failed area of my life; whereas my faith and my relationship with God has just gone from strength to strength. I always speak to God about how I'm feeling emotionally and pray for help and support with all other areas; it [my eating] is one of those areas that I've kept very separate."
>
> [Extract 4, Participant 4]

Some participants felt that the problems they have with food and eating should be something they attempt to deal with themselves first before they take it to God, which further illustrates shame and therefore a deliberate attempt to keep this issue away from God.

> "I've always had the mind-set I'll take it to God, I'll pray about it, but I have to lose weight first."
>
> [Extract 5, Participant 5]

Theme 2:   Beginning to use faith as a resource

The theme 'beginning to use faith as a resource' encompasses the next part of the participants' journey and begins to show how participants engaged with the spiritual element as they progressed through the course; this has been captured through four sub-themes.

Subtheme 1:   Realising God does want to help

From having never relinquished their weight-related struggles to God, participants transitioned to a place where they realised that God does want to help them with their weight-related struggles.

> I ... found the fact that God does want to help me in this [overcoming emotional eating] helpful, because ... it [was] something which I thought was trivial, really not something necessarily that God would be interested in."
>
> [Extract 6, Participant 2]

This acknowledgement meant that participants started to ask God for help with their food issues.

Subtheme 2:   Drawing on faith to achieve a healthier relationship with food

As participants started to understand that God wanted to help them in this area, participants began drawing on their faith and applying their faith in different ways to their eating.

Some of the participants identified how they were not just praying for weight loss, rather they were praying specifically about certain areas they wanted help with in relation to their issues with weight, and noted how they were drawing on strength from God to help them.

> "But obviously, it was not simple as just praying and it happens. Now I realise it's praying for the strength to be able to do [and] fulfil what it [is] that I actually want to happen; so I need the strength to be able to ... make sure I ... exercise regularly [and] make sure I'm content with [the] food I'm eating."
>
> [Extract 7, Participant 6]

Some participants noted how perceiving their relationship with food through the lens of their faith meant they were reading and applying Bible verses in a whole new context. Interpreting their eating behaviours through what Bible scriptures teach led participants to be more mindful about their motives behind eating.

> "God's given us a brain and it's for understanding His word. Overindulgence, selfishness, greed, gluttony, those are things I didn't actually think about when you grew up and have at sort of meals."
>
> [Extract 8, Participant 7]

> "'Everything is permissible but not everything is beneficial' that's given me ... a clearer understanding of how I can stop, think, before I act, consider it, reflect on things, then go do it."
>
> [Extract 9, Participant 7]

Subtheme 3:   God's love as a catalyst for self-love

The content of the programme that considered God's love and acceptance led participants on a journey towards self-love and self-care. The quotes below demonstrate that as participants began to see and love themselves the way God sees and loves them, they experienced a change in their motivation to manage their food and weight.

> "This experience has taught me how to love myself, the love God has for me, and how precious my body is in all aspects—inside and out—so what I put in it is really important."
>
> [Extract 10, Participant 1]

> "God loves me as I am but wants me to love myself and lose some weight to be healthy"
>
> [Extract 11, Participant 2]

Subtheme 4:   No discomfort with, and applicability of, Christian spirituality

Some participants described that despite not belonging to the Christian faith, the Christian spirituality discussed on the programme did not isolate them or pose as a barrier preventing them from participating. Participants reported that they were comfortable with this element and it was not forced on them.

> "I didn't feel pressured, no, I could take it or leave it. If I didn't want to pray—I didn't pray."
>
> [Extract 12, Participant 8]

'I mean I felt even though I'm a non-Christian it was still . . . very applicable...there [was] very general well-being, good stuff . . . I didn't find that a barrier at all."

[Extract 13, Participant 6]

Participants felt that that they could identify with Christian spirituality despite not belonging to the Christian faith group and they could still apply and relate the messages of this element to their eating behaviours.

"A lot the Bible readings were common sense, I mean there were a couple of times when I thought . . . I'm not sure of that one, but I don't think I was the only person, you know, and sometimes we thought, well, actually, no [I] don't really relate to that, and other times you just think, well, actually, you know, that's common sense whether you believe it comes from a God or a universe or whatever—for me it still makes sense."

[Extract 14, Participant 8]

Theme 3: Eating freely was a challenge

Freedom from dietary restrictions formed another novel aspect of Taste & See. The theme 'eating freely was a challenge' explores participants' initial encounter with the 'unconditional permission to eat' element of intuitive eating. The data for this theme was captured using the three sub-themes presented below.

Subtheme 1: Freedom felt dangerous

When participants described their early thoughts about the freedom component of the intervention, participants used phrases like *"Playing with fire"* and *"a license to indulge"* and described how freedom felt like a temptation to eat everything, which seemed counterintuitive to their reasons for joining the programme.

"It was really almost like opening the floodgates and saying right, okay, you can have everything; go and empty Tesco's."

[Extract 15, Participant 8]

Subtheme 2: Freedom felt too good to be true

For many participants, their initial thoughts about the dietary freedom of the programme raised scepticism, as it was going against their existing beliefs about how to lose weight.

"Initially I was a bit sceptical, because it just seems like one of those diets that you see in the *Daily Mail*, like 'oh eat what you want and still lose 5 stone'. . . . It just seemed a bit too good to be true."

[Extract 16, Participant 6]

"'Cos to me, losing weight is deprivation of something; you know, I didn't really see to begin with how you could not do that and lose weight."

[Extract 17, Participant 5]

Subtheme 3: Freedom gave rise to feelings of uncertainty about the programme's success

Whilst practicing intuitive eating, some of the interviews suggested that freedom gave rise to feelings of uncertainty about successful weight loss. As participants ate intuitively, they were convinced they had gained weight, and their accounts suggested that this stemmed from their initial struggles with freedom from dietary restriction.

"I felt like I was eating less but I didn't necessarily feel like I'd lost weight. I weighed myself and I got a real shock because I had actually lost some weight, and I've been trying to lose that weight for 10 years."

[Extract 18, Participant 9]

"That [eating freely] was difficult at the beginning, and of course when you're making free choices about what you're eating you just assume you're going to be putting weight on. So I didn't stand on the scales because I just thought that would stop me and I'd just want to go on a diet again."

[Extract 19, Participant 4]

To address this in the future, one participant suggested that a form of accountability be developed where participants can check in with someone or are provided with an option to weigh themselves to help alleviate these concerns.

Theme 4: There is empowerment and enjoyment in freedom

This theme highlights the positive experiences of participants' engagement with freedom. When engaging with the unconditional permission to eat element, participants started to experience empowerment and enjoyment, which was achieved through liberating themselves from dietary restrictions. This theme is presented through two sub-themes.

Subtheme 1: Freedom teaches you to think for yourself

As participants began to understand the ethos of the freedom message, there was a realization amongst all the participants that freedom is "teaching you to think for yourself". Participants developed a sense of empowerment when engaging with this element as they began thinking of their own ways to manage their eating behaviours. Participants were finding out what worked for them and employing strategies they wanted to use rather than obeying dietary rules that had been provided for them by others.

"I think I was taking responsibility for what I was doing, a little bit more than somebody imposing on me."

[Extract 20, Participant 4]

"It [freedom] teaches you how to think for yourself and not to stick to a schedule."

[Extract 21, Participant 1]

Subtheme 2: Freedom diminishes the negative emotions associated with eating

Throughout the course engaging with the freedom element led participants to feel liberated from negative emotions; there was a realisation that *"Food is not the enemy"*. Participants expressed how the removal of dietary restrictions allowed them to begin to enjoy the foods they previously would have experienced guilt about eating.

"I do eat chocolate still, but I don't crave it, I don't think about it from morning 'til night, which is what I've always done, the whole of my life. It's been almost an obsessive compulsion, so even when I'm dieting successfully I would have that bar of chocolate. I would put it in the cupboard and I would know where it is and I would fixate on it the whole day 'til I was allowed to have it. [Now] days go by when I don't eat chocolate, some days I do, sometimes I eat too much, but it's not [with] that awful guilty [feeling]. I can actually enjoy it whilst I eat it."

[Extract 22, Participant 3]

Some felt they were in a failing battle, with feelings of failure triggering emotional eating. Dietary freedom helped participants to be released from feeling like a failure.

> "I just have whatever I want really. Today I had 2 pieces of toast and honey without too much guilt attached to it, so they weren't horrendous breakfasts but it was really nice to be released from that, because I'm not going through all morning feeling that I've failed already, which is kind of the norm."
>
> [Extract 23, Participant 4]

Theme 5: Addressing more than just a weight problem

Most of the participants were very much aware of their current weight issues, and the implications these have on their wider health, prior to the programme. However, for most of the participants their weight was not the only issue that required addressing. This theme captures how the programme was an opportunity to address more than just their weight as a quantitative measure. The data for this theme has been captured through the three sub-themes presented below.

Subtheme 1: An opportunity to address other issues

As previously described, the course delved into a range of issues around a poor relationship with food (e.g., eating in response to emotion, childhood habits), which provided participants with the opportunity to tackle issues that they had not faced before.

> "I think things that I've never fully accepted or I've found too difficult and I've just hidden, put to one side, thinking it's all about just losing weight but it's the big thing [about] why I've got myself overweight."
>
> [Extract 24, Participant 5]

> "I've found that the week where we were writing letters and kind of really dealing with issues [around] why we have weight gain issues. For me [that] was quite important, it gave me the opportunity to deal with something quite major."
>
> [Extract 25, Participant 3]

Exploring the different issues that can contribute to weight gain gave participants the opportunity to begin understanding their eating behaviours. Some participants had previously identified themselves as emotional eaters. However, following the session around understanding motivations behind eating, they realised they were not emotional eaters but ate in response to feelings of boredom or tiredness. Other participants identified how they had never experienced real physiological hunger and as a result were overeating. In addition, other individuals realised that their issues with food were down to a lack of discipline, which they were now trying to address.

> "The biggest thing for me for was the fact that I thought I was an emotional eater, and I'm not. The reason I'm eating isn't, well it is slightly linked to emotion[s] but it's not linked to me being upset or anxious or stressed, which was what was confusing me. I don't feel that my life is controlled by anxiety and stress at the moment; I'm not in a crisis stage at any point. I'm actually going along quite happily. So, my eating is coming from my boredom and maybe slightly loneliness. I'm used to being surrounded by adults and now I'm at home with the kids and that's a different type of thing. My husband works long hours and quite often long days. [So] I eat 'cos I get bored and fed up and it's something that passes the time. The choices of jobs that need doing aren't necessarily things that interest me or I want to do, [so] it actually hasn't got anything to do with being anxious or stressed or emotionally upset, which is good."
>
> [Extract 26, Participant 4]

Subtheme 2:   Different from previous weight loss attempts

The importance of having the opportunity to address other issues was further emphasised when participants reflected on their previous weight loss attempts. Participants discussed how previously when they tried to lose weight, their focus would be on reducing the number on the weighing scales. Through this they would experience short-term success, but the real issues they had with food remained unaddressed. Participants' accounts illustrated that beginning to address these issues was in some ways more important than weight loss, which was key to participants' journey through the programme.

"What I've found with all other diets and everything else [is that they've] helped in the short term, but I haven't dealt with the underlying reasons why. I've needed to do that."

[Extract 27, Participant 5]

"I think what's important to me [is that] all the way through my life I've gone to diet clubs or followed a diet or whatever. I haven't ever addressed the mindset that I'm in about food, and how I deal with that, and how I feel about it. You've only got to open my fridge [and] realise it's a healthier fridge. You go to my bedroom there isn't a stash, there's nothing to binge on in my bedroom, which is sort of my secret place. That to me at the moment is almost more important than losing the weight; does that make sense?"

[Extract 28, Participant 8]

As participants continued to reflect on their previous weight loss attempts, they described how exploring these issues and actually beginning to address them was valuable in moving forward and developing a more realistic approach to weight management.

"I've learned things about how I'm eating, and the psychological bit of how I am eating, which in some ways is more important because I can't go through life constantly measuring, weighing, adding up points and all the rest of it. It's got to come from somewhere else and that's gonna take time."

[Extract 29, Participant 10]

Subtheme 3:   At times there was too much to take in

Whilst participants credited the intervention with helping them address these complex issues, it was also evident that at times the content of the course could be too much for participants to take in. As participants progressed through the sessions, they found that the course challenged their existing behaviours, provoking them to form new cognitions and attitudes towards food. Whilst this was considered helpful and necessary, this process was at times described as overwhelming.

"We've already had an awful lot of information. You've learned all this, you know what you've been doing wrong, [and] there's going to be more added to it before you get to the end. I found it piled up a bit, you're uncovering some of your weaknesses, and some of the areas that you're not good at...causing you to reflect on your lifestyle."

[Extract 30, Participant 7]

In addition to this, a few participants suggested that the content of the intervention was overwhelming because the solutions were not given to them. There was an expectation amongst most of the participants that they would be provided with rules to follow, akin to other weight management programmes. The aim of the course was to assist participants with finding their own solutions. Whilst most participants could engage with this, some participants would have preferred solutions from the facilitators.

"Sometimes I felt perhaps it was a lot without giving us all the answers, but I realise that's not gonna happen, and that shouldn't happen, [it] can't happen, you've got to do it yourself."

[Extract 31, Participant 5]

Theme 6: Coping with other group members

During each session participants were split into smaller groups of three or four, where they shared their thoughts, feelings and stories. This theme demonstrates how participants felt about this element of the intervention, with participants reporting mixed experiences across their interviews. This has been captured through four sub-themes that are presented below in more detail.

Subtheme 1: The benefits of being in smaller groups

All the participants agreed that separating into small groups of three or four people was a beneficial aspect of the intervention. Being in smaller groups helped to create solidarity, provided a safe environment for discussion and sharing ideas and was a good support system for participants.

"It helps to know that other people go through the same problems [and] the same challenges as you do, and in fact some of them [have] worse challenges."

[Extract 32, Participant 10]

"Yeah I just enjoyed it, it was nice in the discussions to hear how other people were getting on and get other people's input on things, so it was all good."

[Extract 33, Participant 4]

Subtheme 2: People who have bigger issues with eating took over group discussions

Whilst there were benefits to separating into smaller groups, some participants felt that group members who had bigger or deeper issues associated with eating had the tendency to dominate the group discussion.

"Some people have a lot of ... problems and for me that's not particularly helpful. I'm a very selfish person, it has to be said, not wanting to listen to other people's problems.

[Extract 34, Participant 10]

When participants found they could not relate to the discussion, they felt they had to hold back from sharing their experiences, which meant their own issues were not always addressed.

"I felt sometimes there were people with much bigger issues, so I [held] back a little bit with my issues. I think maybe it would have been better to be [in] more similar groups, because I think some people with bigger issues took over the discussion and I felt it didn't really speak to me."

[Extract 35, Participant 11]

Subtheme 3: Different opinions about group consistency

Participants also discussed the consistency of groups and their thoughts on what was most comfortable for them. There were mixed responses on what participants found helpful. For some, keeping groups consistent all the way through was important, as a shared understanding was established and rapport had been built between the group members. By not keeping groups consistent, some participants considered this element was lost.

"When I came in late, I actually sat with a group [where] I didn't know anybody. I really think it's important that if you're going to do a group that the people that you sit with you kind of develop a rapport with and you understand them because they've talked about their past and their problems with food."

[Extract 36, Participant 12]

As well as keeping groups consistent, some participants also felt that participants should be matched according to the issues they have with food, as this gave further common ground for participants to develop rapport.

"I felt the groups needed to be smaller, better or specifically matched together."

[Extract 37, Participant 13]

However, for other participants mixing groups was better for them. For some this was to prevent cliques developing and for others it was so that they could get different ideas and insights.

"I would have liked to be in different groups . . . 'cos otherwise it gets a bit cliquey. You get different ideas off people and where they're coming from and some people are worse than you and you think, 'oh gosh I thought I had problems'."

[Extract 38, Participant 14]

Theme 7: Journeying towards a healthier relationship with food

This theme captures participants' overall experience of the programme and the next part of their journey. This theme has been captured through three sub-themes.

Sub theme 1:   Taste & See has equipped me with tools

Participants acknowledged that the programme had not brought around an instant change but rather equipped them with tools to begin developing a better relationship with food. Many of the participants recognised that they were still at the start of their weight loss journey but moving forward in the right direction.

"What it's given me is [an] understanding [of] the dynamics of eating. Why we eat, what are the triggers, what are the internal triggers, and the external triggers and [how] those influences can negatively affect you and how you can make the wrong choices. [The Bible verse] 'Everything is permissible but not everything is beneficial' [has] given me a clearer understanding of how I can stop [and] think before I act, consider it, reflect on things then go do it. It doesn't always work, I'll be honest, it's something you get caught out [with] so it's still breaking those engrained habits and they take time."

[Extract 39, Participant 7]

Subtheme 2:   Starting to move forward

Throughout the course participants learned about their own eating behaviours. At the end of the course, participants identified that they are at the next stage of their journey where they are beginning to use their tools and apply the things they have learned from the intervention.

"I'm trying not to eat between meals but I haven't got to grips . . . with this"

[Extract 40, Participant 12]

"[I learned that] there is another way out there and that the way I look at food is not necessarily a healthy way of looking at food. I had my eyes opened to a new way of looking at eating and food that I need to grasp and make it become my way of thinking. Does that make sense?"

[Extract 41, Participant 10]

Some participants wanted to repeat the course so they could better consolidate the knowledge they had developed, and make incorporating the intervention into their daily lives easier.

"I really like it and I would love to do it again because I think having got the concept of it, doing it again I'd get a lot more out of it, if that makes any sense? I think it's one of these things you need to do more than once."

[Extract 42, Participant 10]

Sub-theme 3:   Final thoughts on the Taste & See programme

Overall participants highly commended the programme, meriting the use of spirituality and intuitive eating as approaches towards weight management.   The following quotes illustrate participants' final thoughts about the programme.

"I would say I would recommend it to everyone; yeah, I would recommend it to everyone"

[Extract 43, Participant 14]

"I was in a much worse place than I actually really thought I was, and I recognise that I needed to address it [and] I found it hard to address it . . . Spirituality and education about healthy eating works."

[Extract 44, Participant 15]

The development of codes into sub-themes and themes is illustrated in Figure 1.

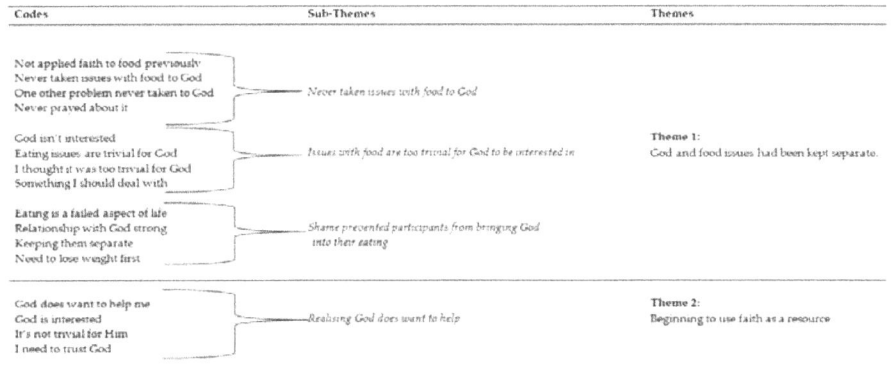

Figure 1. *Cont.*

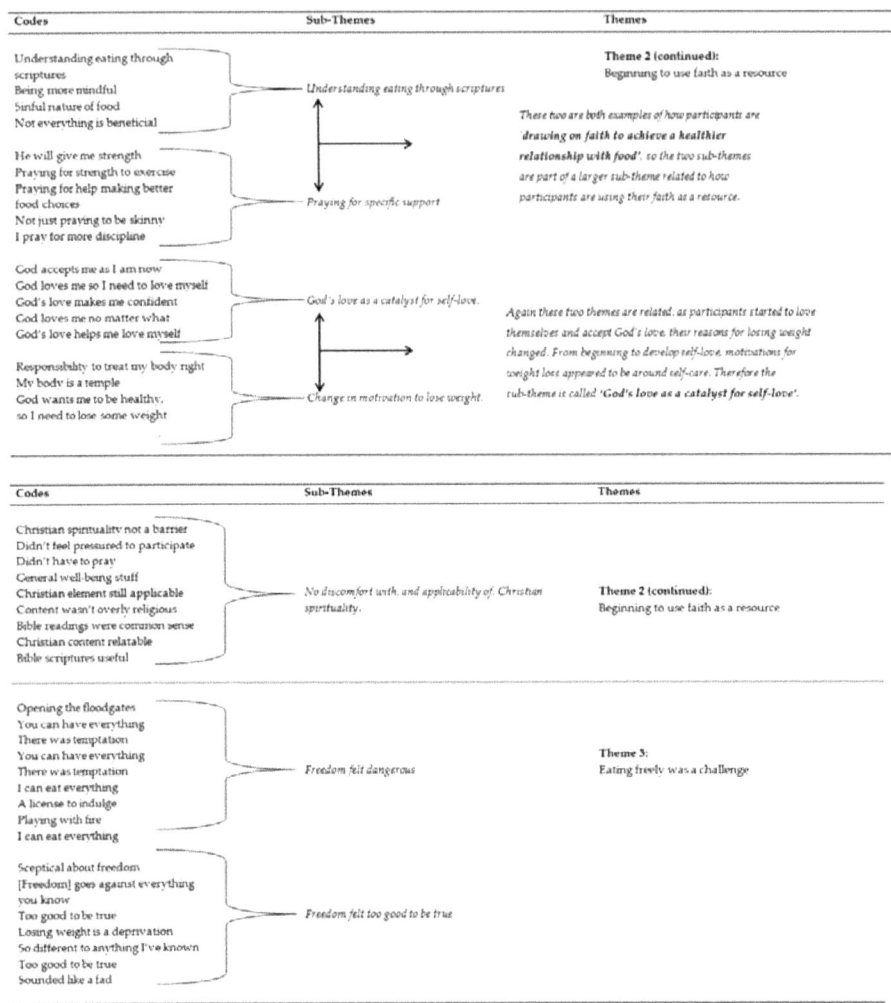

Figure 1. *Cont.*

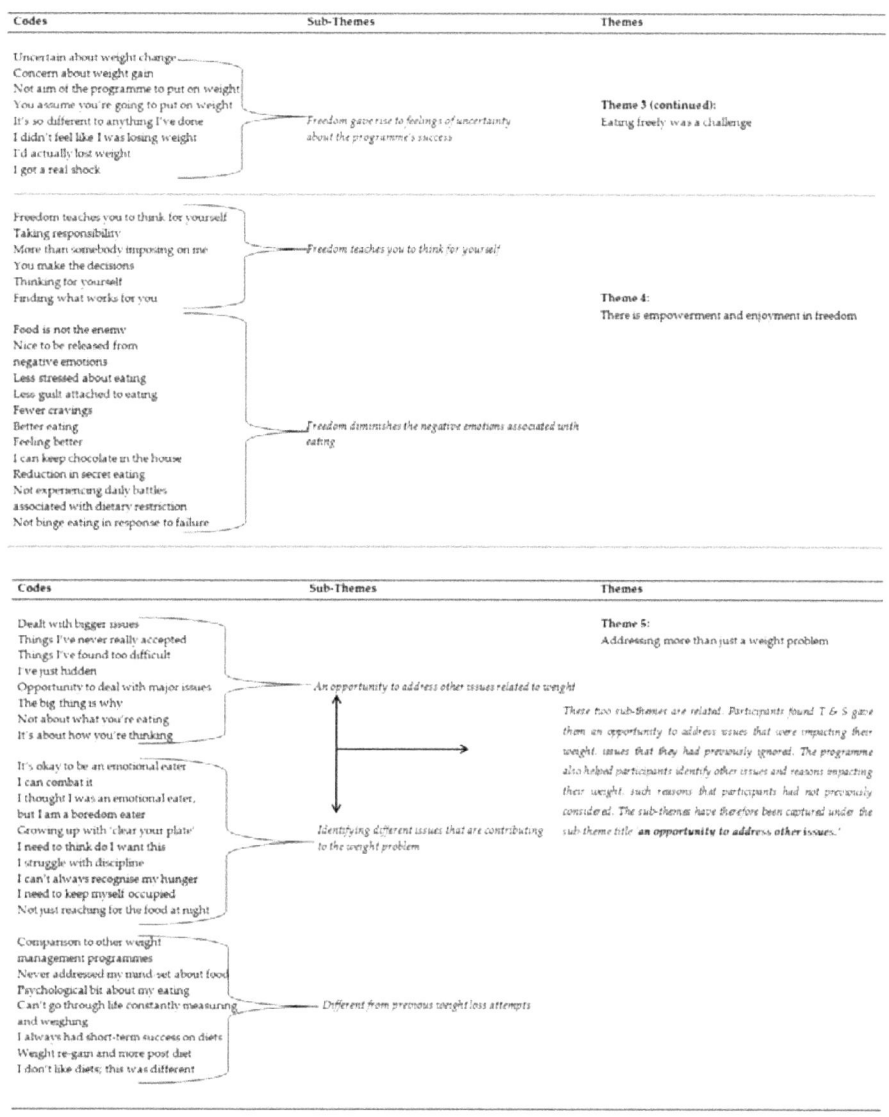

Figure 1. *Cont.*

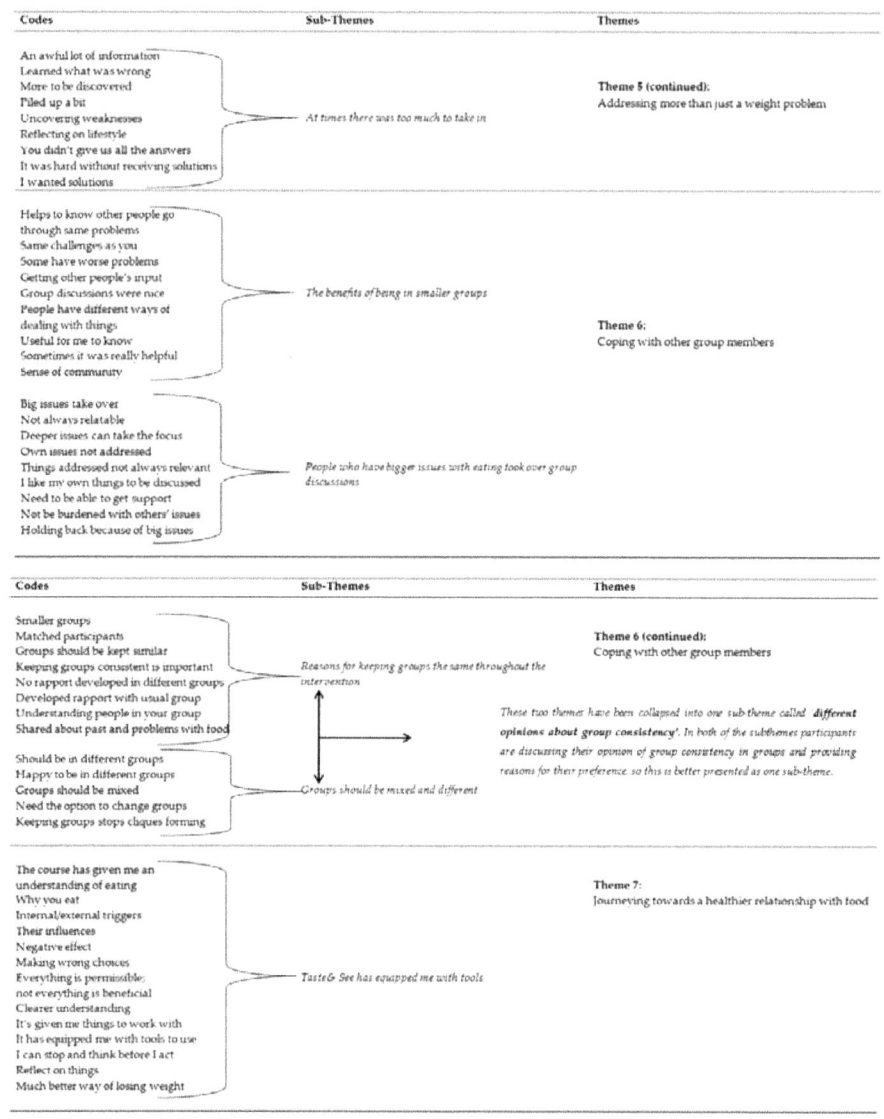

Figure 1. *Cont.*

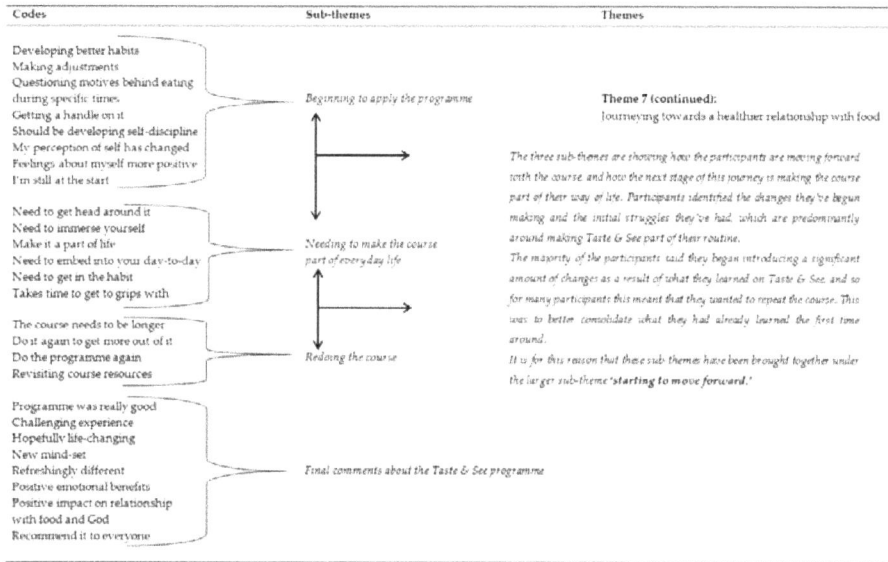

Figure 1. Thematic map of the analysis process displaying how codes were translated into themes.

5. Discussion

5.1. Summary of the Results

The present study explored how acceptable participants found the Taste & See intervention, and further explored how they engaged with the different components. The study is part of a feasibility trial; a full report of the trial is reported elsewhere. The Christian weight management programme was a unique and welcome experience for the participants. For most of the participants, the idea of bringing God into their eating was not something they had previously considered despite experiencing considerable struggles with their weight. Participants identified that engaging with the spiritual content of the intervention took them on a journey towards accepting God's help, using their faith as a resource and learning to love themselves the way God loves them. The latter part of the journey formed an important foundation for changing motives to manage their weight post-intervention. Participants found exploring other reasons to eat and how to challenge these behaviours useful, particularly in terms of listening to feelings of hunger and fullness. Similar to their journey with the spiritual element, the freedom element took participants on a journey where early challenges with freedom were related to difficulties in understanding dietary freedom, and fears of weight gain. The freedom element helped participants experience release from the negative emotions associated with food and eating. Participants identified that there were several benefits to being in smaller groups, which included building rapport and developing solidarity through sharing experiences with one another. However, some participants found small group discussions that were dominated by those with deeper emotional issues unhelpful. On the whole, participants felt that the programme helped them take the next step in their journey towards developing a healthier attitude towards food, suggesting acceptance of and engagement with the programme.

5.2. Strengths and Limitations of the Study

There are several strengths to the current study. Most of the participants in the feasibility trial took part in the interviews. Our findings have provided unique insights into participants' experiences, which has enabled us to gain a fuller understanding of how this intervention worked and illuminated the quantitative findings of our trial. As discussed below, the findings of our study are consistent with previous findings in this area, which increases the credibility of our findings. Furthermore, we reported on the researcher's background, considered the impact this would have on the findings, and took measures to minimize any influence over the results produced. Thematic analysis was used appropriately to answer the research question, and, as described in the methods, through using peer review and keeping an audit trail the rigour of our study was enhanced.

The main limitation of the present study is the small homogenous sample, which limits the transferability of the findings. The participants knew the researchers (Riya Patel and Deborah Lycett) who conducted the interviews; this could have introduced an element of social desirability in the responses participants provided. However, it was emphasized that honest feedback was required from the participants and that this was crucial for the development of the programme.

5.3. Interpretation of Findings and Consistency with Other Findings

Previous studies exploring the acceptability of and engagement with interventions of this nature are scarce. The findings of this qualitative study are, however, consistent with the existing literature within this area. Considering the themes around the intuitive eating component, Kidd et al. [16] conducted a one-group pre-test/post-test design mixed methods feasibility study of obese women's lived experience of a mindful eating group intervention. This intervention, although broader in its mindfulness approach, focused on self-regulation theory and encompassed intuitive eating components. The findings of this study echoed the findings of our study, where women in the study highlighted their initial struggles with freedom and being mindful about their eating behaviours. Kidd et al. [16] identified two themes related to mindful eating: 'Feeling the burden, and then the freedom' and 'Bringing control back'. Collectively, these two themes show how participants initially felt burdened by the concept of eating mindfully but, as they began practicing it, they gradually felt more in control of their eating behaviours. Participants' accounts reflect how they became more aware of the social and environmental cues and how these affect their eating. They also reported feelings of increased self-efficacy and positive emotional gains through eating mindfully. This was like the participants in our study, as identified through our themes *'Eating freely was a challenge'* and *'There is empowerment and enjoyment in freedom'*, where there were initial reports of struggle with freedom, but over time participants felt more in control of their eating and experienced increased enjoyment of their food. Kidd et al. [16] also reported findings around the benefits and support of the smaller groups, and how this was a source of encouragement and bonding, which is consistent with the findings of our theme *'coping with other group members'*. Kidd et al. [16] also discussed a theme 'Moving from thinking the principles to living the principles'; this particular theme mirrors the findings of our final theme, *'Moving forward in their journey towards a healthier relationship with food'*, which explored how participants were moving forward with a new way of thinking about eating and taking steps to incorporate what they had learned on the Taste & See programme into their daily lives. This demonstrates the trustworthiness of our findings.

Our themes around the spiritual element and participants' engagement with this element were similar to those of the participants in Yeary et al. [17]. Yeary et al. [17] described how the connection between participants' faith and health motivated them to change their health behaviours as a sign of devotion to God. Reicks et al. [18] also conducted a qualitative study exploring spirituality in a weight loss programme. Consistent with our findings, Reicks et al. [18] identified how women in the study drew on their relationship with God through praying for help to overcome emotional eating and using Biblical scriptures to understand eating behaviour, which then encouraged women to change their motives for eating. Similarly, the findings of a recent focus group study of participants who had previously participated in a church-based weight loss programme mirrored the findings of our study [19]. Seale et al. [19] concluded that participants anchored themselves on key scriptures, for example 1 Corinthians 6:19, where the body is described as a temple of the Holy Spirit—this provided them with a conscious awareness to treat their bodies better, which in turn motivated them to maintain the behavioural changes learned on the interventions. Participants in our study also anchored themselves on specific scriptures including this one when navigating through their daily lives post-intervention. For example, certain scriptures served as prompts for participants to think about their eating behaviour motives, whilst other scriptures encouraged participants to make better choices around food. Furthermore, Seale et al. [19] also found that participants were actively collaborating with God to seek help and find strength beyond their own means to successfully address the struggles they experienced with their weight. This is discussed in our theme *'beginning to use faith as a resource'*, where participants used the resources available to them through their faith to achieve the lifestyle changes they sought to implement. Collectively, these findings begin to identify what the spiritual component adds to a weight management programme, and how addressing the spiritual needs of the individual during such programmes can be beneficial.

Findings unique to our study were the themes around guilt and shame causing participants to hide their struggles with food and eating from God. When faced with health-related struggles including diagnosis of, or adjustment to, a chronic condition, turning to one's faith and harnessing spiritual beliefs to assist with coping has been observed in the literature [20,21]. It might be that our participants may not perceive obesity as a chronic condition with an immediate health threat, as for example with diabetes or cardiovascular diseases. Furthermore, it could be suggested that these findings are specific to the population under study, as much of the previous research derives from participants of African-American descent, who typically position God centrally in all aspects of their health [22,23] and make the church leader the first port of call for health issues [24,25]; in the United Kingdom, the first port of call for most Christians is the National Health Service. In addition, while the health message about food and diet is central in certain Christian denominations such as Seventh-Day Adventists [26], it is considered much less, and perhaps even not at all, in many other denominations of Christianity. In fact, it has been suggested that overindulgence in food (although not promoted) is overlooked as a 'lesser evil' in comparison to alcohol and smoking [27]. Many religious functions within the church use food, rather than alcohol, as the celebratory good to be consumed [28]. This seems to fit with our findings demonstrated in the subtheme 'drawing on faith to achieve a healthier relationship with food', where food, for some, was not thought about in relation to overindulgence and gluttony prior to completing the Taste & See programme. Despite this, it is interesting to note that guilt, shame and hiding from God characterised many participants' relationship with food; therefore, it may be that the failure to address these aspects of life spiritually is particularly important in the U.K. population.

6. Conclusions and Implications

This is the first study to incorporate intuitive eating and Christian spirituality and the first study to be conducted in a U.K. context. We have shown that participants successfully engaged with a Christian church-based intuitive eating programme. The findings illustrate that the intervention was acceptable to the participants of the study, and support further exploration of interventions of this nature. The rich level of evaluation provided by the participants will be used to improve and enhance the intervention design and evaluation process.

Acknowledgments: We would like to thank the participants who took their time to take part in this study. We gratefully acknowledge the funding of Coventry University. The views expressed here are the opinions of the authors and not of Coventry University.

Author Contributions: D.L. conceived, designed and executed the study, supervised data collection, analysis and the writing of the paper; R.P collected, analysed the data and drafted the paper; A.C. and A.T contributed to the design of the study and drafting of the paper.

Conflicts of Interest: The authors declare no conflict of interest.

References

1. Frühbeck, Gema, and Volkan Yumuk. "Obesity: A Gateway Disease with a Rising Prevalence." *Obesity Facts* 7 (2014): 33–36. [CrossRef] [PubMed]

2. Tan, Min-Min, Carina KY Chan, and Daniel D. Reidpath. "Religiosity, dietary habit, intake of fruit and vegetables, and vegetarian status among Seventh-Day Adventists in West Malaysia." *Journal of Behavioral Medicine* 39 (2016): 675–686. [CrossRef] [PubMed]

3. Tan, Min-Min, Carina KY Chan, and Daniel D. Reidpath. "Religiosity and spirituality and the intake of fruit, vegetable, and fat: A systematic review." *Evidence-Based Complementary and Alternative Medicine* 2013 (2013): article 146214. [CrossRef] [PubMed]

4. Obisesan, Thomas, Ivor Livingston, Harld Dean Trulear, and Frank Gillum. "Frequency of attedance at religious services, cardiovascular disease, metabolic risk factors and dietary intake in Americans: An age stratified exploratory analysis." *International Journal of Psychiatry in Medicine* 36 (2006): 435–48. [CrossRef] [PubMed]

5. Lancaster, Kristie, Lori Carter-Edwards, Stephanie Grilo, Chwan Li Shen, and Antoinette Schoenthaler. "Obesity interventions in African American faith-based organizations: A systematic review." *Obesity Reviews* 15 (2014): 159–76. [CrossRef] [PubMed]

6. Timmons, Shirley. "Review and evaluation of faith-based weight management interventions that target African American women." *Journal of Religion and Health* 54 (2015): 798–809. [CrossRef] [PubMed]

7. Craig, Peter, Paul Dieppe, Sally Macintyre, Susan Michie, Irwin Nazareth, and Mark Petticrew. "Developing and Evaluating Complex Interventions: The new Medical Research Council Guidance." *BMJ* 337 (2008): article a1655. [CrossRef] [PubMed]

8. Lycett, Deborah, Riya Patel, Anne Coufopoulos, and Andy Turner. "Protocol of Taste and See: A Feasibility Study of a Church-Based, Healthy, Intuitive Eating Programme." *Religions* 7 (2016): article 41. [CrossRef]

9. Patel, Riya, Deborah Lycett, Anne Coufopoulos, and Andy Turner. "A Feasibility Study of Taste & See: A church-based, programme to develop a healthy relationship with food." under review with Religions.

10. Tong, Allison, Peter Sainsbury, and Jonathan Craig. "Consolidated criteria for reporting qualitative research (COREQ): A 32-item checklist for interviews and focus groups." *International Journal for Quality in Health Care* 19 (2007): 349–57. [CrossRef] [PubMed]

11. Sobh, Rana, and Chad Perry. "Research design and data analysis in realism research." *European Journal of Marketing* 40 (2006): 1194–209. [CrossRef]

12. Maxwell, Joseph A. *A Realist Approach for Qualitative Research*. Thousand Oaks: Sage, 2012.

13. Braun, Virginia, and Victoria Clarke. "Using thematic analysis in psychology." *Qualitative Research in Psychology* 3 (2006): 77–101. [CrossRef]

14. Kacen, Lea, and Julia Chaitin. "'The Times They are a Changing': Undertaking Qualitative Research in Ambiguous, Conflictual, and Changing Contexts." *The Qualitative Report* 11 (2006): 209–28.

15. Drake, Pat. "Grasping at methodological understanding: A cautionary tale from insider research." *International Journal of Research & Method in Education* 33 (2010): 85–99. [CrossRef]

16. Kidd, Lori I., Christine Heifner Graor, and Carolyn J. Murrock. "A mindful eating group intervention for obese women: A mixed methods feasibility study." *Archives of Psychiatric Nursing* 27 (2013): 211–18. [CrossRef] [PubMed]

17. Yeary, Karen Hye-cheon Kim, Carol Cornell, Jerome Turner, Page Moore, Zoran Bursac, Elaine Prewitt, and Delia Smith West. "Feasibility of an evidence-based weight loss intervention for a faith-based, rural, African American population." *Preventing Chronic Disease* 8 (2011): 1–12.

18. Reicks, Marla, Jordan Mills, and Helen Henry. "Qualitative study of spirituality in a weight loss program: Contribution to self-efficacy and locus of control." *Journal of Nutrition Education and Behavior* 36 (2004): 13–19. [CrossRef]

19. Seale, J. Paul, Judith Fifield, Y. Monique Davis-Smith, Rebecca Satterfield, Joy Goens Thomas, Bonnie Cole, Mark J. Atkinson, and John Mark Boltri. "Developing culturally congruent weight maintenance programs for African American church members." *Ethnicity & Health* 18 (2013): 152–67. [CrossRef] [PubMed]

20. Kristeller, Jean L., Virgil Sheets, Tom Johnson, and Betsy Frank. "Understanding religious and spiritual influences on adjustment to cancer: Individual patterns and differences." *Journal of Behavioral Medicine* 34 (2011): 550–61. [CrossRef] [PubMed]

21. Büssing, Arndt, and Harold G. Koenig. "Spiritual needs of patients with chronic diseases." *Religions* 1 (2010): 18–27. [CrossRef]

22. DeHaven, Mark J., Irby B. Hunter, Laura Wilder, James W. Walton, and Jarett Berry. "Health programs in faith-based organizations: Are they effective? " *American Journal of Public Health* 94 (2004): 1030–36. [CrossRef] [PubMed]

23. Holt, Cheryl L., and Stephanie M. McClure. "Perceptions of the religion-health connection among African American church members." *Qualitative Health Research* 16 (2006): 268–81. [CrossRef] [PubMed]

24. Levin, Jeffrey S. "Roles for the black pastor in preventive medicine." *Pastoral Psychology* 35 (1986): 94–103. [CrossRef]

25. Levin, Jeff, Linda M. Chatters, and Robert Joseph Taylor. "Religion, health and medicine in African Americans: Implications for physicians." *Journal of the National Medical Association* 97 (2005): 237–49. [PubMed]

26. Fraser, Gary E. "Diet as primordial prevention in Seventh-Day Adventists." *Preventive Medicine* 29 (1999): S18–S23. [CrossRef] [PubMed]

27. Cline, Krista, and Kenneth F. Ferraro. "Does religion increase the prevalence and incidence of obesity in adulthood? " *Journal for the Scientific Study of Religion* 45 (2006): 269–81. [CrossRef] [PubMed]

28. Sack, Daniel. *Whitebread Protestants: Food and Religion in American Culture.* New York: Palgrave, 2001.

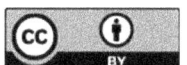

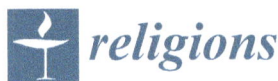

Article

Serenity Spirituality Sessions: A Descriptive Qualitative Exploration of a Christian Resource Designed to Foster Spiritual Well-Being among Older People in Nursing Homes in Ireland

Fiona Timmins [1,*], Suzanne Kelly [2,†], Mary Threadgold [3,†], Michael O'Sullivan [2,4,†] and Bernadette Flanagan [2,†]

1   The School of Nursing and Midwifery, Trinity College, Dublin 2, Ireland
2   All Hallows College, Dublin City University, Gracepark Rd, Drumcondra, Dublin 9, Ireland; suzmarkel@gmail.com (S.K.); bflanagan@allhallows.ie (B.F.)
3   Sonas™ apc, St. Mary's, 201 Merrion Road, Dublin 4, Ireland; marythreadgold@hotmail.com
4   Research Fellow, Department of New Testament, University of the Free State, Bloemfontein, 9300, South Africa; spiritualcapitalireland@gmail.com
*   Author to whom correspondence should be addressed; timminsf@tcd.ie; Tel.: +353-1-896-3699.
†   These authors contributed equally to this work.

Academic Editors: Arndt Büssing and René Hefti
Received: 22 December 2014; Accepted: 13 March 2015; Published: 27 March 2015

Abstract: This paper reports on a descriptive qualitative study that explored the value and benefit of Serenity Spirituality Sessions programme for older nursing home residents. The research was carried out in six nursing homes in the Republic of Ireland. The facilitators of these sessions, who worked in the nursing homes, were interviewed about their experiences of delivering the programme and their views on the impact that the programme had on resident participants. Emergent themes revealed benefits of the intervention for clients, including inducing a calming effect, increased sense of belonging and benefits of ritual use. The programme yielded positive results, and appears suited to the predominantly Christian population, and as such is deemed a useful adjunct to holistic and spiritual care in these settings.

Keywords: spirituality; intervention; older person; nursing home

1. Introduction

There is emerging consensus that spiritual care forms an important role in overall care of older people [1–3]. For many older people, religion and/or spirituality play an important role in their lives [2,3]. It is generally accepted that most people have spiritual needs as well as physical and emotional needs [4]. Spirituality is often a very important coping mechanism when dealing with difficult circumstances or major changes in life, such as moving from independence to dependent care or facing death [2,3]. It is often a core part of the older person's identity and as a result many residential settings for older people support clients' spiritual needs [2]. There are currently more than 20,000 people living in residential nursing home care in Ireland, within more than 450 nursing homes providing care. Many of these provide spiritual care to clients through the use of chaplaincy services. Additionally, a small number of homes also provide access to religious services and/or spiritual care interventions provided by nursing or activities staff. While no national standards exist to support this intervention there is acceptance and recognition that clients have spiritual needs to meet while receiving care (Health Service Executive, and that responsibility for this lies with all health care staff) [4].

2. Providing Spiritual Support to Older People

There is growing consensus that health care can be maximized by providing spiritual care [5]. Reasons for this are outlined in Box 1.

Box 1. Reasons for the provision of spiritual and religious support to patients [6].

(1)	Many patients are religious, and the majority would like their faith to be considered in their health care.
(2)	Religion influences patients' ability to cope with illness.
(3)	Religious beliefs and practices may influence medical outcomes.
(4)	Patients are often isolated from other sources of religious help.
(5)	Religious beliefs and rituals may conflict with or otherwise influence the medical decisions that patients make, particularly when they are seriously ill.
(6)	Religious beliefs and commitments influence the type of health care and monitoring that a patient receives in the community.
(7)	Medical, nursing and psychiatric training programs are now required to ensure that all graduates provide culturally sensitive health care, which includes care that is sensitive to deeply held religious beliefs.

Spiritual needs of older adults are manifestations of the ageing process [7]. It is therefore recommended that that spirituality can be integrated into care in a sensitive and sensible manner by taking a brief spiritual history at the time of admission to a nursing home. Identifying patient needs in this way can provide vital information for the care of the patient [6]. As people age they begin to consider more fully issues of ultimate meaning about life and to prepare for their death [1]. For many, this means a growing concern with responding to ultimate meaning, developing means of transcendence and growing intimacy with God and/or others [1]. There is also a need for forgiveness, to prepare for dying and death and to feel useful [8].

Old age is a life stage where meaning-making is vitally important, a time when the older person can potentially stand back and come to terms with all that has gone before, a time when transcendence is possible. It is suggested that:

> Creating a spiritual life that provides a sense of ultimate meaning gives a resource for putting life events, both positive and negative, in to context, transcending losses and disabilities, creating a sustaining sense of connection with the sacred, and developing the capacity for deep inner peace.

([9], p. 116)

There is also a proposed notion of *gerotranscendence*, which suggests that:

> Spiritual development gradually and steadily increases from middle age onward and results in a shift from materialistic, role-oriented life philosophy to a transcendent, spiritual perspective in late old age.

([9], p. 33)

As such it seems that for some spirituality and aging go hand in hand. This means for some, that healthy aging, requires support to meet the spiritual needs of older people, known as the spiritual tasks of ageing [1] (Box 2).

However, while spiritual needs in older people are being recognised more, there is often reticence around providing or facilitating spiritual care and a focus on doing so in life limiting circumstances [10]. At the same time, recent studies show that older people engage regularly in spiritual activity while at home [11].

Box 2. Spiritual tasks of ageing [1].

- Finding ultimate meaning for themselves—through relationship, reconciliation with family and/or God, dealing with guilt//loss, *etc.*
- Assisting a person in moving from self-centredness to self-transcendence—through acceptance of self, of ageing, of chronic conditions, of anger/grief, *etc.*
- Responding to ultimate meaning with spiritual strategies—through worship, prayer, sacred reading, music, art, *etc.*
- Being "with" the older person, developing intimacy in relationship—though listening, connecting, trusting, caring, honouring, *etc.*
- Moving from provisional life meanings to final meanings—through reminiscence, life-review, finding meaning in growing older, in suffering, in death, *etc.*
- Giving hope—through genuine care, affirmation, support in the dying process, *etc.*

In many nursing homes, caregivers, such as facilitators, can often play a very important role in the life of the resident. They may form very close relationships with residents through daily interaction, often on an intimate level, in terms of bathing, dressing, feeding, sharing concerns, *etc.* They may also provide an intimate listening space to allow residents to relate their personal stories, as form of spiritual reminiscence.

For many older adults in care, ritual has played a huge part in their lives. Ritual provides a sense of continuity, a link with the past, but also to culture and faith [12]. Rituals can take various shapes and forms. For many, the ritual of a Catholic Mass or a similar service can have a dual purpose: it can provide an opportunity to connect with or respond to the resident's concept of the Divine in a familiar setting and provide a space where the resident can feel a sense of community and belonging [1]. While prayer and other rituals may seem quite a religious intervention, these nursing interventions have been found to be popular in other settings [13,14].

This project aims to explore the usefulness of a pre-designed spiritual care programme—the *Serenity Spirituality Sessions*—that was developed by *Sonas apc* Ireland [15]. *Sonas apc* is a charitable (not-for-profit) organisation whose primary aim is to train healthcare staff and family to provide therapeutic support for older people with communication challenges, particularly those with Alzheimer's and dementia. They provide a range of training resources for this purpose, which provide a huge resource in a country that is economically challenged, under resourced, and like the rest of the developed world, has an increasing aging population. The *Serenity Spirituality Sessions* programme was developed in 2011 in response to a growing awareness of the need to provide additional spiritual support to older people. As the majority of people admitted to nursing homes in Ireland are Christian, the package was designed to suit the needs of the majority at this time.

3. The Study

3.1. Aims

To explore the use and value of the *Serenity Spirituality Sessions* programme for older nursing home residents.

3.2. Objectives

The research aimed to:

- To oversee the delivery of the *Serenity Spirituality Sessions* programme to a sample of older nursing home residents.
- To explore the value of using the *Serenity Spirituality Sessions* programme with older nursing home residents from the perspective of the facilitators.

3.3. Method

The Sample

Purposive sampling was used to identify six spiritual care facilitators from six nursing homes in the Republic of Ireland. All participant nursing homes were approved by the Health Information and Quality Authority [16] and were members of Nursing Homes Ireland (NHI). All were privately run. The nursing home residents were generally accepted to be older people and no provision was made to determine or select a nursing home based on demographics.

Purposive sampling determined those nursing homes which appeared to have openness to spiritual care as evidenced from observation of their websites as well as the Nursing Homes Ireland website (NHI 2014). As such, they indicated that spiritual care was important and/or that they offered regular services/visits from various clergy for their residents, and/or that they had an oratory on site. As the intervention is primarily a Christian one, consideration was given to the suitability of its use, namely that residents taking part were Christian and such intervention was deemed consistent with the usual spiritual care component of holistic care at the home.

The nursing homes were either already running the *Serenity Spirituality Sessions* programme for older nursing home residents ($n = 4$) for a short time period (less than one year), or were in agreement to do so. In those four sites where the programme had been running, this was for periods of between seven months and eighteen months. The other two nursing homes ran on a trial basis for the duration of the intervention (four weeks). Inclusion criteria were that both the nursing home and the facilitator needed to be willing to participate and the facilitator needed to provide written consent to take part. Six activity co-ordinators/facilitators in charge of spiritual time/activities were interviewed.

A dedicated activity co-ordinator/facilitator in charge of spiritual time/activities was required to run the intervention. All six facilitators were women. No particular training in either spiritual care delivery or using the programme was required, as the intervention is deemed to be suitable to be used by any adult family member, staff or carers with the capacity to read, understand and conduct sessions. The facilitators self-trained using the "how-to" DVD provided.

3.4. The Serenity Spirituality Sessions

The study comprised the delivery of a specifically devised *Serenity Spirituality Sessions* programme. This programme was developed by *Sonas apc* [15] under the guidance of its founder Sr. Mary Threadgold, a speech and language therapist. Content was selected based on an in-depth expertise in the field and expert advice on other aspects (such as appropriate music) was sought during its development. Sr. Mary Threadgold developed the *Sonas* programme in 1990. She had seen the value of music and touch when working with young people with intellectual disabilities and wanted to design a therapeutic activity for older people who had communication impairment that built on that knowledge. The resultant *Sonas* programme incorporates multi-sensory stimulation within a structured session that involves cognitive, social and emotional stimulation and is now being used frequently in Ireland for people with dementia. The *Serenity Spirituality Sessions* is a specifically designed Christian spiritual support mechanism that can be easily used by staff, family or volunteers who are involved in caring for older people. It is available to purchase at cost of 80 euro [15] and the operation of it is self-explanatory. Those who wish to facilitate spiritual support for older people need only watch the "how-to"-DVD provided with the package. The sessions come as a complete package, which includes a box set of CDs, an information booklet, and a DVD. These materials are visually appealing (Figure 1) and were provided free of charge by *Sonas apc* [15] to participating nursing homes who were not already in possession of the programme.

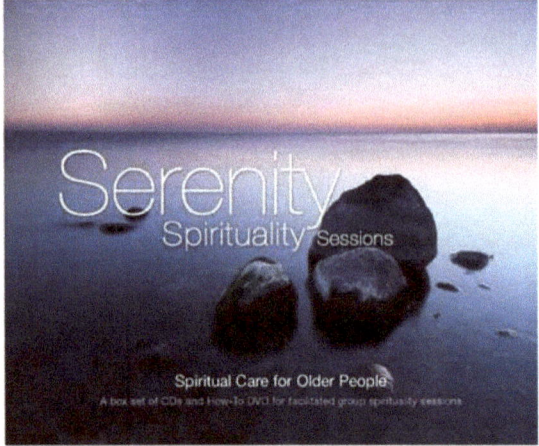

Figure 1. Front cover of *Serenity Spirituality Sessions* explanatory leaflet.

Sonas apc [15] also provide additional assistance, if required, regarding how to use the programme. Sessions usually last between 35 and 45 min and consist of six guided sections (Box 3).

Box 3. Explanation on how the *Serenity Spirituality Sessions* are used.

The *Serenity Spirituality Sessions* box set is a turn-key solution to support the continual nurture of Christian Spirituality for older people in care. A checklist is provided to prepare the way for a successful session. The facilitator is encouraged to keep the group size small (maximum of 8) in order to ensure quality interaction.
Sessions last between 35 and 45 min and consist of 6 guided sections:

(1)   Let's begin,
(2)   Praying with Scripture,
(3)   Prayers and Reflections for Others,
(4)   God's Presence in Nature,
(5)   Personal Prayers,
(6)   Final Blessing and Hymn.

The CDs are played during each session, which gives opportunity to participants to listen to a range of scripture readings, liturgy and music selected by the facilitator. An example of CD content is provided in Box 4. All the material contained in the box set has been carefully selected for older people to be reminiscent of their own Christian prayer throughout their lives. There is a focus on familiar readings, psalms and prayers to facilitate comfortable and easy participation.

In the current study, the facilitator/activities co-ordinator was requested to run the six sessions over a period of three to four weeks, and to participate in a follow-up interview. How the facilitators ran the session varied. Two of them ran the programme on a regular weekly basis, one ran it twice a week and one did not run it on a regular basis at all. All except one nursing home ran it on the same day at the same time in the same place each week. The two facilitators using the programme for the first time ran it once a week for four weeks. In all six cases it was conducted in a sitting room or day room, in the home. Attendance varied from 7 to 12 in general, with up to 20 included in one session in one home. Participants were self-selecting. This choice of numbers was not dictated by the programme but rather according to the needs and facilities of each service.

Box 4. An example of CD content of the *Serenity Spirituality Sessions.*

CD1 Track Listings	
Track 1	Music
Track 2	Church bells ring
Track 3	Hymn—Be Thou My Vision
Track 4	Prayer
Track 5	Scripture Reading
Track 6	Psalm—The Lord's My Shepard
Track 7	Music
Track 8	Hymn—Amazing Grace
Track 9	Scripture reading
Track 10	Music

3.5. Data Collection Measures

Data were collected in 2012. Semi-structured interviews were used to collect data. These interviews comprised a number of open-ended questions, the responses to which were recorded. One-to-one interviews were held in a convenient quiet room in each nursing home site at a time convenient to the participants. Data collection included a seven-item interview schedule. These questions were formulated following consultation with the designers/promoters (Sonas apc, 2014) and in accordance with literature on the topic. Proposed questions were also discussed with some academic peers not participating in the project, in order to establish face and content validity. The questions were sent out to each interviewee in advance to allow time to prepare and contemplate responses. Four of the participants opted to write down some initial preliminary notes to use as an aid in the interview.

3.6. Ethical Considerations

The local College Research Ethics Committee (LCREC) granted ethical approval to conduct the study. A formal request to each nursing home manager determined access. As the nursing homes were already providing Christian spiritual services that residents chose to attend or not, and as the majority of residents at the site were Christian, the ethos of the materials was not deemed inappropriate. Additionally the provision of such a programme, voluntarily attended by residents, was not viewed as coercive by either the managers or the LCREC, as it comprised an extension of usual spiritual service provision. Anonymity and confidentiality, of both the respondents and the sites, were preserved. The method of data collection preserved both of these, and this fact was made clear to respondents. Written information on the study was provided to both the nursing home managers and the facilitators. The nursing home managers acted as gatekeepers and recruited facilitators. Participants also signed a consent form, and were given time in advance to consider and provide consent. Participation in the programme by residents was encouraged in all nursing homes but was voluntary, always respecting the wishes and well-being of the resident.

3.7. Data Analysis

The interviews were audio recorded, transcribed and analysed using thematic analysis [17]. The interview recordings were listened to several times in order to become totally immersed in the data gathered. All recordings were then transcribed in full detail, read through and analysed carefully and finally coded in a thematic manner. The approach used to analyse this data in this research project can be described as one of thematic content analysis. This is an approach widely used in social science research that is useful for identifying rich patterns and trends within the data [18] It follows the 16-step method developed by Burnard [19], with the aim of producing "a detailed and systematic recording of the themes and issues addressed in the interview and to link the themes and interviews together under a reasonably exhaustive category system". The employment of this method meant that notes were taken after each interview regarding the general topic discussed. Interview recordings were listened to several times. Transcripts were then completed and read through several times in order to become immersed in the data and enter the other person's "frame of reference". Unnecessary and repetitious text was removed. Another reading of transcripts identified and noted general headings/themes to categorise the content of the interviews (open coding). The list of categories was then grouped under higher-order headings so as to "collapse" or reduce the number of headings overall and a final list was produced. The next stage involved colour-coding categories and sub-headings. The coded sections were then arranged in appropriate groups. Multiple copies of transcripts were used to ensure the context of the coded sections was maintained.

4. The Findings

Three main themes emerged which can be summarised as follows, benefits and challenges of the sessions, rituals/beliefs to support faith, and a sense of community and belonging.

4.1. Benefits and Challenges of the Sessions

All facilitators expressed the view that the integrated package was a very useful tool to support clients' spirituality. One stated that ([20], p. 39):

> The package is very good. It's very helpful because if I need to do a spiritual session, like praying, I wouldn't know where to start … it's a very good tool to do it.

Another described it as "brilliant, because it's just compact, you know". One facilitator stated that ([20], p. 39):

> It was very easy to follow … because everything is already prepared for you, it cuts out on your preparation time and [having] everything under the one roof is great in an environment like this … it's good to have everything and you can just lift the case and go with it. Put it in your CD player and you know that you've got all the ingredients for a successful group.

Another facilitator mentioned that "an integrated package works, but it needs to kind of stand alone", while another mentioned how it would be a very good tool for someone who was not a native English speaker or not so familiar with Irish culture. Another facilitator expressed the view that the intervention was:

> … easy to manage and to run and it's all there and it explains how to run it. If it wasn't for that, I think it would be quite difficult to kind of come up with something like that yourself, that would be effective and that would have the same impact on older people really.
>
> ([20], p. 39)

All facilitators found it had a huge calming and relaxing effect on the residents. One reported that:

> Two ladies actually on two occasions were very agitated. One of them was looking for home and she wanted her daughter and this, that and the other, and when I brought her up, she sat and she had her hands clasped like this (hands clasped as in prayer) and she tapped in time with the hymns and music and she sang along and she prayed and she became completely, (pause) her whole countenance just changed once she was away from that busy environment, she was just completely calm and relaxed.
>
> ([20], p. 38)

The same facilitator also shared:

The same with another lady, she would pull herself along in the wheelchair, and she was totally out of sorts and when I brought her in here, and just, I think the quiet room, the environment, and she got a lot of joy from it, definitely did and she sang along. She has very poor communication. Now she would have had a stroke and that, and she could only repeat the same words over and over again . . . and she can sing every word of the hymns, and she can sing along with them, so it just taps in to a different part of her memory or her brain . . . very effective for her, particularly her, like I could see just the benefit she got out of that and the other lady that was very restless as well, do you know, it had a great calming effect on them.

([20], p. 38)

One interviewee stated that "residents really feel calm, calm and peaceful after the session". She went on to give a very pertinent example of one lady attending the sessions "who is usually quite agitated . . . and most of the time she settles down, you know". She described another resident who was in another nursing home and was all the time on his own, eating in his room, never out of his room. But that changed:

In our nursing home, with the good work of the care assistants . . . that man is going to have his meals downstairs in the dining room. He comes to Serenity and to Mass. But when you see that he never got out you know, for these things before, it's a great achievement. And he has really enjoyed it.

([20], p. 40)

The same facilitator gave a similar example of another female resident:

she was at home, for a couple of years, she had dementia, she was sitting alone looking at the wall, from day to day . . . When she came here she couldn't participate in anything . . . then Serenity brought her out and then Sonas . . . now she's communicating, she's taking part in all activities, which she would never before. It's just amazing!...she's so happy doing something and not just sitting.

([20], p. 42)

Another facilitator felt "the benefit was the comfort", while a third saw "real benefits in terms of two ladies that were agitated, that were stressed. They calmed down, they were able to sit through the session, they didn't look to leave, which, in other sessions they quite often would look to leave, or still remain agitated. But this they didn't. They stayed calm and remained calm afterwards."

([20], p. 41)

A similar lasting benefit was reported by a fourth facilitator, which underlines the relaxing effect of the sessions: "We've noticed that during the session, as the session is progressing, people become very relaxed. And we noticed that that relaxation carries on then for the rest of the day" ([20], p. 41). Another observed that:

You don't know what effect it has on somebody deep down, really you don't know. It could be subtle . . . it could be something you don't even realise, but tomorrow somebody might notice a change in the person, or that the person is calmer or what have you, so you know, still waters run deep ([20], p. 41). Other direct feedback from the residents given by two more facilitators included comments such as, "That was just beautiful!", "That was lovely", and "When can we do it again?", "Can we do it every evening?"

([20], p. 42)

Several facilitators observed that residents really valued and needed relationship and intimate sharing. A good example of how relationship and intimate caring can benefit the resident was described by one facilitator who felt hymns were so important:

> We've a woman in here, she's blind, but she has her hearing and if you go up to her and sing with her, she'll rock with you, you know, which is brilliant...that's where you need the songs." Another reported that "I think it's nicer because you're giving them more attention, it's more close [sic], there's more closeness, there's more intimacy in it definitely, yeah."
>
> ([20], p. 48)

This emphasis on intimacy resonates with the opinion of Elizabeth MacKinlay ([1] p. 81), who states that "Intimacy is just as important in later life as at any time along the lifespan; perhaps even more so in the frailty of later life, having lost physical or cognitive abilities, the person is even more in need of relationship and love." "For people with dementia" she declares, "relationship is almost synonymous with meaning".

Eileen Shamy ([21], p. 61) also stresses the importance of relationship in her definition of spiritual well-being: "Spiritual well-being is the affirmation of life in a relationship with God, self, community and the environment that nurtures and celebrates wholeness."

This relatedness and connection is illustrated in another facilitator's observation during the trial-run of the Serenity programme:

> I think as a group we all feel very connected, at that time, so allowing myself to connect with the residents in that time, at that level. So including myself as a member of that group, offering my prayers with the residents and sharing something of myself within that group as well, I think that, for me, that is important, that *I feel* and that *the residents feel* that we are connected.
>
> ([20], p. 48)

The importance of the programme for building up relationships and intimacy is demonstrated by another facilitator who reported that "I do feel since I've started this, my relationship with the residents, it's got closer, you know that kind of way. They are opening up a little more about their fears and things like that, which is good." ([20], p. 48).

All facilitators appeared to be very aware of the importance of honouring the personhood of each resident. One stated, "I think before attending to the physical needs of a person, you have to remember that *he is a person* (emphasis participants own)" She went on to describe a common example of carers under time pressure, rushing a resident to get dressed, *etc.* She remarked that carers need to ask themselves if they are performing the task for the resident or for themselves, and declared, "Often you're doing it in your own way, how YOU are used to doing it . . . so before starting any physical needs you should ask how HE would like to do that . . . the main thing to remember is that it's not a piece of meat you're taking care of, you're taking care of a person" ([20], p. 49).

Another facilitator described how her spirituality helps her be a presence for others in the nursing home. She spoke of one man whose wife had died and whose grief was triggered when certain hymns were played; "He'd get upset because it brings back memories, you know which is good, and I'd put my arm around him and say 'but you know it's OK to cry'."([20], p. 49).

Henri Nouwen ([22], p. 19) describes the importance of this compassion when he states, "Yet perhaps our greatest gift is our ability to enter into solidarity with those who suffer. Compassion can never coexist with judgement because judgement creates distance and distinction, which prevents us from really being with the other".

A third interviewee felt that, when caring for older people, being present and giving reassurance in the *Serenity Spirituality Sessions* was vitally important: "older people need an awful lot of reassurance that their life was worth-while, that they spent it well, that we give them a value and a worth at the end of their lives". She understood the importance of being a listening and reassuring presence for those "in spiritual pain"; those worried or even close to death. Her personal experience of watching her own father dying in pain made a deep impact, but also gave her great insight into pain as he revealed to her; "It's all part of the process . . . the beautiful process of dying." She shared that this made her "so conscious, so conscious from that day, that there actually is a process going on for the person who is dying . . . because there isn't a person I sit with that I don't think of him and keep my mouth shut most of the time and just say, 'Listen, I'm here, you're not on your own'." This is a deeply touching example of understanding Personhood and gifting Presence. ([20], p. 49).

The theme of presence was prominent in the literature reviewed and also emerged as a significant theme in the interview data. This is illustrated in a story related by one interviewee concerning a resident who shared after a Serenity session that she was feeling sad and alone. The facilitator recounted how she told the resident "you're not on your own, we're one big family in our community here. We are all here for each other and we're all friends, OK and you're not on your own ([20], p. 50)." She added, "So I was giving her a lot of reassurance, so I told her I loved her and I gave her a big hug, and if she ever needed to talk to somebody, that I was here for her." Then she described how the reassured resident "gave me a big hug and said 'Thank you so much. I feel so much better after that!'" This is another significant example of the healing power of presence. This facilitator showed particular awareness of being present as she declared: "I think it's important, sometimes you know, just sitting there and listening to somebody, it's very important, they need to be able to express how they're feeling." ([20], p. 50).

There were also some challenges with the programme materials. One facilitator mentioned a difficulty she encountered when she noted that "it doesn't really give you a guide as to how do you encourage people to reflect on scripture". This facilitator felt that a template of "just maybe four points on how to reflect" would be useful, because " . . . initially it's difficult to grasp an understanding of what and how you are supposed to say, what do you say? What do I say to a group of elderly people that makes sense to them and that respects their beliefs . . . that was meaningful?" ([20], p. 40). Some facilitators felt that four weeks was too short a time-frame in which to really come to grips with everything involved in running the programme.

In regards to the prayer/hymn booklet, five facilitators felt the format could be improved in various ways for residents with poor eyesight and for those with motor difficulties. For example one wanted to "make it bigger; well make it clearer and [use] bigger font and once you do that, I think that's perfect." ([20], p. 39).

4.2. The Use of Rituals to Support Existent Faith

Maltby [23] maintained that "religious symbols can facilitate the tasks of aging persons by providing a link with the past as well as being a concrete reminder of hope in the future. Even those who have language impairment can frequently sing familiar hymns and become involved in a community ritual".

This view appears to be illustrated well by the *Serenity Spirituality Sessions* experience in terms of examples given by some interviewees. One facilitator described a resident who "has full blown Alzheimer's and she could shout at you and all. And she has her beliefs, so I like her in the group, even if she shouts, but I think it's important that she is in it as well, even though she wouldn't communicate with you, coz there is something there. And yesterday we were singing . . . she was down from me . . . and she was singing along to the CD, and that's great feedback to tell her family." ([20], p. 50).

Another felt the prayers gave great reassurance. She stated, "It gives comfort and they are looking forward to it . . . it gives hope and meaning, yes!" A third facilitator talked about the ritual of weekly prayer together and how "some would pray for their families and praying for this and that and everyone is sharing. I think it brings this feeling of closeness...I think it's very important." ([20], p. 47).

The benefit of ritual prayer and song as a support for clients' spirituality and faith resounded through the findings. One facilitator stated:

I think a lot of our residents have got very strong faith and they like to practise ... they like to come together as a group to pray, it means so much more if you're praying with other people.

([20], p. 42)

Another facilitator said that "the benefit was as well that they knew the hymns ... they were calm and they were getting some peace and joy from it" ([20], p. 41). Another felt that while there was a good Mass service and Communion service in the nursing home, the residents also benefitted from a more informal praying together:

And I think all of the people ... feel very connected when they're together and practising their faith together. So something like this really supports this ... it isn't like an organised religious ceremony or anything, it's kind of quite informal ... and we're coming together to pray because we want to and because they enjoy it.

([20], p. 43)

Another facilitator mentioned the importance of residents being able to express their spirituality during the sessions and how the nursing home provides that continuum of spiritual care:

And they're expressing their spirituality ... it's a ritual they are doing and they need that. They do ... coz religion is very important in peoples' lives you know ... .Like say for example a resident goes to church every morning at 10 o' clock, and you know maybe did the rosary every morning and stuff like that. When they come into a residential home, that option should be there ... that they get that. It's very important, because it was part of their life ... they were doing this ritual all their lives ... You don't come into a residential home and next of all it all stops!

([20], p. 43)

The benefit of ritual prayer and song as a support for clients' spirituality and faith resounded throughout the findings.

4.3. Sense of Community and Belonging

This theme did not appear prominently in the literature reviewed; however, it did surface as a significant theme in all the interviews conducted. All facilitators felt that through the Serenity programme, residents experienced a great sense of community and belonging to the nursing home community, and they felt this was of vital importance to the residents and their sense of spiritual well-being. The fact that all facilitators felt the same way is evidence to support the view of any one of them. These views were illustrated in their comments. One facilitator reported that "I think the programme is a good addition to what's already existing and it's nice for them to come together, there's a sense of community as well, being in a small group." Another felt this sense of community was of great importance because "when you get that sense of belonging you are more brave to go, to step out into the world to do things." ([20], p. 43).

This sense of belonging that facilitators feel is associated with the Serenity programme, and the security and comfort it brings, could also be linked in with Robert Atchley's continuity theory. In this he advocates that "The external aspects of worship—ceremony, music, and religious symbols—all can provide satisfying continuity. It is a repetition that can produce a feeling of comfort and security." ([20], p. 46).

One facilitator found in her experience that the prayers give a lot of comfort; "it gives them some reassurance...it gives comfort and they are looking forward to it ... it gives hope and meaning". She also felt that praying together "brings this feeling of closeness ... and for people who don't have relatives very near, I think this sense of belonging is very important" ([20], p. 47).

Another facilitator commented on the importance of residents being able to participate and share verbally in the Serenity programme. She observed that "the more it went on, they started to give feedback" and while it was different to the ritual of a Mass, she felt that "to actually have to think and then to share, was kind of different ... interesting to see what everyone said, and not often things you're expecting." ([20], p. 47). She added, "They're bringing to mind a family member that they're praying for, which is nice for them to have the opportunity to do that which they mightn't have in a Mass or a Holy Communion service, which I think is nice." ([20], p. 47).

This significance of the practice of sharing was echoed by another facilitator, who found that

> "what we *really* liked about the Serenity actually is sharing. Learning a little bit more about each other and sharing something of ourselves, maybe about our family, you know. When we wanted to pray for a family member or friend, we were able to share that with the group and that was, the residents really enjoyed that. Somebody this morning prayed for a sick relative ... and obviously that was on their mind, so we learned a little bit more about that resident today and their family and where they lived ... and we really learned different things about each other which was nice."

> ([20], p. 47)

She also commented later on some residents who had shared intimate sufferings and loss with the group during prayers and the comfort she felt they received within the group; "He obviously felt comfortable enough to show the group that he did miss his parents and we prayed for them and he got a lot of comfort from that then, when we prayed for his parents and mentioned them in the prayers." Another lady who opened up about the death of her brother "seemed to get a lot of comfort from the fact that we prayed for her brother as a group ... I think they do feel comfortable with each other and it always seemed quite respectful as well. People were allowed the space to talk." ([20], p. 47).

The ability of the sessions to provide a sense of community and belonging among the older residents surfaced as a significant theme in the interviews conducted. All facilitators felt that by using the programme regularly, residents experienced a great sense of community and belonging to the nursing home community. They felt this was of vital importance to the residents and their sense of spiritual well-being.

5. Discussion

Older people residing in nursing homes in Ireland were raised in a society where religion played an important role right throughout their lives. Given the fact that care of older people has changed somewhat over recent years, the appropriateness of religious or spiritual care in these care centres is often unclear. However, these findings shows that spiritual care of older people is not only considered an important aspect of overall care, but that the *Serenity Spirituality Sessions* programme played a very important role within the context of spiritual well-being of older people. The intervention clearly had benefits for older people concerned. Studies of nurses from older people settings reveal that nurses see a clear role in providing spiritual care to their clients. This role is believed to include supporting clients to find meaning and to make connections with others; comfort and reassurance and respect for and/or facilitation of religious beliefs [24]. In keeping with other religious interventions [7] the *Serenity Spirituality Sessions* programme appeared to have beneficial effects.

One unexpected finding was that the intervention seemed to create a space where residents had an increased sense of community and belonging. This was evidenced when facilitators reported that residents sharing and praying with and for each other felt deeper connections within the group. This inherent sense of belonging created a greater sense of peace and well-being. MacKinlay ([1], p. 225) describes the intimate relationship with God and/or others as one of the spiritual tasks of ageing. She states that "relationship is an important aspect of being human" and that "the human spirit longs for connections with others". This is something that was very much evidenced by findings, with several facilitators demonstrating how important they found the development of relationships with and among residents. They all felt this had a very beneficial impact on overall spiritual well-being.

Findings of the research also indicated that rituals of hymn-singing and praying together had a positive impact on the spiritual well-being of residents in nursing homes. Most facilitators described the feedback from residents as extremely positive, with many expressing great joy and peace as a result. Rituals of music and liturgy are identified as playing an important role in how humans may respond to others and can help create a sense of hope [1]. Similarly Atchley's [9] continuity theory indicates the importance of residents having a sense of continuation of spiritual or religious practices while in residential care, which "helps one discover the symbols and themes that are significant and meaning-giving ... and that can serve as resources in adapting to changes", thereby promoting a greater sense of spiritual well-being. Additionally in

> The external aspects of worship—ceremony, music, and religious symbols—all can provide satisfying continuity. It is a repetition that can produce a feeling of comfort and security.

For many older adults in care, ritual has played a huge part in their lives. As Fischer [12] states:

> Ritual is important because it provides a sense of continuity, a link not just with our individual past, but with that of our culture and our faith ... The enactment of ancient ritual brings renewed awareness of where we have come from and who we are. It can help us establish profound emotional connections in terms of our identities as individuals and members of families. In this way we capture the feeling of an old self or a partial self. Ritual is one of the paths to integrity as we age.

Rituals can take various shapes and forms. For many, the ritual of a Catholic Mass or a similar service can have a dual purpose: it can provide an opportunity to connect with or respond to the resident's concept of spiritualty and provide a space where the resident can feel a sense of community and belonging. While overtly religious, older people are drawn towards both the religious and spiritual as they near their end of life and often gain great support from familiar childhood religious ritual [7].

6. Limitations

Although qualitative research makes no claim to generalizability limitations that apply to this approach need to be considered. This is a small-scale study and as such the findings are both limited and context dependent. A follow up larger-scale project that quantitatively measured intervention outcomes using controlled situations would be useful to strengthen preliminary outcomes. The *Serenity Spirituality Sessions* programme was also not used consistently across the homes, a factor which would need to be addressed in any future studies. Another factor that may influence the interpretation of findings is that the residents were self-selecting and chose voluntarily whether or not to attend the sessions. It is likely, therefore, that those attending were more positively disposed towards the concept than those who did not. The use of private nursing homes, homes already using spirituality interventions may have further biased the findings. As four of the six homes were already using *Serenity Spirituality Sessions* this further compounds this bias. The study yielded the facilitator views only, but it would have been useful to also know the residents' views. While the frequency and length of sessions varied from one site to another is an acknowledged limitation of the study, this study was not aiming for methodological rigour or control. This flexibility permitted the Serenity Sessions to be adapted locally to suit each particular group. Obviously, generalising from these findings is difficult; however, the contextual information that arose suggests that the Serenity Sessions is a useful support for older people in residential care, and this study, albeit qualitative and thus subjective, had resoundingly positive results.

7. Conclusions

In an increasingly secular age, it is all too common to see a public diminishing interest in issues of spirituality and religion. However, within the health care setting, and particularly within the care of

Religions **2015**, *6*, 299–316

older people, the aging, those living with chronic illness and nearness of death incline people towards seeking spiritual support. For those with a background of religiosity, solace can be sought in the return to religious rituals. The provision of spiritual support to clients in care is gaining increased international recognition, and in this context the provision of interventions such as the *Serenity Spiritually Sessions* can be a useful adjunct to care. While there are ethical concerns about "omission" (not providing spiritual care) and "commission" (providing spiritual care that might appear coercive) ([25], p. 2099), the provision of faith-based supports to clients who subscribe to, or agree to subscribe although not extensively researched, can be useful [26]. As well as benefits to spiritual well-being there is some emerging evidence that such interventions can improve understandings and control of [25]. As the findings are very positive about the programme's usefulness, we believe that the spirituality sessions ought to be recommended for use in residential settings, for older people and those with dementia, who are willing to participate. However, given the diversity of religious faiths, and increasing secularism, diverse religious interventions are recommended for the sake of meeting the needs of people of other religions. Clearly a one size fits all model may not be the most suitable, so more adaptable and flexible approaches, perhaps using intelligent technology, may be more helpful in this particular domain.

Acknowledgments: The authors thank the Religious Sisters of Charity, Ireland, who provided funding to support the research study.

Author Contributions: The writing committee for this paper included Fiona Timmins, Suzanne Kelly, Mary Threadgold, Michael O' Sullivan and Bernadette Flanagan. Suzanne Kelly, Mary Threadgold, Michael O' Sullivan and Bernadette Flanagan were involved in the overall concept and design of the project. Suzanne Kelly participated in the planning and conducting of the study and its analysis and contributed to the development of the manuscript. Fiona Timmins managed the planning and design of the manuscript. Suzanne Kelly, Mary Threadgold, Michael O' Sullivan and Bernadette Flanagan were involved in manuscript development. Each author has participated sufficiently in the work to take public responsibility for appropriate portions of the content. All authors have read and approved the final version of the article.

Conflicts of Interest: The authors declare no conflict of interest.

References

1. Elizabeth MacKinlay. *Spiritual Growth and Care in the Fourth Age of Life*. London: Jessica Kingsley Publishers, 2006.
2. Elizabeth MacKinlay. *Palliative Care, Aging and Spirituality*. London: Jessica Kingsley Publishers, 2012.
3. Timothy P. Daaleman, and Debra Dobbs. "Religiosity, spirituality, and death attitudes in chronically ill older adults." *Research on Aging* 32 (2010): 224–43.
4. Health Services Executive. "A Question of Faith: The Relevance of Faith and Spirituality in Health Care." Available online: http://www.hse.ie/eng/services/publications/corporate/Your_Service,_Your_Say_Consumer_Affairs/Reports/questionoffaith.pdf (accessed on 13 September 2014).
5. Christina M. Puchalski. "The Role of Spirituality in Health Care." *Baylor University Medical Center Proceedings* 14 (2001): 352–57.
6. Harold G. Koenig. *Spirituality in Patient Care: Why, How, When and What*, 3rd ed. West Conshohocken: Templeton Foundation Press, 2013.
7. Mary Elizabeth O'Brien. *Spirituality in Nursing: Standing on Holy Ground*, 3rd ed. Sudbury: Jones and Bartlett Publishers, 2008.
8. David O. Moberg. *Aging and Spirituality: Spiritual Dimensions of Aging Theory, Research, Practice, and Policy.* New York: The Haworth Pastoral Press, 2001.
9. Robert C. Atchley. *The Continuity of the Spiritual Self in Aging, Spirituality and Religion: A Handbook Volume 1.* Minneapolis: Fortress Press, 2003.
10. Robert M. Lawrence, Julia Head, Georgina Christodoulou, Biljana Andonovska, Samina Karamat, Anita Duggal, Jonathan Hillam, and Sarah Eagger. "Clinicians' attitudes to spirituality in old age psychiatry." *International Psychogeriatrics* 19 (2007): 962–73.
11. Kimberly A. Skarupskiab, Geroge Fitchett, Denis A. Evans, and Carlos F. Mendes de Leona. "Daily spiritual experiences in a biracial, community-based population of older adults." *Aging & Mental Health* 14 (2010): 779–89.

12. Kathleen Fischer. *Winter Grace: Spirituality and Aging*. Nashville: Upper Room Books, 1998.
13. Grant Don. "Spiritual interventions: How, when and why nurses use them." *Holistic Nursing Practice* 18 (2004): 36–42.
14. Inez Tuck, Lisa Pullen, and Debra C. Wallace. "Spirituality and Spiritual Care Provided by Parish Nurses Western." *Journal of Nursing Research* 23 (2001): 441–53.
15. Sonas APC. "Serenity Spirituality Sessions Spiritual Care for Older People." 2015. Available online: http://www.sonasapc.ie/spirituality/124-serenity-spirituality-sessions-spiritual-care-for-older-people.html (accessed on 9 February 2015).
16. "Health Information & Quality Authority (HIQA)." Available online: http://www.hiqa.ie/about-us (accessed on 13 February 2015).
17. Denise F. Polit, and Cheryl Tatano Beck. *Nursing Research: Generating and Assessing Evidence for Nursing Practice*, 9th ed. London: Lippincott Williams & Wilkins, 2012.
18. Virginia Braun, and Victoria Clarke. "Using thematic analysis in psychology." *Qualitative Research in Psychology* 6 (2006): 77–101.
19. Philip Burnard. "A Method of Analysing Interview Transcripts in Qualitative Research." *Nurse Education Today* 11 (1991): 461–62.
20. Suzanne Kelly. *Serenity Spirituality Sessions: A Pilot Study of a Christian Resource Designed to Foster Well-being of Older People in Nursing Homes in Ireland*. Dublin: Sonas Ireland, 2012, Unpublished Report.
21. Eileen Shamy. *A Guide to the Spiritual Dimension of Care for People with Alzheimer's Disease and Related Dementia. More Than Body, Brain, and Breath*. London: Jessica Kingsley Publishers, 2003.
22. Henri J.M. Nouwen. *A Spirituality of Caregiving*. Nashville: Upper Room Books, 2011.
23. Tony Maltby. "Pastoral care of the aging." In *Healthcare Ministry: A Handbook for Chaplains*. Edited by Hayes Helen and Cornelius J. Van Der Poel. New York: Paulist Press, 1990, pp. 98–104.
24. Aru Narayanasamy, Philip Clissett, Logan Parumal, Deborah Thompson, Sam Annasamy, and Richard Edge. "Responses to the spiritual needs of older people." *Journal of Advanced Nursing* 48 (2004): 6–16.
25. Rebecca L. Polzer, and Joan C. Engebretson. "Ethical issues of incorporating spiritual care into clinical practice." *Journal of Clinical Nursing* 21 (2012): 2099–107.
26. Lisa M. Sacco, Mary T. Quinn Griffin, Rita McNulty, and Joyce J. Fitzpatrick. "Use of the Serenity Prayer among adults with type 2 diabetes: A pilot study." *Holistic Nursing Practice* 25 (2011): 192–98.

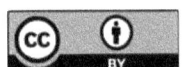

Research Institute for Spirituality and Health (RISH)

Vision and History

The Research Institute for Spirituality and Health (RISH) promotes research and academic training in the interdisciplinary fields of religion, spirituality and health, in Europe and internationally. By linking persons and institutions, it fosters a network of researchers, scholars and health care professionals. European conferences, research workshops and collaborative research projects are important activities of the institute.

The Research Institute for Spirituality and Health was founded in 2005 in parallel with the first research workshop run by Prof. Harold Koenig in Switzerland. The initiative has been handed over to René Hefti MD, Medical Director of the Department for Psychosomatic Medicine at the Clinic SGM Langenthal, a clinic for whole-person medicine and psychiatry.

Scientific Activities

European Conferences on Religion, Spirituality and Health

Annual European Conferences (held since 2008) aim to enhance scientific and interdisciplinary dialogue between medicine, health and life sciences, science of religion, spirituality and theology, covering physical as well as mental health issues. The conferences promote the European and international network as well as collaborative research and training projects.

Research Workshops on Religion, Spirituality and Health

The 4-day research workshops—with Prof. Harold Koenig from the Duke University Medical Center, who is one of the world's leading experts in religion, spirituality and health (RSH) research—offer a unique opportunity to receive comprehensive research training in this field.

The following topics are discussed: Previous research on religion, spirituality and health; importance of definitions; understanding mechanisms and pathways; highest priority studies for future research; strengths and weaknesses of religion and spirituality measures; designing different types of research projects; statistics and statistical modeling; funding your research; writing a grant; managing a research project; writing a research paper for publication.

Teaching Medical Students in "Medicine and Spirituality"

A one-year program has been developed to train medical students in how to integrate religion and spirituality into clinical practice. The course covers the following topics: definitions of religion and spirituality, meaning-making, the extended biopsychosocial model, research on religion, spirituality and physical as well as mental health, religious and spiritual coping, the spiritual care model, opportunities and limitations of the integration, taking a spiritual history, supporting spiritual needs and resources, dealing with spiritual struggles.

Own and Collaborative Research Projects

A regular activity of the research institute is to promote and supervise bachelor-, master-, and doctoral theses in religion, spirituality and health, mainly in medicine and psychology. Specific topics of own and collaborative research are religious and spiritual coping in psychosomatic medicine and psychiatry and its association with the outcome of in- and outpatient treatment; religion and spirituality as moderator of the physiological and psychological stress response (stress buffering), physiological profiles of different "spiritualities" and the attitude of physicians towards the integration of religion and spirituality into clinical practice.

Different Types of Publications

The research institute publishes scientific articles in peer reviewed journals, as well as reviews and CME articles in professional journals. A new series called "RSH-publications" was initiated and a first volume on "religion and mental health" realized. Two books have been published, one a selection of contributions to the first European conferences (Peter Lang Verlag 2012) and one a translation of "Spirituality in Patient Care" (Kohlhammer 2012).

Networking

Regular Newsletters

The research institute publishes two newsletters: An English newsletter that is designed to promote and support the European network, and a German Newsletter as a platform of the working group for spiritual care focusing on Switzerland. Both newsletters can be ordered and downloaded free of charge on the RISH website (www.rish.ch).

Website and E-Letter

The RISH website is a platform to share and distribute information about recent activities and resources related to the research institute and the European network. It is complemented by an e-letter sent out several times a year.

Contact Information

Research Institute for Spirituality and Health RISH, Weissensteinstrasse 30, CH 4900 Langenthal, Phone +41 62 919 23 97, Fax +41 62 919 22 00, info@rish.ch, www.rish.ch

MDPI

St. Alban-Anlage 66

4052 Basel

Switzerland

Tel. +41 61 683 77 34

Fax +41 61 302 89 18

www.mdpi.com

Religions Editorial Office

E-mail: religions@mdpi.com

www.mdpi.com/journal/religions

www.ingramcontent.com/pod-product-compliance
Lightning Source LLC
Chambersburg PA
CBHW041137120626
46547CB00020B/3017